WOMEN IN DRAMA

In the plays selected for this volume, we see the evolving vision of womanhood as it has come down to us from the world of ancient Greece to our own world of struggle and change. We view woman as a creature of passion and vengeance; woman as the voice of sanity raised against the madness of men; woman forced to be an instrument of intrigue and deception; woman as a social rebel; woman twisted and perverted; woman finding her way to fulfillment; and, finally, woman transcending any narrow sexual definition to stand as a universally heroic figure.

MEDEA • LYSISTRATA • WOMEN BEWARE WOMEN • THE LADY FROM THE SEA • MISS JULIE • MRS. WARREN'S PROFESSION • TRIFLES • APPROACHING SIMONE

HARRIET KRIEGEL, a native New Yorker who earned her M.A. in Theater from Hunter College, both acted in and directed Off-Broadway theater productions. She has taught English and Drama in the New York City schools, and, in 1974, completed a film, *Domestic Tranquility*, under the sponsorship of Women Make Movies. She is currently working on another film project.

MENTOR Books of Special Interest

WOMEN
⤫ IN ⤫
DRAMA

AN ANTHOLOGY

EDITED BY

Harriet Kriegel

Ⓜ

A MENTOR BOOK
NEW AMERICAN LIBRARY

TIMES MIRROR
NEW YORK AND SCARBOROUGH, ONTARIO
THE NEW ENGLISH LIBRARY LIMITED, LONDON

Library of Congress Catalog Card Number: 74-32635

ACKNOWLEDGMENTS

APPROACHING SIMONE: Megan Terry. Copyright © by Megan Terry, 1970. Reprinted by permission of Elisabeth Marton, 96 Fifth Avenue, New York, N. Y. 10011.

THE LADY FROM THE SEA: Henrik Ibsen. Translated by Rolf Fjelde. Copyright © 1970 by Rolf Fjelde. Reprinted by permission of The New American Library, Inc.

LYSISTRATA: Aristophanes. Translated by C. T. Murphy. From the book *Greek Literature in Translation* by Murphy, Guinagh, and Oates. Copyright 1947 by C. T. Murphy. Published by Longmans Green and Company. Reprinted by permission of the David McKay Company, Inc.

MEDEA: Euripides. Translated by Rex Warner. First published 1944. Reprinted by permission of The Bodley Head Limited and The New American Library, Inc.

MISS JULIE: August Strindberg. Translated by C. D. Locock. From *Lucky Peter's Travels.* Reprinted by permission of Jonathan Cape Limited.

MRS. WARREN'S PROFESSION: George Bernard Shaw. Acknowledgment is made to The Society of Authors on behalf of the Bernard Shaw Estate.

TRIFLES: Susan Glaspell. From *Plays* by Susan Glaspell. Copyright 1920 by Dodd, Mead & Company, Inc. Copyright renewed 1948 by Susan Glaspell. Reprinted by permission of Dodd, Mead & Company, Inc.

NOTE: *Application in reproducing the plays in this volume protected by copyright against any unauthorized performance or publication, in whole or in part, in any medium, should be made to the copyright holders.*

SIGNET, SIGNET CLASSICS, MENTOR, PLUME and MERIDIAN BOOKS are published *in the United States* by The New American Library, Inc., 1301 Avenue of the Americas, New York, New York 10019, *in Canada* by The New American Library of Canada Limited, 81 Mack Avenue, Scarborough, Ontario M1L 1M8, *in the United Kingdom* by The New English Library Limited, Barnard's Inn, Holborn, London, E.C. 1, England

FIRST MENTOR PRINTING, APRIL, 1975

2 3 4 5 6 7 8 9 10

PRINTED IN THE UNITED STATES OF AMERICA

To Lenny, Mark, and Bruce

Acknowledgments

I should like to thank my husband, Leonard Kriegel, for his critical reading of the Introduction as well as for his help and encouragement. My thanks to Harold Clurman for his consistently stimulating ideas about theater and society. I am also grateful to Reva Mark Kriegel who knows that liberation requires the willingness of women to help each other.

Contents

WOMEN
IN
DRAMA

Introduction

This anthology has a dual purpose: It is intended to depict attitudes toward women as they are reflected in dramatic literature as well as to portray the changing roles women have assumed and the ways drama itself has influenced some of those changes. Most of the plays have long since been "classics" of theater, with all the dubious distinction that word endows. But none of these plays is stale. And if they seem to possess an even greater vitality today than when they were written, that can be attributed to the new tensions surrounding women in our time. The new feminism—a less jaundiced term than women's liberation—is only one in a multitude of changing role definitions, but may be, at least at present, the most interesting and very possibly the most "radical" to Western society.

Perhaps no other art form allows us to view our myths in a clearer light than does dramatic literature. And to examine the portrayals of women in the dramatic literature of the past is to be made aware of how our present concerns are the culmination of a complex legacy—the manner in which women in the Western world have been treated and expected to function.*

So much of dramatic literature deals with exactly that subject. To examine the shifts in the territory women occupy in the Western mind is especially fascinating in a time such as ours, when women are the focus of a culture that has been—and still is—politically, economically, socially, and psychologically dominated by men. To watch the dramatic record unfold is to be made aware of how the roles of women have changed, shifting so that at times women race against the current, only to be forced back ultimately into the

---

*I do not mean to imply that Western women have been treated more harshly than women in other parts of the world. Whatever oppression they may have faced, they have fared considerably better than their counterparts elsewhere. But the literature with which we are concerned is specifically Western—both in its origins and the problems it treats.

conventions and subterfuges demanded by a world in which the holy virgin battles the temple prostitute for dominance in the minds of men. In such a world, to be a woman is inevitably to be a creature of extremes.

The plays included here make up a very small part of the record. Where, one might ask, is the urbanity of the women in Restoration comedy or the plays of Molière? Where is Chekhov, whose women struggle with the imminent upheavals of their society? Where is García Lorca, whose women are among the most powerful in contemporary drama? It would be easy enough to name scores of other plays and playwrights that might have been included. I chose, instead, to focus on certain plays from ancient Greece, Elizabethan England, nineteenth- and twentieth-century Europe, and contemporary America. In all these societies, the roles women were permitted to play were rooted in the conception of what women were permitted to be. The correlation between how women were portrayed in drama and how women functioned in society is overwhelming. In periods in which they find room for development in their lives, they are self-sufficient, reasonable, sometimes courageous, often inspiring. In periods in which they are constricted within the confines provided by social pressures, they can be demonic or they can be caricature. What they rarely can be is human.

Classical Greek Theater

No greater roles have been created for women than those written by the classical Greek playwrights. Never since has there been an era in which women have been portrayed with such extraordinary depth and range. The richness of Greek myth created the basis for Greek drama. Clytemnestra, Electra, Medea, Hecuba, Iphigenia, Antigone, Alcestis, Phaedra, and Andromache—such women are capable of great heroism and passion. Motivated by complex emotions, they struggle against fate and determine their own destinies as men do. Not until Elizabethan theater will women on stage possess the bravura and intelligence of a Praxagora; not until Ibsen will they crave the independence of an Antigone; not until Shaw will their wit and strength combine in a potential for heroism to match that of Lysistrata.

Seldom do the Greek heroines act for the sake of love—almost the sole motivation of the modern heroine. Their struggles are rooted in honor, country, family, ideals. They possess a solid basis for their nobility, and they are able to live courageously, even without the comfort of love.

Exactly why the Greek dramatists were able to view women as they did remains something of a mystery. With all that we know about the Greek world, we still know relatively little about the actual conditions of women. We do know, of course, something about their legal status. They could not own property, and they possessed few legal rights other than to divorce and to testify under oath. We also know that the state attempted to protect them from poverty and actively sought to arrange marriages for women who had been orphaned.

But none of this tells us very much about the actual conception of women held by Greek culture. Women were very much part of a society in which public and private life were not as divided as they are today. Often well-educated and talented, they shared in the religious life of the family and of the state. Contrary to what is commonly believed, homosexuality was viewed as an aberration, practiced by anti-democratic circles in Athens and by the warrior communities of Sparta and Thebes that believed it more encouraging to the martial spirit than loving a woman. In fact, domestic life was of prime importance in Athenian society, and wives and mothers were esteemed. It is probably this, more than any other single factor, that accounts for women in Greek drama being so vigorously delineated. Often more resourceful than their men, they display intelligence, passion, and strength of purpose. An Antigone, an Electra, an Iphegenia—all were figures who aroused strong empathy in their audience (both male and female).* And empathy cannot be aroused if an audience is unable to connect with what it has witnessed.

While it is not certain whether a true matriarchy existed before the Golden Age, there is evidence that the earlier inhabitants of Greece, as was usual for primitive, agricultural peoples, worshiped a mother goddess and revered femininity as the source of life. Women played an important role in that society, perhaps a dominant one. The early Minoan culture, for example, was matrilineal, authority being achieved through the female line, a tradition which was evident for a long time.† Eventually, the older matriarchal chthonian religion of the peasants combined with the newer patriarchal Olympian religion of the Achaean invaders. Significantly, dramatists dealing with the ancient legends depict women in a dominant role. It has been suggested that the dramatization

---

*Women in ancient Athens had no difficulty in viewing with equanimity the comedies of Aristophanes, which is more than many of their modern-day counterparts can claim.

† Oedipus becomes ruler of Thebes because he marries Jocasta.

↳ But this isn't matrilineal

of the Orestes myth purposefully enhanced the authority of
the newer religion by illustrating how patriarchal loyalty
transcended matriarchal devotion.

Greek drama remains richer in heroines than any drama
that followed it. Offered a wealth of plays from which to
choose, the *Medea* of Euripides and the *Lysistrata* of Aristophanes were selected because they provide so striking a contrast of the portrayal of women; taken together, they reflect
the essence of the Greek attitude toward women. Both Medea and Lysistrata are unusually resourceful, manipulative,
and intelligent. Medea is the sorceress capable of unleashing
wanton destruction; Lysistrata the rationalist intent on saving
man from his follies.

And yet, of all the heroines of classical Greek drama, Medea can be said to be the least Greek—or the least Athenian,
at any rate. She is a Colchian princess, which was enough to
explain to her audience her penchant for barbarism. Ironically enough, she is motivated by love, performs the most
terrible deeds for its sake, and is the most "romantic" of all
Greek heroines. Other heroines manage their emotions better;
Medea abandons all for love of Jason. For love of Jason, she
deceives her father, kills her own brother, and destroys his
uncle. Her emotions are violent and intemperate; her passion
Byronic and unmastered. Her grief is merely the obverse of
her passionate nature. Overcome by the knowledge that she
has been used and that Jason's love is illusory, she indulges in
a full-blown display of grief, demonstrating a *sturm und
drang* intensity which nothing will contain or comfort. An
all-consuming love is transformed into an all-consuming desire for vengeance. Where she was once overwhelmed by her
love, she is now overwhelmed by the passion to inflict pain.
She remains a creature of absolutes.

She is also the most modern of Greek heroines, the figure
with whom contemporary women can best identify. She lives
a life in which she is manipulated by extremes. She can be
one thing or the other, mistress or murderess. Not only does
she articulate the injustices done to her sex, she also represents those extremes through which women have been vic-
timized. Just as, in a single decade, our own culture passed
from the vise of "togetherness" and the mystique of domesticity to the denunciation of the family and the most violent
rhetoric, so Medea passes from her fierce love to her fiercer
hate.

> . . . For in other ways a woman
> Is full of fear, defenceless, dreads the sight of cold

> Steel; but, when once she is wronged in the matter
>   of love,
> No other soul can hold so many thoughts of blood.

The speech in which she describes the inequities suffered by
women has a remarkably contemporary ring.

> It was everything to me to think well of one man,
> And he, my own husband, has turned out wholly vile.
> Of all things which are living and can form a judgement
> We women are the most unfortunate creatures.
> Firstly, with an excess of wealth it is required
> For us to buy a husband and take for our bodies
> A master; for not to take one is even worse.
> And now the question is serious whether we take
> A good or bad one; for there is no easy escape
> For a woman, nor can she say no to her marriage.
> She arrives among new modes of behaviour and manners,
> And needs prophetic power, unless she has learnt
>   at home,
> How best to manage him who shares the bed with her.
> And if we work out all this well and carefully,
> And the husband lives with us and lightly bears his
>   yoke,
> Then life is enviable.

The very essence of modernity, she recognizes that she can
achieve her ends only if she can meet the price. Skeptical
enough to know that whatever bargain she makes will be a
poor one, she willingly trades knowledge and craft for freedom. By endowing Aigeus with fertility, she ensures her escape from Corinth. She seduces her enemies, dooming them
with golden gifts. She knows, as does Claire Zachanassian of
Dürrenmatt's *The Visit*, that anyone can purchase accom-
plices if she remains knowledgeable about the marketplace of
morality. When she cannot dominate the world by natural
means, she willingly turns to sorcery.

But Medea's weapons are not merely her craft and intelligence. She employs her children, too. Centuries after Euripides, writers will argue that a trained mind *and* the ability to
produce children endow women with too much power. Medea is what they had in mind. She possesses the ability to
confer life or death. She can destroy her enemies, bestow the
gift of fertility on her friends and allies. She can give birth to
children, she can kill her children. She is the embodiment of
the contradictory impulses which categorize women. On the

one hand, to act instinctually or violently is to be "unsexed."
(Shakespeare's Lady Macbeth and Aeschylus's Clytemnestra
come to mind here.) On the other hand, it is in the very
"nature" of women to act without reflection, to be violent,
tempestuous, childish.

It is difficult to think of Euripides as a misogynist since he
created so many powerful and complex roles for women. But
at least one of his fellow Athenians had no such difficulty.
Aristophanes seems to have enjoyed satirizing Euripides's
work, particularly his treatment of women. His *The Thesmo-
phoriazusae* (*The Women at Demeter's Festival*) is a comedy
in which the Athenian women plot to punish Euripides for his
notorious misogyny; the man "it pleases to put all the vile
women who ever were on the stage" is indicted for having
tarnished the reputation of their sex. In *The Ecclesiazusae*
(*The Women of Parliament*), Aristophanes suggests that the
state might be in better hands if it were entrusted to women.
His heroine, Praxagora, convinces the Senate to preempt its
own powers and hand the running of the state over to
women; as mothers, they will spare the blood of the soldiers
(and incidentally, see that they are better fed). It is a theme
of *Lysistrata*, too.

Aristophanes's view of women anticipates that of the great
Victorian dramatist, George Bernard Shaw. Like Shaw, Aristophanes viewed women as able to manage their household
affairs in a society where their men made a mess of the affairs of state. But where Shaw was the victim of the inhibitions of Victorianism, Aristophanes created a much broader,
overtly sexual comedy. Like Shaw's heroines, however, the
Lysistrata whom we see here is bossy and domineering, but
capable of both good humor and intelligent leadership. She
holds her legions in line—admittedly with difficulty—and she
stands up to all those who get in her way. Her competence
and good sense are illuminated by the very humor of her situation. If Aristophanes, like Shaw, recognized that the striving for Utopia often made human beings ridiculous, he is also
concerned with the problems of peace and justice.

As Shaw's good friend, the eminent classical scholar, Gil-
bert Murray, pointed out, Lysistrata "dominates every group,
male or female, in which she finds herself." And if she is
dominating, she is also remarkably resourceful, unfazed by
the emergencies which she must confront; she is the general
rallying her troops. Aristophanes respects her. Unlike the
other characters in the play, she never loses her dignity nor is
she ever placed in a compromising moral position. Her language is not coarse and she does not indulge in the game of

making sexual double entendres. For her, vulgarity is a gesture of candor, not a joke. Her powers of persuasion can be seen in the support she receives. She has no trouble in enlisting support from the women of all the warring Greek states.

What is perhaps most striking about *Lysistrata* is that women suffer, as much as their men do, from sexual deprivation. In all of Western dramatic literature, there are few other plays in which women so vigorously seize the opportunity to enjoy their sexuality. And there is perhaps no other play in which sexuality offers women as much pleasure as it offers men. For Aristophanes, sex is not a prurient activity to be enjoyed only by men or by women of dubious reputation; it is, rather, to be enjoyed without shame, apology, or coyness by respectable men and women. In *Lysistrata*, it is esteemed matrons, not ladies of the street, who have difficulty in taking the oath of sexual restraint. Nor are they considered salacious because they possess appetite. They believe in sexuality, but unlike the women of Restoration comedy, they seek their pleasure in the marriage bed. Behind its farcical humor, *Lysistrata* suggests that men and women can deal with sex rationally, as a source of pleasure to be actively pursued and enjoyed.

Edith Hamilton once wrote that the Greeks "had no real taste for embroidery, and they detested exaggeration." True to the demands of their culture, the Greek playwrights did not exaggerate the characteristics of their women characters any more than they indulged in other exaggerations. Reality created its own demands. Their women could be heroic but not godly, wicked but not demonic. Unfortunately, it was a lesson lost in the teaching.

Elizabethan Drama

As medieval feudalism began to break up, Everyman (that allegorical figure whose very name precluded women from the higher concerns of life) grew less concerned about the state of his soul as he grew more concerned about the state of his pocketbook. A new class was born, the bourgeoisie, for whom the accumulation of goods and wealth assumed immense importance. The family gained a new centrality, and the role of the wife grew correspondingly stronger. (Medieval women had already begun to assume greater responsibilities as well as enjoy greater freedom, acting as assistants to their husbands in small businesses and often taking over these enterprises entirely when their husbands died.

They had even been admitted to some craft guilds on an equal basis with men.)

In England, Henry VIII's break with the Church of Rome led to further questioning of the traditional attitude toward domestic relations and women. The Puritans glorified the virtues of domestic life and no longer held to the belief that virginity was the highest good. Rather, chastity in marriage was the virtue most praised. The new attitudes enhanced the woman's role. Concerned with the continuity of the family's property and the frugal use of its resources, the maintenance of harmony in the home was a serious matter to the rising mercantile classes; scores of books and pamphlets were published with this object in mind. While the poets of the court entertained their ladies with pretty praises, writers of the middle class concerned themselves with determining women's true merit and rightful role.

A great deal of energy was expended in the controversy arising from the new woman. Pamphlets and sermons began to appear on the dangers and the advantages of feminine freedom. While some preachers felt such freedom was a symptom of the evil of the age, others were quick to come to women's defense, creating an early feminist literature.

Once they assumed wider roles and insisted on the right to make their own decisions, women found themselves victims of parody and satire. Not the least of these was a vitriolic document by John Knox in 1558, *The Monstrous Regiment of Women*. Counterattacks followed. Actually, much of this literature was politically motivated. Those who wished to seek the favor of Queen Elizabeth praised women extravagantly; those who wished to undermine her influence emphasized woman's weakness and folly—though few were as bold as Knox. Attacks on women were far more virulent both before and after Elizabeth's reign than during it.

That the ruler of England was a woman had immense social and political implications. If medieval women had made certain advances, Christianity still regarded them as the embodiment of sin and temptation, daughters of Eve who possessed few redeeming qualities, justifiably subservient to their husbands. (Women of the court fared somewhat better. Medieval Mariolatry and courtly poetry created a less restricted ambience.) Attitudes toward women changed as the middle class assumed power, but it was Elizabeth, a woman in a position of unusual power and visibility, who demonstrated to all that women were politically competent. Displaying the governing virtues traditionally attributed to men, she became the outstanding monarch of her age.

If Shakespeare had no other model for feminine greatness, he had her. But Shakespeare lived in an age which was relatively benevolent to women, and other interesting models were not difficult to come by. His women are of a high order—intelligent, interesting, self-willed. As a rule, the women of his comedies are witty, charming, bright, and self-possessed. They frequently control their own property and rule their own lives; they command those who serve them authoritatively. Even the shrew, Kate, is accorded better treatment than might be expected. Petruchio does not tame his wife by amply beating her as does the popular hero of the ballad on which Shakespeare based his plot; he tames her through persuasion and manipulation.

The controversy over women continued throughout Elizabeth's reign, though it grew somewhat muted during her last two decades. But after the ascendancy of James I, the antifeminist faction in England launched its attack with renewed ferocity. James himself disliked independent women. The women who had been appointed by Elizabeth to positions at court were soon relieved of their posts. James discouraged learning in women altogether, a prejudice invigorated by a series of court scandals. Women also made themselves vulnerable to attack by their ostentatious dress, a major means of displaying a rise in social status, at a time when Puritanism, which frowned on such display, was becoming more and more powerful. To the Puritan, exhibitionism in dress was the very antithesis of modesty and thrift; it bespoke the sin of pride.

Puritanism itself, which had been instrumental in the improved status of women, now looked on them with increasing disapproval. In a system which took the myth of Adam and Eve to its theological bosom, it was probably inevitable that women ultimately be viewed as instruments of pleasure. The combination of the rise of Puritanism with its ever-increasing antagonism to the pleasurable and a new monarch who preferred the older Catholic traditions conspired to threaten all the gains women had made under Elizabeth.

The dramatic literature of the period clearly demonstrated these changes. While women were not always shown in the most positive light during Elizabeth's reign—the morality and mystery plays had left too deep an impression for such a radical change—there were roles in which women embodied both private and public virtues. Aristocratic and learned ladies in particular were portrayed to advantage. It was obviously safer to deal with the shortcomings of middle-class wives than with the shortcomings of the women of the court while Elizabeth was on the throne, and it had been the change in status of middle-class women that particularly aroused the ire of the more conservative members of society. Characteristically, Shakespeare dealt fairly with both sexes of *all* classes. The heroines of *The Merry Wives of Windsor,* for example, are intelligent middle-class women with whom the women of London could cheerfully identify.

But even Shakespeare began to reflect a less benevolent attitude towards women after the coronation of James. In part, this was a reflection of the growing pessimism of the age, which accompanied the increasing tendency to question the values of a mercantile society. In Shakespeare's case such cynical influences could be detected earlier; all of his comedies have their darker side. And tragedies such as *Troilus and Cressida* and *Hamlet,* written just before the death of the old queen, reflected this darkening spirit.

But Shakespeare's women become considerably more sinister after the death of Queen Elizabeth in 1603. They are demonic in *King Lear* (1605-06), power hungry in *Macbeth* (1606), and irresponsible to the point of losing an empire for the satisfaction of sensual desire in *Antony and Cleopatra* (1607). We might well imagine Shakespeare's inhibitions in creating a Lady Macbeth while Elizabeth was on the throne. Nor could he be completely comfortable in depicting a sovereign such as Cleopatra, who was renowned for her unpredictability and self-indulgence.

Though some playwrights, notably Thomas Heywood, remained champions of the new class and its women, the general trend grew increasingly critical. Thomas Middleton's *Women Beware Women,* for example, is striking in the way it reflects the misogynistic and cynical attitudes of its time. Livia is Middleton's warning to other women. Her machinations ultimately lead to the destruction of all the principal characters in the play. Like Cleopatra, manipulation is her means to autonomy. In a world controlled by men, she survives through devious skills in the management of others. When power cannot be confronted directly, it is not unusual to develop circuitous methods of dealing with it. This is not a particularly feminine trait, yet control through deceit came to be regarded as a typically feminine characteristic, perhaps because women traditionally found themselves in untenable and powerless positions. When a man contrives situations which have unfortunate consequences, he is a villain. When women act similarly, all women are deceivers. Iago is an evil man. Livia is representative of her sex.

Gaining favor of those in power is the ultimate aim of a

sycophantic society. Livia, therefore, as an important member of the Florentine court, has everything to gain by contriving Bianca's seduction with the Duke. By so doing Guardiano becomes indebted to her for his improved position at court, and she herself has improved her own position with the Duke by maneuvering the seduction he so sorely desires.

Women Beware Women is not a particularly appropriate name for Middleton's play. Indeed, the men act as reprehensively as the women. For example, while it is true that Livia is guilty of lying to Isabella by informing her that Hippolito is not truly her uncle, one wonders why Hippolito is not equally contemptible for his eagerness to take part in the incestuous union. Nor should it be forgotten that Livia's action is prompted by compassion for a niece faced with a lifetime of marriage to a fool. And certainly Guardiano is as responsible as Livia for setting up Bianca's seduction.

There are few seduction scenes in dramatic literature which possess a comparable ruthlessness to the seduction in this play. With the power of his office and the drive of his desire, the Duke threatens Bianca and ultimately traps her. With veiled threats, he makes his entreaties.

It is not mere lust which Middleton condemns but the conversion of sexual desire into a commodity which can be exchanged for political and economic advantage. Guardiano improves his political position by offering Bianca to the Duke. Fabrico provides a most unsuitable husband for his daughter Isabella for financial gain. When Leantio attempts to exact revenge on Bianca by becoming Livia's paramour, his desire is made even more palatable by his improved surroundings and his more elegant clothes. Ironically, Livia, the villainess, finds Leantio personally attractive on his own merit.

Middleton indicates that Bianca is not properly resistant to the Duke because she is overcome by the wealth and aura of royalty. The meanness of her husband's home supposedly fills her with contempt after her seduction. This, however, is never entirely convincing. It is true that the Duke attempts to appeal to her by offering her wealth and honor, but we cannot dismiss the threats that go with the bartering. Nor are we convinced that a woman so in love with her husband at the beginning of the play that she willingly renounces family and social position could so quickly grow enamored of material advantages. There are no hints at the beginning of the play that she finds her husband's home repellent. That she would be agitated by her experience is obvious, and that she might vent her distress on her mother-in-law, who has innocently acted as pawn in Bianca's misadventure, also makes sense. It is even possible that her sexual appetite may have been aroused by the Duke. But money and improved status do not seem an accurate motivation for Bianca's behavior, nor does Bianca's complete change in character seem convincing.

The play has superb scenes, eloquent language, and fascinating characters. However, it is marred by Middleton's rather strained effort to illustrate the failings of women and the corruption of his time. When he permits his characters to develop naturally, they are interesting, vigorous people with the intriguing complications that humans possess. But his play suffers from an ending which is unbelievable; he is too anxious to instruct us in the evils of humankind. Consequently, he forces his characters to behave with spurious motives.

The forces calling women's reputations into question were similar to the forces which eventually led to the closing down of the theaters. Court entertainments continued to flourish, but the theater reflected the growing cleavage between aristocratic and bourgeois ideals. English theater began to lose a certain vitality because it had lost a wide audience. While Puritan relations with theater were dubious at best, it had nevertheless been tolerated as historically instructive, even morally edifying, when it glorified the middle class. When drama began to attack that class with ever-increasing fervor, there was no reason for members of the bourgeoisie to pay good money to see themselves reviled. As a result, an important portion of the population withdrew its support. Ultimately, civil war closed the theaters altogether in 1642. It was not until 1660 that the theaters were reopened for a Restoration drama that portrayed upper-class wives as suitable subjects for seduction.

Modern European Drama

The Industrial Revolution and the Enlightenment were eighteenth-century cultural and political phenomena whose impact on two succeeding centuries still cannot be adequately measured. Inevitably the Industrial Revolution created the modern family; the agrarian family diminished in importance as cultivable land became less available and as opportunities for factory employment brought increasing throngs into the cities. The demands of industry, which required men to be removed from the daily life of their families, changed not only their roles but their wives' as well. Traditional structures broke down; once again the proper function of women was questioned, especially when they, too, began to work in the factories and the mines in order to supplement the meager wages of the men.

Reformists, imbued with the spirit of the time and distressed by the inequities of the age, began to agitate for the improvement of those conditions which continued to enslave mankind. The themes of liberation and self-realization, fundamental to the work of Ibsen, were primary tenets to the philosophers of the Enlightenment. Social theorists such as Montesquieu and Rousseau, primarily concerned with the problem of self-realization rather than of women's rights, nevertheless illustrated their beliefs by depicting the position of women in society. Though contradictory about women's place, Rousseau's *Social Contract* contains the seeds of women's liberation, as it contains the principles of liberation for all oppressed people. Rousseau's just society is of neither patriarchal nor divine origin, but is based upon a contract of equals in a state of nature. He questions the authority of the strongest who, by sheer physical compulsion, asserts the right to rule and then reinforces command through such abstract demands as duty to authority and obedience to higher powers. Opposing slavery, Rousseau insists on liberty as the fundamental condition of the state of nature to which society must return. But it was not until Mary Wollstonecraft wrote her famous *Vindication* that "inalienable human rights" and "the pursuit of happiness" were conceived of as the rights of woman as well as the "Rights of Man."

Romanticism ushered in the nineteenth century by claiming for freedom and equality an absolute prerogative and by questioning not only the order of society but the order of the universe as well. Goethe, Schiller, and the English Romanticists left an indelible mark on Ibsen's Europe. Rousseau, Kant, and Hegel, along with the Danish Paludan-Müller and Kierkegaard, strongly influenced Ibsen. In Paludan-Müller he found the suffering individual who compromises his ideals while achieving external success; in Kierkegaard, the questioning of organized Christianity and the sanctity of marriage. Nietzsche, Marx, and Darwin added their disturbing voices to the attack on the status quo. For Ibsen, to attack the complacency of middle-class society by questioning the marriage relationship and espousing the still-radical idea of self-fulfillment was inevitable.

Even earlier, however, Scandinavian women writers were already turning public taste toward the new realism. Lacking university training, ignorant both of the classical disciplines and the requirements of Romanticism, they wrote simply about a world they knew. Some were novelists, though more frequently they were regular contributors to periodicals which found in their work an alternative for a public grown weary of Norse sagas. One of Norway's first realistic novelists and one of its earliest feminists, Camilla Collett, savagely attacked the social inequities of marriage. She demanded freedom and self-determination for women, and had a lasting influence on Ibsen. But it was not until the publication of John Stuart Mill's *The Subjection of Women* in 1869, translated into the Danish by Georg Brandes in the same year, that women's rights became one of the leading issues of the day in Scandinavia. Women began to organize, hoping to find both intellectual stimulation and economic opportunity in the school system and civil service.

Primarily concerned with self-realization, Ibsen found himself embroiled in the struggle for women's rights. In *Pillars of Society*, for example, he asks that men and women strive to be true to themselves rather than adopt a role imposed by society. Asta Hansteen, one of the leading feminists of the day, was his model for Lona Hessel. Ibsen saw her as a woman who possessed the courage and independence to rebel against stifling convention. He thought women were particularly suited for this because they remained in touch with their inner feelings and were spontaneous and intuitive. In *Pillars of Society*, not only does Lona speak out against the unequal position women occupy in society, but Dina Dorf defies that society as well. In an earlier play, *The League of Youth*, Ibsen's forerunner of Nora, Selma Bratsberg, complains of being infantilized—dressed like a doll, played with like a child, and prevented from undertaking even the semblance of responsible behavior. After *Pillars of Society*, the problem of women's place in society inevitably became one of Ibsen's major themes.

Concerned with the freedom of the individual and the potential for self-realization rather than a specific program of women's rights, Ibsen wrote *A Doll House** in 1879, bringing notoriety to what had up to that time been an eminently successful career. Before that, conservative Norwegian society delighted in *The League of Youth*, which attacked "liberals" for unthinkingly adopting the ideas of the young. *Pillars of Society* attacked that portion of the community which was so bent on profit that it used "floating coffins" (unsafe sailing vessels) to ship goods. But *A Doll House* was an attack on the very foundation of society, the family.

---

*The title of this play is often translated as *A Doll's House*; however, the more accurate translation is without the possessive.

While it has become fashionable to charge Ibsen with being essentially unsympathetic to the feminist cause (a dubious notion, at best), a significant number of his plays deal specifically with the problems of women. The tragedy of *Ghosts*, for example, occurs when a woman does not rely on her own instincts and remains within societal conventions. *Hedda Gabler* illustrates the consequences of a woman's inability to fulfill herself in any meaningful way. *The Lady from the Sea* treats the happiness of a woman allowed to make choices for herself.

Hedda Gabler is most frequently quoted as an example of Ibsen's disillusionment with woman's emancipation. The play was written eleven years after *A Doll House*, after he himself had become identified as a public champion of women. Ibsen found himself linked in the public mind to a phenomenon which he did not wholly approve of: the "new woman" who seemed emancipated but who was as chained as her less liberated sisters. Finding the doll's house too stultifying and the prospect of freedom too threatening, she made inordinate demands on men. Unable to live her own life, she leaned more heavily on men than did those women who continued to seek traditional roles. *Hedda Gabler* is not a play about a woman who becomes destructive because she has too much freedom; rather, it is a play about a woman who cannot make her escape once the door is open.

Ibsen's conviction that freedom and responsibility were essential for all human beings is illustrated in *The Lady from the Sea*. Ellida's struggle for freedom underscores Ibsen's belief in woman's self-realization. The female self, like its male counterpart, must seize what it desires.

The subplots parallel Ellida's conflicts. Lyngstrand, the ailing artist, believes that what makes a man strong is his work, and infuriates Bolette by suggesting that a woman's sole function is to supply the man with inspiration and emotional support.

In *The Lady from the Sea* three women realize their potential. Not only does Ellida find freedom and responsibility—Bolette, too, discovers a way out of her predicament. She agrees to marry Arnholm, who promises to educate her. If women today find the play's solutions too paternalistic, the fact is that women were far more dependent on the largesse of men in 1888 than they are now. Even Hilda, the younger daughter, achieves her measure of happiness through Ellida, who now becomes the mother Hilda so sorely wanted.

Not only is *The Lady from the Sea* about freedom, it is about conjugal responsibility as well—wives and husbands share in providing happiness for each other. Human commitment is the demand which must be met if human happiness is to be achieved.

While most playwrights are content to deal with rather singular views of women, Ibsen gives us an entire gallery of different women. What is peculiar to modern drama is that succeeding playwrights have chosen just two of his women as models for their plays: Nora and Hedda. His other women characters have been ignored. Only Shaw took up the banner for Nora, the rational woman, who desires to discover who she is and who wishes to determine her own destiny. Why twentieth-century dramatists derive their women from Hedda rather than Nora and Strindberg's Miss Julie rather than Ibsen's Ellida is a question that encapsulates woman's struggle in drama. The dramatic dominance of the destructive female was a pattern already adopted in the nineteenth century, and no man was more responsible for that than August Strindberg. Strindberg was obsessed with the possibilities of human domination. The destinies of his people are determined by their strengths and weaknesses. Circumstance is almost incidental. In his plays, two individuals of almost equal strength are pitted against each other in a struggle to determine who is the stronger: This alone provides the dramatic basis for his works. The stronger person is always more ruthless, possesses the greater will and determination, and has little or no tenderness. The struggle for domination is usually depicted as a sexual struggle, although it often has decisive class overtones.

Infuriated by Ibsen's championing of the woman's cause, Strindberg went to great lengths to illustrate the madness of woman's emancipation. George Bernard Shaw describes *The Creditors* as "the terrible play with which Strindberg wreaked the revenge of the male for *A Doll's House* . . . it is the man who is the victim of domesticity, and the woman who is the tyrant and soul destroyer. Thus *A Doll's House* did not dispose of the question: it only brought on the stage the endless recrimination of idealistic marriage." But for all of Strindberg's misogyny in *The Creditors*, the portraits of the two men, Gustav and Adolf, are far more terrible than that of the wife, Tekla. Using the language of commerce to describe the paucity of human relationships, Strindberg's people owe debts to each other through guilt; thus they become "creditors." They are speculators not only in business but in human souls, like Hummel in *The Ghost Sonata*. Reciprocal acts of cruelty cancel each other out.

Professed misogynist though he is, Strindberg provides ample motivation even for his most predatory women. In *The Father*, Laura, the most destructive of his female characters, is given cause to act as she does. The enormous limitations imposed upon her by marriage inflame her rage and strengthen her determination to control the destiny of her daughter. Living in an economic straitjacket, having lost her birthright when she married, her individuality ignored, she passionately affirms her daughter's talent as a means of expressing her own repressed ambitions. It is over the daughter that the battle is fought, and it is the Captain's own neurotic nature which enables Laura ultimately to achieve her devastating victory.

In recoiling from Laura, we may forget that in many of Strindberg's other plays it is men, as well as women, who ruthlessly take advantage of their victims. In *The Creditors*, Gustav exhibits far greater cruelty than Tekla. In *The Dance of Death*, Strindberg portrays a wretched marriage filled with hatred and cruelty, where both partners enjoy indulging their passion for vindictiveness, but the greatest burden of destructiveness lies with the male. In *The Ghost Sonata*, it is Hummel, the male, who is the prime life-destroyer. Miss Julie, victim of her own repressed sexuality, finds it necessary to humiliate a suitor of her own class, but is compulsively attracted to Jean, her father's valet. While Miss Julie throws herself with abandon at the young man and purposefully arouses him, Jean responds to her with ruthless opportunism, employing her weakness to his own advantage. Like Hedda, Miss Julie is unable to deal with her sexuality and she destroys herself. In spite of Strindberg's misogyny (and in spite of his hatred of the decaying aristocracy), he portrays Miss Julie's sufferings with greater compassion than he probably intended.

To view Strindberg's misogyny either as the totality of his view of women or as an extension of general misanthropy is to take a peculiarly narrow view of what his actual achievement was. In *The Father* there is a parody of Shylock's "Does not a Jew bleed" speech, in which man's right to emotional display is brilliantly defended. But just as Shakespeare, undoubtedly without intending to, created out of the figure of the wretched Jewish miser what remains to this very day perhaps the most impassioned defense of the Jew's peripheral position in Western Christian society, so in Strindberg the presence of masculine cruelty, along with the ceaseless masculine quest for ego and dominance, offers, however unintentionally, a most powerful plea that women be granted the dignity they demand. For the very fact that Strindberg's men are so demeaned is what brutalizes their women.

Strindberg is the dramatist from whom most succeeding playwrights take their inspiration, and Miss Julie is the archetypal heroine, both victim and destroyer. George Bernard Shaw, however, does not follow Strindberg. A society such as ours, which romanticizes the primitive, inevitably undervalues the theater of Shaw. His was a drama of ideas, carefully articulated and wittily expressed; it provided a more stimulating theater than the calculatingly "theatrical" offerings to which we have recently been exposed. In a world which limits the value of women to physical pulchritude, Shaw's women may seem abrasive, even threatening. They are, in fact, physically attractive, open, and remarkably successful in employing their charms to achieve their ends. Shaw was anxious to tear away romantic ideas about women. While *Mrs. Warren's Profession* may not be his best play, it is probably his most revolutionary, and caused an enormous outcry when first produced. He scandalized his audience not only by questioning the value of marriage but by depicting prostitution as one more business venture in a capitalistic society. Prostitution was frequently depicted in Victorian theaters, but the sullied heroines had the decency to die in their lovers' arms or suffer other melodramatic misfortunes. Even the sanctity of motherhood is questioned in *Mrs. Warren's Profession*. Shaw offers one of the early portraits of the domineering, theatrically devoted mother. Vivie Warren is the prototype of the Shavian heroine: self-possessed, determined, strong, disciplined, capable of resisting claims made upon her by her lover, her mother, and her society.

All Shaw's women hold steadfastly to what they view as the best in themselves. A woman such as Candida, who has a conventional role in life, assumes that role with wit, originality, and intelligence, confident of the special function she fulfills. Women are exhorted, as Cleopatra is, to give up their childishness and assume their worthwhile place in the world. Working-class women are encouraged to improve themselves and overcome the restrictions imposed by their class, as Eliza Doolittle does in *Pygmalion*. Shaw urges them to hold fast to their common sense and not give in to romantic notions. A young woman need not be forever beholden to her mentor; *Pygmalion* ends quite differently from *My Fair Lady*. Major Barbara and Saint Joan insist on a mission in life. Not only do Shaw's women feel the exhilaration of purpose, they possess the skill, the courage, the tenacity, and the energy to carry out their intentions.

Believing that men and women were capable of bringing order to their lives through their intelligence and will, Shaw espoused ̤socialism as a means of creating an orderly economy and a rational social structure in which the talents and energies of *all* people would be utilized. Capitalism was an evil particularly harmful to women, exploiting them, wasting their potential.

American Drama

After Shaw, the rational woman all but disappears from drama. Of course, a case can be made that rational man disappears as well. Having lost his belief in God and in a meaningful future, man's faith in his own powers and abilities begins to dissipate. But contemporary dramatists depict the important questions of the day through men, while women, if they are dealt with at all, not only lose their rational identities but are usually predators bordering on caricature. In American drama, for example, Eugene O'Neill essentially deals with psychological types beset by psychic demons, women who are destructive to others as well as to themselves. Tennessee Williams offers a devastating view of American society through his pitiful women, beings who have no control over their destinies, who are maimed and mutilated by the world, who are overwhelmed by loneliness and weakness. Arthur Miller's major concern is what responsibility men owe each other, a question which hardly touches his women at all. Not until after his disastrous marriage to Marilyn Monroe did he attempt a portrait of a woman as woman. In Europe, Bertolt Brecht contrasts the instinctual mother with her enormous capacity for survival with the predatory and avaricious woman who is similar to her male counterpart. Dürrenmatt shows the greediness and corruptibility of humankind through the designs of a predatory woman. Albee's women are castrating; in Le Roi Jones's *Dutchman*, the white woman is pathologically destructive; in Kopit, mothers gobble fathers and sons whole; in Pinter, women are particularly sinister in their sexual attractions and appetites; and in Beckett they hardly seem to exist at all, except as memories of past pleasures. Estragon and Vladimir wait for Godot, while Shelagh Delaney's characters are unable to extricate themselves from the morass and disorder of their lives.

And successful women playwrights have depicted members of their own sex as cruelly as their male counterparts have. *The Women* by Clare Boothe Luce shows women pecking away at one another like hens anxious to get at the prize rooster. The play, in fact, might be interpreted as the story of how women are diminished by their symbiotic dependence on men for economic survival and social status. Lillian Hellman is also not known for her flattering women characters. Concerned with the ills and greed of our time, she does not deal with either sex generously, but her women demonstrate an even greater talent for viciousness and rapacity than her men.

Though America began to develop a native theater long before 1920, it was not until that year that Eugene O'Neill became known to the general public with the Broadway production of *Beyond the Horizon*. Nineteen-twenty was a significant year for the women of America as well; it was the year they were granted suffrage. Ironically, their very victory signaled the death blow for the women's movement for a long time to come. Having received the vote, women no longer possessed a focus for their cause, and American dramatists, never having shown an appreciable interest in feminism to begin with, saw no necessity to deal with the problem now that the American woman ostensibly had what she wanted. Eugene O'Neill came of age artistically at precisely that moment when women seemed to enjoy unprecedented political and sexual freedom.

Along with suffrage, women in America had to deal with a popularized psychology rooted in Freudianism. Basic instinctual drives, Oedipal and Electra complexes, fear of domination by women, penis envy, castration fears, anxiety over the "proper" sexual responses of women—in short, all the neurotic impulses dramatized earlier by Strindberg were grafted upon the American psyche under the aegis of psychoanalysis. It is no more than fitting that Strindberg had so great an influence on O'Neill. Driven by forces over which they felt little control, both playwrights used their craft to exorcise past ghosts, imparting emotions so powerful to their drama that they overcame weaknesses inherent in the writing.

O'Neill's women are instinctual creatures. Often maternal, though frequently sinister in their maternity; often fragile, though destructive in their fragility, they are driven by emotions which they are usually incapable of either understanding or articulating. They can dominate and possess men as Nina does in *Strange Interlude*, or arouse men with their instinctual desires as Abbie Putnam does in *Desire Under the Elms*. They are undependable, dangerous creatures, tormented by unconscious drives and conflicts. They have "strange devious intuitions that tap the hidden currents of life," and can trap a man, urge him to act against his own best interests, and prevent him from fulfilling his destiny.

Other American playwrights succumbed to popularized

Freudianism. George Kelly offered a neurotic, compulsive housewife in *Craig's Wife*, and Sidney Howard, in *The Silver Cord*, was among the first to take a shot at that creature who was to anchor so many American traumas, the overpossessive mother. Two women playwrights, however, continued to write sympathetically about women and their problems. One was Susan Glaspell, co-founder of the Provincetown Players, the theatrical group responsible for the discovery of O'Neill; the other was Sophie Treadwell, whose *Machinal* is an expressionistic description of a suffering woman caught between a grasping, mechanistic society and an impersonal, empty marriage.

Susan Glaspell's *Trifles* is a one-act play whose seemingly casual surface belies the strong feelings of its characters and the play's ultimate impact. It illustrates the willingness of women to act as allies in times of crisis. It is significantly different from other plays—even those written by women—since it represents a departure from the cliché that women betray their own sex. Instead, the women in *Trifles* demonstrate their sympathy with and understanding of another woman's plight when they are confronted with her violent retaliation against her husband's domination and brutality.

As the nation nursed its economic ills in the thirties and entered another world war in the forties, feminism seemed a hopelessly shopworn issue. During the Depression, women had been expected to stay out of the job market so that what few jobs there were would be available to men. The reverse was true during the war, when women were called upon to fill vacancies in American industry and commerce. It was with mixed feelings that many women gave up their jobs when their men returned from war. Nevertheless, the nation engaged in building families with virtual ferocity. Having been formerly occupied with world tensions, attention now was directed to the private world, and the preoccupations of the late forties developed into the "feminine mystique" of the fifties and early sixties. New cultural heroines were created, and women, as well as men, had a hard time choosing between the grotesque sexuality of a Marilyn Monroe or Jayne Mansfield and the antiseptic virginity of a Debbie Reynolds or June Allyson. The decade's obsession with virginity was symptomatic of the Neo-Victorianism of the time, reflected in such popular fare as *The Moon Is Blue* or *Marjorie Morningstar*.

Tennessee Williams, whose discipleship extended from Strindberg to D. H. Lawrence and who was deeply marked by that peculiar American polarity between sensual need and

Puritan denial, wrote plays that reflected society's most schiz-ophrenic impulses. Goaded by the Hollywood glorification of sex, aroused by the erotic in literature and advertising, spurred by psychoanalysis to give up sublimation and express instinctual drives, America was thrown into sexual hysteria. Unable to decide whether it wanted its women to be seduc-tive or chaste, it ultimately excoriated them for being both.

Williams's own spiritual and emotional conflicts mirror those of the nation. His homosexuality intensified the conflict and is probably responsible for the extent to which he roman-ticizes sexual passion. He rages against repressive dictums which insist that men remain good little boys, yet is disgusted by the female who threatens men with her prurient desires. He is shocked at the brutality of men, yet seems to take vicarious delight in inflicting sexual humiliation upon his he-roines. His fantasies of rape take the form of a punishment intensely desired by the sexually repressed. Williams's own need to inflict such punishment against the "pure" woman who denies the existence of sexual feeling (in itself a form of castration) can be seen as a homosexual's experiencing the violence and humiliation of rape. Healthy sexual appetites are generally reserved for foreign women (Spanish or Italian); native American women are consumed by lust or dry up like withered leaves.

The cleavage between spiritual and sexual aspiration is best expressed in *Summer and Smoke*. In *A Streetcar Named De-sire*, revenge is once again exacted from the lady who poses as "pure." As in *Miss Julie*, it is a working-class male who is responsible for the destruction of the debilitated aristocrat. Dramatizing myths held dear by the nation, Williams equates the white working class with virility, and brutality with sexual prowess.

Amanda Wingfield of *The Glass Menagerie* is in some re-spects not terribly different from Alex Portnoy's mother, despite her WASP background and D.A.R. qualifications. Nagging at her son, Tom, she imposes a code of behavior in-imical to him, insisting that he behave like a "gentleman," modeled on the "gentlemen callers" she remembers so vividly from her youth. A complex character, she is silly, irritating, frequently given to fantasy, yet she arouses our pity and compassion and forces us to recognize the severe limitations imposed by the Southern myth of female gentility.

Though appearing sympathetic to women, Williams betrays a misogynistic strain. But no writer has embodied the sense of victimization and the dramatic misogyny of Strindberg more powerfully than has Edward Albee in *Who's Afraid of*

Virginia Woolf? The power of Albee's play derives in part from a perverse sympathy with what Martha's life and environment have made of her. Martha directs her self-loathing against others, particularly against her husband, George. The clawing anger with which George and Martha torment each other serves as a substitute for sexual orgasm. Their sterile marriage is symptomatic of their sterile lives. Martha attempts to fill the emptiness with the futile sex play which leads to further frustration, drink, quarreling, and the need for illusion.

In spite of her vulgarity, Martha is as much a victim of conventional opinion as Miss Julie or Hedda Gabler. She is doomed to failure in her attempts to meet the popular view of womanhood—mother, homemaker, and glamour girl. Unable to attain status in her own right, possessing only a superficial education from a girls' finishing school, defensive about her intellect in an academic environment, sexually undesirable, unable to have children, Martha is trapped and lacks the resources needed to escape her sense of worthlessness. Incapable of meeting life courageously, she must depend upon the acquiescence of her husband to maintain her fantasies.

It is ironic that it was during the fifties and early sixties (Albee's play was first produced in 1962), when women were attempting to adapt to the "feminine mystique," that phrases such as "penis envy" and "momism" came into popular use. It would seem that when women inhibited their own creativity and directed their ambitions through others, they became destructive and envious of their husbands and offspring. While many women overcame the myths of the time, most of the heroines of modern drama do not. Our interest in them lies in their desire to overcome limitations which seem endemic to being born female.

With the rise of the new feminism, new voices began to make themselves heard in theater. Women have come to insist on their right to speak for themselves and to create their own portraits. New models are demanded. And it was out of the desire to create new heroines for women that Megan Terry wrote her tribute to Simone Weil, *Approaching Simone.*

Approaching Simone is the product of a number of new trends in drama. It mirrors the political pessimism of our age by questioning whether any government or any political system is capable of ruling without cruelty. Like many of Megan Terry's own generation, Simone, originally active in major social causes, ultimately withdraws from society to seek spiritual salvation.

Of more interest in terms of its theatricality is that Terry's Simone Weil represents a departure from recent heroines. She is a throwback to the Greeks. By exhibiting physical, intellectual, and spiritual courage, she deals with both internal conflicts and political struggles. She is an adult female being. Her battles are not sexually determined; they do not arise because of her relationships with men. She is a Marxist who believes in working in factories and an intellectual who attempts to mold her insights to reality, to the "what is" of existence rather than the "what should be." Her pervasive sense of guilt, however, makes her ultimately a passive hero, not the model more militant women are seeking today. Nevertheless, she is radically different from the sort of woman we usually find represented in the theater, a woman who not only possesses intellectual stature but attempts in her own sacrifice to endow Christ's sacrifice with a specific meaning. If the new feminism fulfills its promise, new heroines will continue to emerge and the image of woman in theater be revitalized.

There have been outbursts of feminism in the past, many of them as vital as our own. For this reason, if for no other, we must question where the new feminism is going. Women may still find themselves dehumanized on the stage, mythicized out of proportion and out of nature as well. It may be that only a "realistic" drama can treat women as people. And the anti-feminist bias may yet evolve into a new dimension because of the very heightened consciousness which the new feminism demands. If in the past playwrights depicted women as predators, they were working within a well-established tradition. The great dramatic portraits of women offer us faces in a picture gallery of domination—women trapped by economics, by inferior education, by inadequate training, by social and even biological expectations which simply cannot be met.

MEDEA

Euripides

Characters

MEDEA, *princess of Colchis and wife of*
JASON, *son of Aeson, king of Iolcos*
TWO CHILDREN *of Medea and Jason*
KREON, *king of Corinth*
AIGEUS, *king of Athens*
NURSE *to Medea*
TUTOR *to Medea's children*
MESSENGER
and
CHORUS OF CORINTHIAN WOMEN

(In front of Medea's house in Corinth. Enter from the house Medea's NURSE.)

NURSE: How I wish the Argo never had reached the land
Of Colchis, skimming through the blue Symplegades,
Nor ever had fallen in the glades of Pelion
The smitten fir-tree to furnish oars for the hands
Of heroes who in Pelias's name attempted
The Golden Fleece! For then my mistress Medea
Would not have sailed for the towers of the land of Iolcos,
Her heart on fire with passionate love for Jason,
Nor would she have persuaded the daughters of Pelias
To kill their father, and now be living here
In Corinth with her husband and children. She gave
Pleasure to the people of her land of exile,
And she herself helped Jason in every way.
This is indeed the greatest salvation of all,—
For the wife not to stand apart from the husband.
But now there's hatred everywhere. Love is diseased.
For, deserting his own children and my mistress,
Jason has taken a royal wife to his bed,
The daughter of the ruler of this land, Kreon.
And poor Medea is slighted, and cries aloud on the
Vows they made to each other, the right hands clasped
In eternal promise. She calls upon the gods to witness
What sort of return Jason has made to her love.
She lies without food and gives herself up to suffering,
Wasting away every moment of the day in tears.
So it has gone since she knew herself slighted by him.
Not stirring an eye, not moving her face from the ground,
No more than either a rock or surging sea water
She listens when she is given friendly advice.
Except that sometimes she twists back her white neck
        and
Moans to herself, calling out on her father's name,

[3]

<u>And her land, and her home betrayed when she came</u>
    <u>away with</u>
A man who <u>now is determined to dishonour</u> her.
Poor creature, she has discovered by her sufferings
What it means to one not to have lost one's own country.
She has turned from the children and does not like to see
        them.
I am afraid she may think of some dreadful thing,
For her heart is violent. She will never put up with
The treatment she is getting. I know and fear her
Lest she may sharpen a sword and thrust to the heart,
Stealing into the palace where the bed is made,
Or even kill the king and the new-wedded groom,
And thus bring a greater misfortune on herself.
She's a strange woman. I know it won't be easy
To make an enemy of her and come off best.
But here the children come. They have finished playing.
They have no thought at all of their mother's trouble.
Indeed it is not usual for the young to grieve.

(*Enter from the right the slave who is the* TUTOR *to Medea's
two small children. The children follow him.*)

TUTOR: You old retainer of my mistress's household,
Why are you standing here all alone in front of the
Gates and moaning to yourself over your misfortune?
Medea could not wish you to leave her alone.
NURSE: Old man, and guardian of the children of Jason,
If one is a good servant, it's a terrible thing
When one's master's luck is out; it goes to one's heart.
So I myself have got into such a state of grief
That a longing stole over me to come outside here
And tell the earth and air of my mistress's sorrows.
TUTOR: Has the poor lady not yet given up her crying?
NURSE: Given up? She's at the start, not half-way through
    her tears.
TUTOR: Poor fool,—if I may call my mistress such a
    name,—
How ignorant she is of trouble more to come.
NURSE: What do you mean, old man? You needn't fear to
    speak.
TUTOR: Nothing. I take back the words which I used just
    now.
NURSE: Don't, by your beard, hide this from me, your fel-
    low-servant.
If need be, I'll keep quiet about what you tell me.

TUTOR: I heard a person saying, while I myself seemed
Not to be paying attention, when I was at the place
Where the old draught-players sit, by the holy fountain,
That Kreon, ruler of the land, intends to drive
These children and their mother in exile from Corinth.
But whether what he said is really true or not
I do not know. I pray that it may not be true.

NURSE: And will Jason put up with it that his children
Should suffer so, though he's no friend to their mother?

a good question

TUTOR: Old ties give place to new ones. As for Jason, he
No longer has a feeling for this house of ours.

NURSE: It's black indeed for us, when we add new to old
Sorrows before even the present sky has cleared.

TUTOR: But you be silent, and keep all this to yourself.
It is not the right time to tell our mistress of it.

NURSE: Do you hear, children, what a father he is to you?
I wish he were dead,—but no, he is still my master.
Yet certainly he has proved unkind to his dear ones.

Jason

TUTOR: What's strange in that? Have you only just dis-
    covered
That everyone loves himself more than his neighbour?
Some have good reason, others get something out of it.
So Jason neglects his children for the new bride.

NURSE: Go indoors, children. That will be the best thing.
And you, keep them to themselves as much as possible.
Don't bring them near their mother in her angry mood
For I've seen her already blazing her eyes at them
As though she meant some mischief and I am sure that
She'll not stop raging until she has struck at someone.
May it be an enemy and not a friend she hurts!

(MEDEA *is heard inside the house.*)

MEDEA: Ah, wretch! Ah, lost in my sufferings,
I wish, I wish I might die.

NURSE: What did I say, dear children? Your mother
Frets her heart and frets it to anger.
Run away quickly into the house,
And keep well out of her sight.
Don't go anywhere near, but be careful
Of the wildness and bitter nature
Of that proud mind.
Go now! Run quickly indoors.
It is clear that she soon will put lightning
In that cloud of her cries that is rising
With a passion increasing. Oh, what will she do,

the sense of absolute certainty that she will translate her grief into violent action —

Proud-hearted and not to be checked on her course,
A soul bitten into with wrong?

(*The* TUTOR *takes the children into the house.*)

MEDEA: Ah, I have suffered
What should be wept for bitterly. I hate you,
Children of a hateful mother. I curse you
And your father. Let the whole house crash.
NURSE: Ah I pity you, you poor creature.
How can your children share in their father's
Wickedness? Why do you hate them? Oh children,
How much I fear that something may happen!
Great people's tempers are terrible, always
Having their own way, seldom checked,
Dangerous they shift from mood to mood.
How much better to have been accustomed
To live on equal terms with one's neighbours.
I would like to be safe and grow old in a
Humble way. What is moderate sounds best,
Also in practice *is* best for everyone.
Greatness brings no profit to people.
God indeed, when in anger, brings
Greater ruin to great men's houses.

(*Enter, on the right, a* CHORUS OF CORINTHIAN WOMEN.
They have come to enquire about MEDEA *and to attempt to
console her.*)

CHORUS: I heard the voice, I heard the cry
Of Colchis' wretched daughter.
Tell me, mother, is she not yet
At rest? Within the double gates
Of the court I heard her cry. I am sorry
For the sorrow of this home. O, say, what has happened?
NURSE: There is no home. It's over and done with.
Her husband holds fast to his royal wedding,
While she, my mistress, cries out her eyes
There in her room, and takes no warmth from
Any word of any friend.
MEDEA: Oh, I wish
That lightning from heaven would split my head open.
Oh, what use have I now for life?
I would find my release in death
And leave hateful existence behind me.
CHORUS: O God and Earth and Heaven!

CHORUS: Did you hear what a cry was that
Which the sad wife sings?
Poor foolish one, why should you long
For that appalling rest?
The final end of death comes fast.
No need to pray for that.
Suppose your man gives honour
To another woman's bed.
It often happens. Don't be hurt,
God will be your friend in this.
You must not waste away
Grieving too much for him who shared your bed.

[handwritten: The moderate voice, conseling Reason — But is Medea's situation "normal"?]

MEDEA: Great Themis, lady Artemis, behold
The things I suffer, though I made him promise,
My hateful husband. I pray that I may see him,
Him and his bride and all their palace shattered
For the wrong they dare to do me without cause.
Oh, my father! Oh, my country! In what dishonour
I left you, killing my own brother for it.

[handwritten: Did all tho for love, for Jason]

NURSE: Do you hear what she says, and how she cries
On Themis, the goddess of Promises, and on Zeus,
Whom we believe to be the Keeper of Oaths?
Of this I am sure, that no small thing
Will appease my mistress's anger.

CHORUS: Will she come into our presence?
Will she listen when we are speaking
To the word we say?
I wish she might relax her rage
And temper of her heart.
My willingness to help will never
Be wanting to my friends.
But go inside and bring her
Out of the house to us,
And speak kindly to her: hurry,
Before she wrongs her own.
This passion of hers moves to something great.

NURSE: I will, but I doubt if I'll manage
to win my mistress over.
But still I'll attempt it to please you.
Such a look she will flash on her servants
If any comes near with a message,
Like a lioness guarding her cubs.
It is right, I think, to consider
Both stupid and lacking in foresight
Those poets of old who wrote songs
For revels and dinners and banquets,

The Greek articulation of the
TRAGIC *aspects of life*
WOMEN IN DRAMA

Pleasant sounds for men living at ease;
But none of them all has discovered
How to put to an end with their singing
Or musical instruments grief,
Bitter grief, from which death and disaster
Cheat the hopes of a house. Yet how good
If music could cure men of this! But why raise
To no purpose the voice at a banquet? For *there* is
Already abundance of pleasure for men
With a joy of its own.

(*The* NURSE *goes into the house.*)

CHORUS: I heard a shriek that is laden with sorrow.
Shrilling out her hard grief she cries out
Upon him who betrayed both her bed and her marriage.
Wronged, she calls on the gods,
On the justice of Zeus, the oath sworn,
Which brought her away
To the opposite shore of the Greeks
Through the gloomy salt straits to the gateway
Of the salty unlimited sea.

(MEDEA, *attended by servants, comes out of the house.*)

MEDEA: Women of Corinth, I have come outside to you
Lest you should be indignant with me; for I know
That many people are overproud, some when alone,
And others when in company. And those who live
Quietly, as I do, get a bad reputation.
For a just judgement is not evident in the eyes
When a man at first sight hates another, before
Learning his character, being in no way injured:
And a foreigner especially must adapt himself.
I'd not approve of even a fellow-countryman
Who by pride and want of manners offends his neigh-
          bours.
But on me this thing has fallen so unexpectedly,
It has broken my heart. I am finished. I let go
All my life's joy. My friends, I only want to die.
It was everything to me to think well of one man,
And he, my own husband, has turned out wholly vile.
Of all things which are living and can form a judgement
We women are the most unfortunate creatures.
Firstly, with an excess of wealth it is required
For us to buy a husband and take for our bodies

The woman's fate: ALL Wmn.
not just MEDEA

[handwritten top margin: for Centuries: the need of a master bec. fate of single wmn is worse]

A master; for not to take one is even worse.
And now the question is serious whether we take
A good or bad one; for there is no easy escape
For a woman, nor can she say no to her marriage.
She arrives among new modes of behaviour and manners,
And needs prophetic power, unless she has learnt at
  home,
How best to manage him who shares the bed with her.
And if we work out all this well and carefully,
And the husband lives with us and lightly bears his yoke,
Then life is enviable. If not, I'd rather die.
A man, when he's tired of the company in his home,
Goes out of the house and puts an end to his boredom
And turns to a friend or companion of his own age.
But we are forced to keep our eyes on one alone.
What they say of us is that we have a peaceful time
Living at home, while they do the fighting in war.
How wrong they are! I would very much rather stand
Three times in the front of battle than bear one child.
Yet what applies to me does not apply to you.
You have a country. Your family home is here.
You enjoy life and the company of your friends.
But I am deserted, a refugee, thought nothing of
By my husband,—something he won in a foreign land.
I have no mother or brother, nor any relation
With whom I can take refuge in this sea of woe.
This much then is the service I would beg from you:
If I can find the means or devise any scheme
To pay my husband back for what he has done to me,—
Him and his father-in-law and the girl who married
  him,—
Just to keep silent. For in other ways a woman
Is full of fear, defenceless, dreads the sight of cold
Steel; but, when once she is wronged in the matter of
  love,
No other soul can hold so many thoughts of blood.

  CHORUS: This I will promise. You are in the right, Medea,
In paying your husband back. I am not surprised at you
For being sad.
            But look! I see our king Kreon
Approaching. He will tell us of some new plan.

  (*Enter, from the right,* KREON, *with attendants.*)

  KREON: You, with that angry look, so set against your hus-
    band,

[handwritten margin annotations: Husband is shackled in marriage but only so far; Challenges the east; woman's life; tales on the myth; woman as outsider; PAY BACK; Chorus sides w/ Medea]

Medea, I order you to leave my territories
An exile, and take along with you your two children,
And not to waste time doing it. It is my decree,
And I will see it done. I will not return home
Until you are cast from the boundaries of my land.

MEDEA: Oh, this is the end for me. I am utterly lost.
Now I am in the full force of the storm of hate
And have no harbour from ruin to reach easily.
Yet still, in spite of it all, I'll ask the question:
What is your reason, Kreon, for banishing me?

KREON: I am afraid of you,—why should I dissemble it?—
Afraid that you may injure my daughter mortally.
Many things accumulate to support my feeling.
You are a clever woman, versed in evil arts,
And are angry at having lost your husband's love.
I hear that you are threatening, so they tell me,
To do something against my daughter and Jason
And me, too. I shall take my precautions first.
I tell you, I prefer to earn your hatred now
Than to be soft-hearted and afterwards regret it.

MEDEA: This is not the first time, Kreon. Often previously
Through being considered clever I have suffered much.
A person of sense ought never to have his children
Brought up to be more clever than the average.
For, apart from cleverness bringing them no profit,
It will make them objects of envy and ill-will.
If you put new ideas before the eyes of fools
They'll think you foolish and worthless into the bargain;
And if you are thought superior to those who have
Some reputation for learning, you will become hated.
I have some knowledge myself of how this happens;
For being clever, I find that some will envy me,
Others object to me. Yet all my cleverness
Is not so much. Well, then, are you frightened, Kreon,
That I should harm you? There is no need. It is not
My way to transgress the authority of a king.
How have you injured me? You gave your daughter
        away
To the man you wanted. O, certainly I hate
My husband, but you, I think, have acted wisely;
Nor do I grudge it you that your affairs go well.
May the marriage be a lucky one! Only let me
Live in this land. For even though I have been wronged,
I will not raise my voice, but submit to my betters.

KREON: What you say sounds gentle enough. Still in my
        heart
I greatly dread that you are plotting some evil,
And therefore I trust you even less than before.
A sharp-tempered woman, or for that matter a man,
Is easier to deal with than the clever type
Who holds her tongue. No. You must go. No need for
        more
Speeches. The thing is fixed. By no manner of means
Shall you, an enemy of mine, stay in my country.

MEDEA: I beg you. By your knees, by your new-wedded girl.

KREON: Your words are wasted. You will never persuade me.

MEDEA: Will you drive me out, and give no heed to my
        prayers?

KREON: I will, for I love my family more than you.

MEDEA: O my country! How bitterly now I remember you!

KREON: I love my country too,—next after my children.

MEDEA: O what an evil to men is passionate love!

KREON: That would depend on the luck that goes along
        with it.

MEDEA: O God, do not forget who is the cause of this!

KREON: Go. It is no use. Spare me the pain of forcing you.

MEDEA: I'm spared no pain. I lack no pain to be spared me.

KREON: Then you'll be removed by force by one of my men.

MEDEA: No, Kreon, not that! But do listen, I beg you.

KREON: Woman, you seem to want to create a disturbance.

MEDEA: I *will* go into exile. *This* is not what I beg for.

KREON: Why then this violence and clinging to my hand?

MEDEA: Allow me to remain here just for this one day,
So I may consider where to live in my exile,
And look for support for my children, since their father
Chooses to make no kind of provision for them.
Have pity on them! You have children of your own.
It is natural for you to look kindly on them.
For myself I do not mind if I go into exile.
It is the children being in trouble that I mind.

KREON: There is nothing tyrannical about my nature,
And by showing mercy I have often been the loser.
Even now I know that I am making a mistake.
All the same you shall have your will. But this I tell you,
That if the light of heaven tomorrow shall see you,
You and your children in the confines of my land,
You die. This word I have spoken is firmly fixed.
But now, if you must stay, stay for this day alone.
For in it you can do none of the things I fear.

a schemed, now a calculating user

(*Exit* KREON *with his attendants.*)

CHORUS: Oh, unfortunate one! Oh, cruel!
Where will you turn? Who will help you?
What house or what land to preserve you
From ill can you find?
Medea, a god has thrown suffering
Upon you in waves of despair.

MEDEA: Things have gone badly every way. No doubt of
        that.
But not these things this far, and don't imagine so.
There are still trials to come for the new-wedded pair,
And for their relations pain that will mean something.
Do you think that I would ever have fawned on that man
Unless I had some end to gain or profit in it?
I would not even have spoken or touched him with my
        hands.
But he has got to such a pitch of foolishness
That, though he could have made nothing of all my plans
By exiling me, he has given me this one day
To stay here, and in this I will make dead bodies
Of three of my enemies,—father, the girl and my hus-
        band.
I have many ways of death which I might suit to them,
And do not know, friends, which one to take in hand;
Whether to set fire underneath their bridal mansion,
Or sharpen a sword and thrust it to the heart,
Stealing into the palace where the bed is made.
There is just one obstacle to this. If I am caught
Breaking into the house and scheming against it,
I shall die, and give my enemies cause for laughter.
It is best to go by the straight road, the one in which
I am most skilled, and make away with them by poison
So be it then.
And now suppose them dead. What town will receive
        me?
What friend will offer me a refuge in his land,
Or the guarantee of his house and save my own life?
There is none. So I must wait a little time yet,
And if some sure defence should then appear for me,
In craft and silence I will set about this murder.
But if my fate should drive me on without help,
Even though death is certain, I will take the sword
Myself and kill, and steadfastly advance to crime.
It shall not be,—I swear it by her, my mistress,
Whom most I honour and have chosen as partner,

*Look at how she plots her
choices: Either murder & save
herself or murder & die too.
NEVER CONSIDERS NO MURDER*

Hecate, who dwells in the recesses of my hearth,—
That any man shall be glad to have injured me.
Bitter I will make their marriage for them and mournful,
Bitter the alliance and the driving me out of the land.
Ah, come, Medea, in your plotting and scheming
Leave nothing untried of all those things which you
        know.
Go forward to the dreadful act. The test has come
For resolution. You see how you are treated. Never
Shall you be mocked by Jason's Corinthian wedding,
Whose father was noble, whose grandfather Helios.
You have the skill. What is more, you were born a
        woman,
And women, though most helpless in doing good deeds,
Are of every evil the cleverest of contrivers.

CHORUS: Flow backward to your sources, sacred rivers,
And let the world's great order be reversed.
It is the thoughts of men that are deceitful,
Their pledges that are loose.
Story shall now turn my condition to a fair one,
Women are paid their due.
No more shall evil-sounding fame be theirs.

Cease now, you muses of the ancient singers,
To tell the tale of my unfaithfulness.
For not on us did Phoebus, lord of music,
Bestow the lyre's divine
Power, for otherwise I should have sung an answer
To the other sex. Long time
Has much to tell of us, and much of them.

You sailed away from your father's home,
With a heart on fire you passed
The double rocks of the sea.
And now in a foreign country
You have lost your rest in a widowed bed,
And are driven forth, a refugee
In dishonour from the land.

Good faith has gone, and no more remains
In great Greece a sense of shame.
It has flown away to the sky.
No father's house for a haven
Is at hand for you now, and another queen
Of your bed has dispossessed you and
Is mistress of your home.

(*Enter* JASON, *with attendants.*)

JASON: This is not the first occasion that I have noticed
How hopeless it is to deal with a stubborn temper
For, with reasonable submission to our ruler's will, *true?*
You might have lived in this land and kept your home.
As it is you are going to be exiled for your loose speak-
          ing.
Not that I mind myself. You are free to continue
Telling everyone that Jason is a worthless man.
But as to your talk about the king, consider
Yourself most lucky that exile is your punishment.
I, for my part, have always tried to calm down
The anger of the king, and wished you to remain.
But you will not give up your folly, continually
Speaking ill of him, and so you are going to be banished.
All the same, and in spite of your conduct, I'll not desert
My friends, but have come to make some provision for
          you, *NOT, NOTICE, TO PREVENT EXILE*
So that you and the children may not be penniless
Or in need of anything in exile. Certainly
Exile brings many trouble with it. And even
If you hate me, I cannot think badly of you.
    MEDEA: O coward in every way,—that is what I call you,
why? With bitterest reproach for your lack of manliness,
You have come, you, my worst enemy, have come to me!
Bury It is not an example of over-confidence
them Or of boldness thus to look your friends in the face,
off Friends you have injured,—no, it is the worst of all
Human diseases, shamelessness. But you did well
To come, for I can speak ill of you and lighten
My heart, and you will suffer while you are listening.
And first I will begin from what happened first.
I saved your life, and every Greek knows I saved it,
Who was a ship-mate of yours aboard the Argo,
When you were sent to control the bulls that breathed
          fire
And yoke them, and when you would sow that deadly
          field.
Also that snake, who encircled with his many folds
The Golden Fleece and guarded it and never slept,
I killed, and so gave you the safety of the light.
And I myself betrayed my father and my home,
And came with you to Pelias' land of Iolcos.
And then, showing more willingness to help than wisdom,
I killed him, Pelias, with a most dreadful death

*Medea makes a potent point —
She has alienated family & friends
For Jason so now she has nowhere
to go —*

At his own daughters' hands, and took away your fear.
This is how I behaved to you, you wretched man,
And you forsook me, took another bride to bed
Though you had children; for, if that had not been,
You would have had an excuse for another wedding.
Faith in your word has gone. Indeed I cannot tell
Whether you think the gods whose names you swore by
        then
Have ceased to rule and that new standards are set up,
Since you must know you have broken your word to me.
O my right hand, and the knees which you often clasped
In supplication, how senselessly I am treated
By this bad man, and how my hopes have missed their
        mark!
Come, I will share my thought as though you were a
        friend,—
You! Can I think that you would ever treat me well?
But I will do it, and these questions will make you
Appear the baser. Where am I to go? To my father's?
Him I betrayed and his land when I came with you.
To Pelias' wretched daughters? What a fine welcome
They would prepare for me who murdered their father!
For this is my position,—hated by my friends
At home, I have, in kindness to you, made enemies
Of others whom there was no need to have injured.
And how happy among Greek women you have made me
On your side for all this! A distinguished husband
I have,—for breaking promises. When in misery
I am cast out of the land and go into exile,
Quite without friends and all alone with my children,
That will be a fine shame for the new-wedded groom,
For his children to wander as beggars and she who saved
        him.
O God, you have given to mortals a sure method
Of telling the gold that is pure from the counterfeit;
Why is there no mark engraved upon men's bodies,
By which we could know the true ones from the false
        ones?
        CHORUS: It is a strange form of anger, difficult to cure
When two friends turn upon each other in hatred.
    JASON: As for me, it seems I must be no bad speaker.
But, like a man who has a good grip of the tiller,
Reef up his sail, and so run away from under
This mouthing tempest, woman, of your bitter tongue.
Since you insist on building up your kindness to me,
My view is that Cypris was alone responsible

Risked euth for him & he betrayed her

what of Jason's argument

JASON:

Of men and gods for the preserving of my life.
You are clever enough,—but really I need not enter
Into the story of how it was love's inescapable
Power that compelled you to keep my person safe.
On this I will not go into too much detail.
In so far as you helped me, you did well enough.
But on this question of saving me, I can prove
You have certainly got from me more than you gave.
Firstly, instead of living among barbarians,
You inhabit a Greek land and understand our ways,
How to live by law instead of the sweet will of force.
And all the Greeks considered you a clever woman.
You were honoured for it; while, if you were living at
The ends of the earth, nobody would have heard of you.
For my part, rather than stores of gold in my house
Or power to sing even sweeter songs than Orpheus,
I'd choose the fate that made me a distinguished man.
There is my reply to your story of my labours.
Remember it was you who started the argument.
Next for your attack on my wedding with the princess:
Here I will prove that, first, it was a clever move,
Secondly, a wise one, and, finally, that I made it
In your best interests and the children's. Please keep
        calm.
When I arrived here from the land of Ioxcos,
Involved, as I was, in every kind of difficulty,
What luckier chance could I have come across than this,
An exile to marry the daughter of the king?
It was not,—the point that seems to upset you—that I
Grew tired of your bed and felt the need of a new bride;
Nor with any wish to outdo your number of children.
We have enough already. I am quite content.
But,—this was the main reason—that we might live well,
And not be short of anything. I know that all
A man's friends leave him stone-cold if he becomes poor.
Also that I might bring my children up worthily
Of my position, and, by producing more of them
To be brothers of yours, we would draw the families
Together and all be happy. You need no children.
And it pays me to do good to those I have now
By having others. Do you think this is a bad plan?
You wouldn't if the love question hadn't upset you.
But you women have got into such a state of mind
That, if your life at night is good, you think you have
Everything; but, if in that quarter things go wrong,
You will consider your best and truest interests

Most hateful. It would have been better far for men
To have got their children in some other way, and
    women
Not to have existed. Then life would have been good.
  CHORUS: Jason, though you have made this speech of yours
    look well,
Still I think, even though others do not agree,
You have betrayed your wife and are acting badly.
  MEDEA: Surely in many ways I hold different views
From others, for I think that the plausible speaker
Who is a villain deserves the greatest punishment.
Confident in his tongue's power to adorn evil,
He stops at nothing. Yet he is not really wise.
As in your case. There is no need to put on the airs
Of a clever speaker, for one word will lay you flat.
If you were not a coward, you would not have married
Behind my back, but discussed it with me first.
  JASON: And you, no doubt, would have furthered the
    proposal,
If I had told you of it, you who even now
Are incapable of controlling your bitter temper.
  MEDEA: If was not that. No, you thought it was not
    respectable
As you got on in years to have a foreign wife.
  JASON: Make sure of this: it was not because of a woman
I made the royal alliance in which I now live,
But, as I said before, I wished to preserve you
And breed a royal progeny to be brothers
To the children I have now, a sure defence to us.
  MEDEA: Let me have no happy fortune that brings pain with
    it,
Or prosperity which is upsetting to the mind!
  JASON: Change your ideas of what you want, and show
    more sense.
Do not consider painful what is good for you,
Nor, when you are lucky, think yourself unfortunate.
  MEDEA: You can insult me. You have somewhere to turn to.
But I shall go from this land into exile, friendless.
  JASON: It was what you chose yourself. Don't blame others
    for it.
  MEDEA: And how did I choose it? Did I betray my husband?
  JASON: You called down wicked curses on the king's family.
  MEDEA: A curse, that is what I am become to your house
    too.

Is this admirable or not

JASON: I do not propose to go into all the rest of it;
But, if you wish for the children or for yourself
In exile to have some of my money to help you,
Say so, for I am prepared to give with open hand,
Or to provide you with introductions to my friends
Who will treat you well. You are a fool if you do not
Accept this. Cease your anger and you will profit.

MEDEA: I shall never accept the favours of friends of yours,
Nor take a thing from you, so you need not offer it.
There is no benefit in the gifts of a bad man.

JASON: Then, in any case, I call the gods to witness that
I wish to help you and the children in every way,
But you refuse what is good for you. Obstinately
You push away your friends. You are sure to suffer for it.

MEDEA: Go! No doubt you hanker for your virginal bride,
And are guilty of lingering too long out of her house.
Enjoy your wedding. But perhaps,—with the help of
        God—
You will make the kind of marriage that you will regret.

(JASON *goes out with his attendants.*)

CHORUS: When love is in excess
It brings a man no honour
Nor any worthiness.
But if in moderation Cypris comes,
There is no other power at all so gracious.
O goddess, never on me let loose the unerring
Shaft of your bow in the poison of desire.

1st

Let my heart be wise.
It is the gods' best gift.
On me let mighty Cypris
Inflict no wordy wars or restless anger
To urge my passion to a different love.
But with discernment may she guide women's weddings,
Honouring most what is peaceful in the bed.

2nd

O country and home,
Never, never may I be without you,
Living the hopeless life,
Hard to pass through and painful,
Most pitiable of all.
Let death first lay me low and death
Free me from this daylight.

ck. translation

There is no sorrow above
The loss of a native land.

I have seen it myself,
Do not tell of a secondhand story.
Neither city nor friend
Pitied you when you suffered
The worst of sufferings.
O let him die ungraced whose heart
Will not reward his friends,
Who cannot open an honest mind
No friend will he be of mine.

(*Enter* AIGEUS, *king of Athens, an old friend of* MEDEA.)

AIGEUS: Medea, greeting! This is the best introduction
Of which men know for conversation between friends.
MEDEA: Greeting to you too, Aigeus, son of King Pandion,
Where have you come from to visit this country's soil?
AIGEUS: I have just left the ancient oracle of Phoebus.
MEDEA: And why did you go to earth's prophetic centre?
AIGEUS: I went to inquire how children might be born to me.
MEDEA: Is it so? Your life still up to this point childless?
AIGEUS: Yes. By the fate of some power we have no children.
MEDEA: Have you a wife, or is there none to share your
bed?
AIGEUS: There is. Yes, I am joined to my wife in marriage.
MEDEA: And what did Phoebus say to you about children?
AIGEUS: Words too wise for a mere man to guess their
meaning.
MEDEA: Is it proper for me to be told the god's reply?
AIGEUS: It is. For sure what is needed is cleverness.
MEDEA: Then what was his message? Tell me, if I may
hear.
AIGEUS: I am not to loosen the hanging foot of the wine-
skin ... *Don't drink so much*
MEDEA: Until you have done something, or reached some
country?
AIEGUS: Until I return again to my hearth and house.
MEDIA: And for what purpose have you journeyed to this
land?
AIGEUS: There is a man called Pittheus, king of Troezen.
MEDEA: A son of Pelops, they say, a most righteous man.
AIGEUS: With him I wish to discuss the reply of the god.
MEDEA: Yes. He is wise and experienced in such matters.

AIGEUS: And to me also the dearest of all my spear-friends.

MEDEA: Well, I hope you have good luck, and achieve your will.

AIGEUS: But why this downcast eye of yours, and this pale cheek?

MEDEA: O Aigeus, my husband has been the worst of all to me.

AIGEUS: What do you mean? Say clearly what has caused this grief.

MEDEA: Jason wrongs me, though I have never injured him.

AIGEUS: What has he done? Tell me about it in clearer words.

MEDEA: He has taken a wife to his house, supplanting me.

AIGEUS: Surely he would not dare to do a thing like that.

MEDEA: Be sure he has. Once dear, I now am slighted by him.

AIGEUS: Did he fall in love? Or is he tired of your love?

MEDEA: He was greatly in love, this traitor to his friends.

AIGEUS: Then let him go, if, as you say, he's so bad.

MEDEA: A passionate love,—for an alliance with the king.

AIGEUS: And who gave him his wife? Tell me the rest of it.

MEDEA: It was Kreon, he who rules this land of Corinth.

AIGEUS: Indeed, Medea, your grief was understandable.

MEDEA: I am ruined. And there is more to come: I am banished.

AIGEUS: Banished? By whom? Here you tell me of a new wrong.

MEDEA: Kreon drives me an exile from the land of Corinth.

AIGEUS: Does Jason consent? I cannot approve of this.

MEDEA: He pretends not to, but he will put up with it.
Ah, Aigeus, I beg and beseech you, by your beard
And by your knees I am making myself your suppliant,
Have pity on me, have pity on your poor friend,
And do not let me go into exile desolate,
But receive me in your land and at your very hearth.
So may your love, with God's help, lead to the bearing
Of children, and so may you yourself die happy.
You do not know what a chance you have come on here.
I will end your childlessness, and I will make you able
To beget children. The drugs I know can do this.

AIGEUS: For many reasons, woman, I am anxious to do
This favour for you. First, for the sake of the gods,
And then for the birth of children which you promise,
For in that respect I am entirely at my wits' end.

Medea Extracts promise of refuge from Aiegeus (handwritten annotation)

But this is my position: if you reach my land,
I, being in my rights, will try to befriend you.
But this much I must warn you of beforehand:
I shall not agree to take you out of this country;
But if you by yourself can reach my house, then you
Shall stay there safely. To none will I give you up.
But from this land you must make your escape yourself,
For I do not wish to incur blame from my friends.

  MEDEA: It shall be so. But, if I might have a pledge from you
For this, then I would have from you all I desire.

  AIGEUS: Do you not trust me? What is it rankles with you?

  MEDEA: I trust you, yes. But the house of Pelias hates me,
And so does Kreon. If you are bound by this oath,
When they try to drag me from your land, you will not
Abandon me; but if our pact is only words,
With no oath to the gods, you will be lightly armed,
Unable to resist their summons. I am weak,
While they have wealth to help them and a royal house.

  AIGEUS: You show much foresight for such negotiations.
Well, if you will have it so, I will not refuse.
For, both on my side this will be the safest way
To have some excuse to put forward to your enemies,
And for you it is more certain. You may name the gods.

  MEDEA: Swear by the plain of Earth, and Helios, father
Of my father, and name together all the gods. . . .

  AIGEUS: That I will act or not act in what way? Speak.

  MEDEA: That you yourself will never cast me from your land,
Nor, if any of my enemies should demand me,
Will you, in your life, willingly hand me over.

  AIGEUS: I swear by the Earth, by the holy light of Helios,
By all the gods, I will abide by this you say.

  MEDEA: Enough. And, if you fail, what shall happen to you?

  AIGEUS: What comes to those who have no regard for
    heaven.

  MEDEA: Go on your way. Farewell. For I am satisfied,
And I will reach your city as soon as I can,
Having done the deed I have to do and gained my end.

(AIGEUS *goes out.*)

  CHORUS: May Hermes, god of travellers,
Escort you, Aigeus, to your home!
And may you have the things you wish
So eagerly; for you
Appear to me to be a generous man.

MEDEA: God, and God's daughter, justice, and light of
 Helios!
Now, friends, has come the time of my triumph over
My enemies, and now my foot is on the road.
Now I am confident they will pay the penalty.
For this man, Aigeus, has been like a harbour to me
In all my plans just where I was most distressed.
To him I can fasten the cable of my safety
When I have reached the town and fortress of Pallas.
And now I shall tell to you the whole of my plan.
Listen to these words that are not spoken idly.
I shall send one of my servants to find Jason
And request him to come once more into my sight.
And when he comes, the words I'll say will be soft ones.
I'll say that I agree with him, that I approve
The royal wedding he has made, betraying me.
I'll say it was profitable, an excellent idea.
But I shall beg that my children may remain here:
Not that I would leave in a country that hates me
Children of mine to feel their enemies' insults,
But that by a trick I may kill the king's daughter.
For I will send the children with gifts in their hands
To carry to the bride, so as not to be banished,—
A finely woven dress and a golden diadem.
And if she takes them and wears them upon her skin
She and all who touch the girl will die in agony;
Such poison will I lay upon the gifts I send.
But there, however, I must leave that account paid.
I weep to think of what a deed I have to do.
Next after that, for I shall kill my own children.
My children, there is none who can give them safety.
And when I have ruined the whole of Jason's house,
I shall leave the land and flee from the murder of my
Dear children, and I shall have done a dreadful deed.
For it is not bearable to be mocked by enemies.
So it must happen. What profit have I in life?
I have no land, no home, no refuge from my pain.
My mistake was made the time I left behind me
My father's house, and trusted the words of a Greek,
Who, with heaven's help, will pay me the price for that.
For those children he had from me he will never
See alive again, nor will he on his new bride
Beget another child, for she is to be forced
To die a most terrible death by these my poisons.
Let no one think me a weak one, feeble-spirited,
A stay-at-home, but rather just the opposite,

One who can hurt my enemies and help my friends;
For the lives of such persons are most remembered.
   CHORUS: Since you have shared the knowledge of your
      plans with us,
I both wish to help you and support the normal
Ways of mankind, and tell you not to do this thing.
   MEDEA: I can do no other thing. It is understandable
For you to speak thus. You have not suffered as I have.
   CHORUS: But can you have the heart to kill your flesh and
      blood?
   MEDEA: Yes, for this is the best way to wound my hus-
      band.
   CHORUS: And you too. Of women you will be most un-
      happy.
   MEDEA: So it must be. No compromise is possible.

(*She turns to the* NURSE.)

Go, you, at once, and tell Jason to come to me.
You I employ on all affairs of greatest trust.
Say nothing of these decisions which I have made,
If you love your mistress, if you were born a woman.
   CHORUS: From of old the children of Erechtheus are
Splendid, the sons of blessed gods. They dwell
In Athen's holy and unconquered land,
Where famous Wisdom feeds them and they pass gaily
Always through that most brilliant air where once, they
     say,
That golden Harmony gave birth to the nine
Pure Muses of Pieria.

And beside the sweet flow of Cephisos' stream,
Where Cypris sailed, they say, to draw the water,
And mild soft breezes breathed along her path,
And on her hair were flung the sweet-smelling garlands
Of flowers of roses by the Lovers, the companions
Of Wisdom, her escort, the helpers of men
In every kind of excellence.

How then can these holy rivers
Or this holy land love you,
Or the city find you a home,
You, who will kill your children,
You, not pure with the rest?
O think of the blow at your children
And think of the blood that you shed.

O, over and over I beg you,
By your knees I beg you do not
Be the murderess of your babes!
O where will you find the courage *[BEAUTIFUL LANGUAGE + RHYTHM]*
Or the skill of hand and heart,
When you set yourself to attempt *[c.f. p27]*
A deed so dreadful to do?
How, when you look upon them,
Can you tearlessly hold the decision
For murder? You will not be able,
When your children fall down and implore you,
You will not be able to dip
Steadfast your hand in their blood.

(*Enter* JASON *with attendants.*)

JASON: I have come at your request. Indeed, although you
        are
Bitter against me, this you shall have: I will listen
To what new thing you want, woman, to get from me.
    MEDEA: Jason, I beg you to be forgiving towards me
For what I said. It is natural for you to bear with
My temper, since we have had much love together.
I have talked with myself about this and I have
Reproached myself. 'Fool,' I said, 'why am I so mad?
Why am I set against those who have planned wisely?
Why make myself an enemy of the authorities
And of my husband, who does the best thing for me
By marrying royalty and having children who
Will be as brothers to my own? What is wrong with me?
Let me give up anger, for the gods are kind to me.
Have I not children, and do I not know that we
In exile from our country must be short of friends?'
When I considered this I saw that I had shown
Great lack of sense, and that my anger was foolish. Now
I agree with you. I think that you are wise
In having this other wife as well as me, and I
Was mad. I should have helped you in these plans of
        yours,
Have joined in the wedding, stood by the marriage bed,
Have taken pleasure in attendance on your bride.
But we women are what we are,—perhaps a little
Worthless; and you men must not be like us in this,
Nor be foolish in return when we are foolish.
Now I give in, and admit that then I was wrong.

[Medea woos Jason]
[women = worthless]

I have come to a better understanding now.

(*She turns towards the house.*)

Children, come here, my children, come outdoors to us!
Welcome your father with me, and say goodbye to him,
And with your mother, who just now was his enemy,
Join again in making friends with him who loves us.

(*Enter the children, attended by the* TUTOR.)

We have made peace, and all our anger is over.
Take hold of his right hand,—O God, I am thinking
Of something which may happen in a secret future.
O children, will you just so, after a long life,
Hold out your loving arms at the grave? O children,
How ready to cry I am, how full of foreboding!
I am ending at last this quarrel with your father,
And, look, my soft eyes have suddenly filled with tears.
     CHORUS: And the pale tears have started also in my eyes.
O may the trouble not grow worse than now it is!
   JASON: I approve of what you say. And I cannot blame you
Even for what you said before. It is natural
For a woman to be wild with her husband when he
Goes in for secret love. But now your mind has turned
To better reasoning. In the end you have come to
The right decision, like the clever woman you are.
And of you, children, your father is taking care.
He has made, with God's help, ample provision for you.
For I think that a time will come when you will be
The leading people in Corinth with your brothers.
You must grow up. As to the future, your father
And those of the gods who love him will deal with that.
I want to see you, when you have become young men,
Healthy and strong, better men than my enemies.
Medea, why are your eyes all wet with pale tears?
Why is your cheek so white and turned away from me?
Are not these words of mine pleasing for you to hear?
   MEDEA: It is nothing. I was thinking about these children.
   JASON: You must be cheerful. I shall look after them well.
   MEDEA: I will be. It is not that I distrust your words,
But a woman is a frail thing, prone to crying.
   JASON: But why then should you grieve so much for these
     children?
   MEDEA: I am their mother. When you prayed that they
     might live,

I felt unhappy to think that these things will be.
But come, I have said something of the things I meant
To say to you, and now I will tell you the rest.
Since it is the king's will to banish me from here,—
And for me too I know that this is the best thing,
Not to be in your way by living here or in
The king's way, since they think me ill-disposed to them,—
I then am going into exile from this land;
But do you, so that you may have the care of them,
Beg Kreon that the children may not be banished.
    JASON: I doubt if I'll suceed, but I'll attempt it.
    MEDEA: Then you must tell your wife to beg from her father
That the children may be reprieved from banishment.
    JASON: I will, and with her I shall certainly succeed.
    MEDEA: If she is like the rest of us women, you will.
And I too will take a hand with you in this business,
For I will send her some gifts which are far fairer,
I am sure of it, than those which now are in fashion,
A finely-woven dress and a golden diadem,
And the children shall present them. Quick, let one of you
Servants bring here to me that beautiful dress.

(*One of her attendants goes into the house.*)

She will be happy not in one way, but in a hundred,
Having so fine a man as you to share her bed,
And with this beautiful dress which Helios of old,
My father's father, bestowed on his descendants.

(*Enter attendant carrying the poisoned dress and diadem.*)

There, children, take these wedding presents in your hands.
Take them to the royal princess, the happy bride,
And give them to her. She will not think little of them.
    JASON: No, don't be foolish, and empty your hands of these.
Do you think the palace is short of dresses to wear?
Do you think there is no gold there? Keep them, don't
            give them
Away. If my wife considers me of any value,
She will think more of me than money, I am sure of it.
    MEDEA: No, let me have my way. They say the gods them-
        selves
Are moved by gifts, and gold does more with men than
        words.
Hers is the luck, her fortune that which god blesses;
She is young and a princess; but for my children's reprieve

I would give my very life, and not gold only.
Go children, go together to that rich palace,
Be suppliants to the new wife of your father,
My lady, beg her not to let you be banished.
And give her the dress,—for this is of great importance,
That she should take the gift into her hand from yours.
Go, quick as you can. And bring your mother good news
By your success of those things which she longs to gain.

(JASON *goes out with his attendants, followed by the* TUTOR
and the children carrying the poisoned gifts.)

CHORUS: Now there is no hope left for the children's lives.
Now there is none. They are walking already to murder.
The bride, poor bride, will accept the curse of the gold,
Will accept the bright diadem. *EXAMPLE OF RYTHM*
Around her yellow hair she will set that dress
Of death with her own hands.
The grace and the perfume and the glow of the golden robe
Will charm her to put them upon her and wear the wreath,
And now her wedding will be with the dead below,
Into such a trap she will fall.
Poor thing, into such a fate of death and never
Escape from under that curse.

JASON'S RESPONSIBILITY

You too, O wretched bridegroom, making your match
    with kings,
You do not see that you bring
Destruction on your children and on her,
Your wife, a fearful death. — *JASON WILL "FALL"*
Poor soul, what a fall is yours!

In your grief too I weep, mother of little children,
You who will murder your own,
In vengeance for the loss of married love
Which Jason has betrayed
As he lives with another wife.

(*Enter the* TUTOR *with the children.*)

TUTOR: Mistress, I tell you that these children are reprieved,
And the royal bride has been pleased to take in her hands
Your gifts. In that quarter the children are secure.
But come,
Why do you stand confused when you are fortunate?

Medea greets the news of the successfully delivered gifts. She is stricken

Why have you turned round with your cheek away from
  me?
Are not these words of mine pleasing for you to hear?

MEDEA: Oh! I am lost!

TUTOR: That word is not in harmony with my tidings.

MEDEA: I am lost, I am lost!

TUTOR: Am I in ignorance telling you
Of some disaster, and not the good news I thought?

MEDEA: You have told what you have told. I do not blame
  you.

TUTOR: Why then this downcast eye, and this weeping of
  tears?

MEDEA: Oh, I am forced to weep, old man. The gods and I,
I in a kind of madness have contrived all this.

TUTOR: Courage! You too will be brought home by your
  children.

MEDEA: Ah, before that happens I shall bring others home.

TUTOR: Others before you have been parted from their
  children.
Mortals must bear in resignation their ill luck.

MEDEA: This is what I shall do. But go inside the house.
And do for the children your usual daily work.

  (*The* TUTOR *goes into the house.* MEDEA *turns to her children.*)

O children, O my children, you have a city,
You have a home, and you can leave me behind you,
And without your mother you may live there for ever.
But I am going in exile to another land
Before I have seen you happy and taken pleasure in you,
Before I have dressed your brides and made your mar-
      riage beds,
And held up the torch at the ceremony of wedding.
Oh, what a wretch I am in this my self-willed thought!
What was the purpose, children, for which I reared you?
For all my travail and wearing myself away?
They were sterile, those pains I had in the bearing of you.
O surely once the hopes in you I had, poor me,
Were high ones: you would look after me in old age,
And when I died would deck me well with your own
      hands;
A thing which all would have done. O but now it is gone,
That lovely thought. For, once I am left without you,
Sad will be the life I'll lead and sorrowful for me.
And you will never see your mother again with

impt. that Medea waver

Your dear eyes, gone to another mode of living.
Why, children, do you look upon me with your eyes?
Why do you smile so sweetly that last smile of all?
Oh, Oh, what can I do? My spirit has gone from me,
Friends, when I saw that bright look in the children's eyes.
I cannot bear to do it. I renounce my plans
I had before. I'll take my children away from
This land. Why should I hurt their father with the pain
They feel, and suffer twice as much of pain myself?
No, no, I will not do it. I renounce my plans.
Ah, what is wrong with me? Do I want to let go
My enemies unhurt and be laughed at for it?
I must face this thing. Oh, but what a weak woman
Even to admit to my mind these soft arguments.
Children, go into the house. And he whom law forbids
To stand in attendance at my sacrifices,
Let him see to it. I shall not mar my handiwork.
Oh! Oh!
Do not, O my heart, you must not do these things!
Poor heart, let them go, have pity upon the children.
If they live with you in Athens they will cheer you.
No! By Hell's avenging furies it shall not be,—
This shall never be, that I should suffer my children
To be the prey of my enemies' insolence.
Every way is it fixed. The bride will not escape.
No, the diadem is now upon her head, and she,
The royal princess, is dying in the dress, I know it.
But,—for it is the most dreadful of roads for me
To tread, and them I shall send on a more dreadful still—
I wish to speak to the children.

   (*She calls the children to her.*)
                              Come, children, give
Me your hands, give your mother your hands to kiss them.
O the dear hands, and O how dear are these lips to me,
And the generous eyes and the bearing of my children!
I wish you happiness, but not here in this world.
What is here your father took. O how good to hold you!
How delicate the skin, how sweet the breath of children!
Go, go! I am no longer able, no longer
To look upon you. I am overcome by sorrow.

   (*The children go into the house.*)

I know indeed what evil I intend to do,

But stronger than all my afterthoughts is my fury,
Fury that brings upon mortals the greatest evils.

(*She goes out to the right, towards the royal
palace.*)

THE CHORUS IS FEMALE

CHORUS: Often before
I have gone through more subtle reasons,
And have come upon questionings greater
Than a woman should strive to search out.
But we too have a goddess to help us
And accompany us to wisdom.
Not all of us. Still you will find
Among many women a few,
who can attain wisdom
And our sex is not without learning.
This I say, that those who have never
Had children, who know nothing of it,
In happiness have the advantage
Over those who are parents.
The childless, who never discover
Whether children turn out as a good thing
Or as something to cause pain, are spared
Many troubles in lacking this knowledge.
And those who have in their homes
The sweet presence of children, I see that their lives
Are all wasted away by their worries.
sounds like a radical fem view
First they must think how to bring them up well and
How to leave them something to live on.
And then after this whether all their toil
Is for those who will turn out good or bad,
Is still an unanswered question.
or a planned parenthood tract-
And of one more trouble, the last of all,
That is common to mortals I tell.
For suppose you have found them enough for their living,
Suppose that the children have grown into youth
And have turned out good, still, if God so wills it,
Death will away with your children's bodies,
And carry them off into Hades.
What is our profit, then, that for the sake of
Children the gods should pile upon mortals
After all else
This most terrible grief of all?

(*Enter* MEDEA, *from the spectators' right.*)

MEDEA: Friends, I can tell you that for long I have waited

For the event. I stare towards the place from where
The news will come. And now, see one of Jason's servants
Is on his way here, and that laboured breath of his
Shows he has tidings for us, and evil tidings.

(*Enter, also from the right, the* MESSENGER.)

MESSENGER: Medea, you who have done such a dreadful
    thing,
So outrageous, run for your life, take what you can,
A ship to bear you hence or chariot on land.
    MEDEA: And what is the reason deserves such flight as
        this?
    MESSENGER: She is dead, only just now, the royal princess,
And Kreon dead too, her father, by your poisons.
    MEDEA: The finest words you have spoken. Now and
        hereafter
I shall count you among my benefactors and friends.
    MESSENGER: What! Are you right in the mind? Are you
        not mad,
Woman? The house of the king is outraged by you.
Do you enjoy it? Not afraid of such doings?
    MEDEA: To what you say I on my side have something too
To say in answer. Do not be in a hurry, friend,
But speak. How did they die? You will delight me twice
As much again if you say they died in agony.
    MESSENGER: When those two children, born of you, had
        entered in,
Their father with them, and passed into the bride's house,
We were pleased, we slaves who were distressed by your
        wrongs.
All through the house we were talking of but one thing,
How you and your husband had made up your quarrel.
Some kissed the children's hands and some their yellow
        hair,
And I myself was so full of my joy that I
Followed the children into the women's quarters.
Our mistress, whom we honour now instead of you,
Before she noticed that your two children were there,
Was keeping her eye fixed eagerly on Jason.
Afterwards however she covered up her eyes,
Her cheek paled and she turned herself away from him,
So disgusted was she at the children's coming there.
But your husband tried to end the girl's bad temper,
And said 'You must not look unkindly on your friends.
Cease to be angry. Turn your head to me again.

Have as your friends the same ones as your husband has.
And take these gifts, and beg your father to reprieve
These children from their exile. Do it for my sake.'
She, when she saw the dress, could not restrain herself.
She agreed with all her husband said, and before
He and the children had gone far from the palace,
She took the gorgeous robe and dressed herself in it,
And put the golden crown around her curly locks,
And arranged the set of the hair in a shining mirror,
And smiled at the lifeless image of herself in it.
Then she rose from her chair and walked about the room,
With her gleaming feet stepping most soft and delicate,
All overjoyed with the present. Often and often
She would stretch her foot out straight and look along it.
But after that it was a fearful thing to see.
The colour of her face changed, and she staggered back,
She ran, and her legs trembled, and she only just
Managed to reach a chair without falling flat down.
An aged woman servant who, I take it, thought
This was some seizure of Pan or another god,
Cried out 'God bless us,' but that was before she saw
The white foam breaking through her lips and her rolling
The pupils of her eyes and her face all bloodless.
Then she raised a different cry from that 'God bless us,'
A huge shriek, and the women ran, one to the king,
One to the newly wedded husband to tell him
What had happened to his bride; and with frequent sound
The whole of the palace rang as they went running.
One walking quickly round the course of a race-track
Would now have turned the bend and be close to the goal,
When she, poor girl, opened her shut and speechless eye,
And with a terrible groan she came to herself.
For a two-fold pain was moving up against her.
The wreath of gold that was resting around her head
Let forth a fearful stream of all-devouring fire,
And the finely-woven dress your children gave to her,
Was fastening on the unhappy girl's fine flesh.
She leapt up from the chair, and all on fire she ran,
Shaking her hair now this way and now that, trying
To hurl the diadem away; but fixedly
The gold preserved its grip, and, when she shook her hair,
Then more and twice as fiercely the fire blazed out.
Till, beaten by her fate, she fell down to the ground,
Hard to be recognised except by a parent.
Neither the setting of her eyes was plain to see,
Nor the shapeliness of her face. From the top of

Her head there oozed out blood and fire mixed together.
Like the drops on pine-bark, so the flesh from her bones
Dropped away, torn by the hidden fang of the poison.
It was a fearful sight; and terror held us all
From touching the corpse. We had learned from what had
    happened.
But her wretched father, knowing nothing of the event,
Came suddenly to the house, and fell upon the corpse,
And at once cried out and folded his arms about her,
And kissed her and spoke to her, saying 'O my poor child,
What heavenly power has so shamefully destroyed you?
And who has set me here like an ancient sepulchre,
Deprived of you? O let me die with you, my child!'
And when he had made an end of his wailing and crying,
Then the old man wished to raise himself to his feet;
But, as the ivy clings to the twigs of the laurel,
So he stuck to the fine dress, and he struggled fearfully.
For he was trying to lift himself to his knee,
And she was pulling him down, and when he tugged hard
He would be ripping his aged flesh from his bones.
At last his life was quenched and the unhappy man
Gave up the ghost, no longer could hold up his head.
There they lie close, the daughter and the old father,
Dead bodies, an event he prayed for in his tears.
As for your interests, I will say nothing of them,
For you will find your own escape from punishment.
Our human life I think and have thought a shadow,
And I do not fear to say that those who are held
Wise amongst men and who search the reasons of things
Are those who bring the most sorrow on themselves.
For of mortals there is no one who is happy.
If wealth flows in upon one, one may be perhaps
Luckier than one's neighbour, but still not happy.

(Exit.)

JASON "DESERVED
THIS"

CHORUS: Heaven, it seems, on this day has fastened many
Evils on Jason, and Jason has deserved them.
Poor girl, the daughter of Kreon, how I pity you
And your misfortunes, you who have gone quite away
To the house of Hades because of marrying Jason.
MEDEA: Women, my task is fixed: as quickly as I may
To kill my children, and start away from this land,
And not, by wasting time, to suffer my children
To be slain by another hand less kindly to them.
Force every way will have it they must die, and since

This must be so, then I, their mother, shall kill them.
O arm yourself in steel, my heart! Do not hang back
From doing this fearful and necessary wrong.
O come, my hand, poor wretched hand, and take the
       sword,
Take it, step forward to this bitter starting point,
And do not be a coward, do not think of them,
How sweet they are, and how you are their mother. Just for
This one short day be forgetful of your children,
Afterwards weep; for even though you will kill them,
They were very dear,—O, I am an unhappy woman!

(With a cry she rushes into the house.)

CHORUS: O Earth, and the far shining
Ray of the Sun, look down, look down upon
This poor lost woman, look, before she raises
The hand of murder against her flesh and blood.
Yours was the golden birth from which
She sprang, and now I fear divine
Blood may be shed by men.
O heavenly light, hold back her hand,
Check her, and drive from out the house
The bloody Fury raised by fiends of Hell.

Vain waste, your care of children;
Was it in vain you bore the babes you loved,
After you passed the inhospitable strait
Between the dark blue rocks, Symplegades?
O wretched one, how has it come,
This heavy anger on your heart,
This cruel bloody mind?
For God from mortals asks a stern
Price for the stain of kindred blood
In like disaster falling on their homes.

(A cry from one of the children is heard.)

CHORUS: Do you hear the cry, do you hear the children's
       cry?
O you hard heart, O woman fated for evil!
ONE OF THE CHILDREN *(from within)*: What can I do and
    how escape my mother's hands?
ANOTHER CHILD *(from within)*: O my dear brother, I can-
    not tell. We are lost.
CHORUS: Shall I enter the house? O surely I should

Defend the children from murder.

A CHILD (*from within*): O help us, in God's name, for now
we need your help.

Now, now we are close to it. We are trapped by the sword.

CHORUS: O your heart must have been made of rock or
steel,

You who can kill
With your own hand the fruit of your own womb.
Of one alone I have heard, one woman alone
Of those of old who laid her hands on her children,
Ino, sent mad by heaven when the wife of Zeus
Drove her out from her home and made her wander;
And because of the wicked shedding of blood
Of her own children she threw
Herself, poor wretch, into the sea and stepped away
Over the sea-cliff to die with her two children.
What horror more can be? O women's love,
So full of trouble,
How many evils have you caused already!

(*Enter* JASON *with attendants.*)

JASON: You women, standing close in front of this dwelling,
Is she, Medea, she who did this dreadful deed,
Still in the house, or has she run away in flight?
For she will have to hide herself beneath the earth,
Or raise herself on wings into the height of air,
If she wishes to escape the royal vengeance.
Does she imagine that, having killed our rulers,
She will herself escape uninjured from this house?
But I am thinking not so much of her as for
The children,—her the king's friends will make to suffer
For what she did. So I have come to save the lives
Of my boys, in case the royal house should harm them
While taking vengeance for their mother's wicked deed.

CHORUS: O Jason, if you but knew how deeply you are
Involved in sorrow, you would not have spoken so.

JASON: What is it? That she is planning to kill me also?

CHORUS: Your children are dead, and by their own own
mother's hand.

JASON: What! This is it? O woman, you have destroyed me.

CHORUS: You must make up your mind your children are
no more.

JASON: Where did she kill them? Was it here or in the
house?

CHORUS: Open the gates and there you will see them murdered.

JASON: Quick as you can unlock the doors, men, and undo
The fastenings and let me see this double evil,
My children dead and her,—O her I will repay.

(*His attendants rush to the door.* MEDEA *appears above the
house in a chariot drawn by dragons. She has the dead bodies
of the children with her.*)

MEDEA: Why do you batter these gates and try to unbar
them,
Seeking the corpses and for me who did the deed?
You may cease your trouble, and, if you have need of me,
Speak, if you wish. You will never touch me with your
hand, *are the Gods on her side?*
Such a chariot has Helios, my father's father,
Given me to defend me from my enemies.
JASON: You hateful thing, you woman most utterly loathed
By the gods and me and by all the race of mankind,
You who have had the heart to raise a sword against
Your children, you, their mother, and left me childless,—
You have done this, and do you still look at the sun
And at the earth, after these most fearful doings?
I wish you dead. Now I see it plain, though at that time
I did not, when I took you from your foreign home
And brought you to a Greek house, you, an evil thing,
A traitress to your father and your native land.
The gods hurled the avenging curse of yours on me.
For your own brother you slew at your own hearthside,
And then came aboard that beautiful ship, the Argo.
And that was your beginning. When you were married
To me, your husband, and had borne children to me,
For the sake of pleasure in the bed you killed them.
There is no Greek woman who would have dared such
deeds.
Out of all those whom I passed over and chose you
To marry instead, a bitter destructive match,
A monster not a woman, having a nature
Wilder than that of Scylla in the Tuscan sea.
Ah! no, not if I had ten thousand words of shame
Could I sting you. You are naturally so brazen.
Go, worker in evil, stained with your children's blood.
For me remains to cry aloud upon my fate,
Who will get no pleasure from my newly-wedded love,
And the boys whom I begot and brought up, never

Shall I speak to them alive. Oh, my life is over!

MEDEA: Long would be the answer which I might have
    made to
These words of yours, if Zeus the father did not know
How I have treated you and what you did to me.
No, it was not to be that you should scorn my love,
And pleasantly live your life through, laughing at me;
Nor would the princess, nor he who offered the match,
Kreon, drive me away without paying for it.
So now you may call me a monster, if you wish,
O Scylla housed in the caves of the Tuscan sea
I too, as I had to, have taken hold of your heart.

JASON: You feel the pain yourself. You share in my sor-
    row.

MEDEA: Yes, and my grief is gain when you cannot mock it.

JASON: O children, what a wicked mother she was to you!

MEDEA: They died from a disease they caught from their
    father.

JASON: I tell you it was not my hand that destroyed them.

MEDEA: But it was your insolence, and your virgin wed-
    ding.

JASON: And just for the sake of that you chose to kill
    them.

MEDEA: Is love so small a pain, do you think, for a
    woman?

JASON: For a wise one, certainly. But you are wholly evil.

MEDEA: The children are dead. I say this to make you suf-
    fer.

JASON: The children, I think, will bring down curses on
    you.

MEDEA: The gods know who was the author of this sor-
    row.

JASON: Yes, the gods know indeed, they know your loath-
    some heart.

MEDEA: Hate me. But I tire of your barking bitterness.

JASON: And I of yours. It is easier to leave you.

MEDEA: How then? What shall I do? I long to leave you
    too.

JASON: Give me the bodies to bury and to mourn them.

MEDEA: No, that I will not. I will bury them myself,
Bearing them to Hera's temple on the promontory;
So that no enemy may evilly treat them
By tearing up their grave. In this land of Corinth
I shall establish a holy feast and sacrifice
Each year for ever to atone for the blood guilt.
And I myself go to the land of Erechtheus

To dwell in Aigeus' house, the son of Pandion.
While you, as is right, will die without distinction,
Struck on the head by a piece of the Argo's timber,
And you will have seen the bitter end of my love.
   JASON: May a Fury for the children's sake destroy you,
And justice. Requiter of blood.
   MEDEA: What heavenly power lends an ear
To a breaker of oaths, a deceiver?
   JASON: O, I hate you, murderess of children.
   MEDEA: Go to your palace. Bury your bride.
   JASON: I go, with two children to mourn for.
   MEDEA: Not yet do you feel it. Wait for the future.
   JASON: Oh, children I loved!
   MEDEA: I loved them, you did not.
   JASON: You loved them, and killed them.
   MEDEA: To make you feel pain.
   JASON: Oh, wretch that I am, how I long
To kiss the dear lips of my children!
   MEDEA: Now you would speak to them, now you would
     kiss them.
Then you rejected them.
   JASON: Let me, I beg you,
Touch my boys' delicate flesh.
   MEDEA: I will not. Your words are all wasted.
   JASON: O God, do you hear it, this persecution,
These my sufferings from this hateful
Woman, this monster, murderess of children?
Still what I can do that I will do:
I will lament and cry upon heaven,
Calling the gods to bear me witness
How you have killed my boys and prevent me from
Touching their bodies or giving them burial.
I wish I had never begot them to see them
Afterwards slaughtered by you.

   CHORUS: Zeus in Olympus is the overseer
Of many doings. Many things the gods
Achieve beyond our judgement. What we thought
Is not confirmed and what we thought not God
Contrives. And so it happens in this story.

LYSISTRATA

Aristophanes

Characters*

LYSISTRATA ⎫
  CALONICE   ⎬ *Athenian women*
MYRRHINE ⎭
LAMPITO, *a Spartan woman*
LEADER OF THE CHORUS OF OLD MEN
CHORUS OF OLD MEN
LEADER OF THE CHORUS OF OLD WOMEN
CHORUS OF OLD WOMEN
ATHENIAN MAGISTRATE
THREE ATHENIAN WOMEN
CINESIAS, *an Athenian, husband of Myrrhine*
SPARTAN HERALD
SPARTAN AMBASSADORS
ATHENIAN AMBASSADORS
TWO ATHENIAN CITIZENS
CHORUS OF ATHENIANS
CHORUS OF SPARTANS

---

*As is usual in ancient comedy, the leading characters have sig-
nificant names. LYSISTRATA is "She who disbands the armies"; MYRR-
HINE's name is chosen to suggest *myrton*, a Greek word meaning
pudenda muliebria; LAMPITO is a celebrated Spartan name; CINESIAS,
although a real name in Athens, is chosen to suggest a Greek verb
kinein, to move, then *to make love, to have intercourse,* and the
name of his deme, Paionidai, suggests the verb *paiein,* which has
about the same significance.

SCENE. *In Athens, beneath the Acropolis. In the center of the stage is the Propylaea, or gate-way to the Acropolis; to one side is a small grotto, sacred to Pan. The Orchestra represents a slope leading up to the gate-way.*

It is early in the morning. LYSISTRATA *is pacing impatiently up and down.*

LYSISTRATA If they'd been summoned to worship the God of Wine, or Pan, or to visit the Queen of Love, why, you couldn't have pushed your way through the streets for all the timbrels. But now there's not a single woman here—except my neighbour; here she comes.

(*Enter* CALONICE.) *Cal - oN - ICE*

Good day to you, Calonice.

CALONICE: And to you, Lysistrata. (*Noticing* LYSISTRATA'S *impatient air*) But what ails you? Don't scowl, my dear; it's not becoming to you to knit your brows like that.

LYSISTRATA (*sadly*): Ah, Calonice, my heart aches; I'm so annoyed at us women. For among men we have a reputation for sly trickery—

CALONICE: And rightly too, on my word!

LYSISTRATA: —but when they were told to meet here to consider a matter of no small importance, they lie abed and don't come.

CALONICE: Oh, they'll come all right, my dear. It's not easy for a woman to get out, you know. One is working on her husband, another is getting up the maid, another has to put the baby to bed, or wash and feed it.

LYSISTRATA: But after all, there are other matters more important than all that.

CALONICE: My dear Lysistrata, just what is this matter you've summoned us women to consider? What's up? Something big?

[41]

LYSISTRATA: Very big.

CALONICE (*interested*): Is it stout, too?

LYSISTRATA (*smiling*): Yes indeed—both big and stout.

CALONICE: What? And the women still haven't come?

LYSISTRATA: It's not what you suppose; they'd have come soon enough for *that*. But I've worked up something, and for many a sleepless night I've turned it this way and that.

CALONICE (*in mock disappointment*): Oh, I guess it's pretty fine and slender, if you've turned it this way and that.

LYSISTRATA: So fine that the safety of the whole of Greece lies in us women.

CALONICE: In us women? It depends on a very slender reed then.

LYSISTRATA: Our country's fortunes are in our hands; and whether the Spartans shall perish—

CALONICE: Good! Let them perish, by all means.

LYSISTRATA: —and the Boeotians shall be completely annihilated.

CALONICE: Not completely! Please spare the eels.

LYSISTRATA: As for Athens, I won't use any such unpleasant words. But you understand what I mean. But if the women will meet here—the Spartans, the Boeotians, and we Athenians— then all together we will save Greece.

CALONICE: But what could women do that's clever or distinguished? We just sit around all dolled up in silk robes, looking pretty in our sheer gowns and evening slippers.

LYSISTRATA: These are just the things I hope will save us: these silk robes, perfumes, evening slippers, rouge, and our chiffon blouses.

CALONICE: How so?

LYSISTRATA: So never a man alive will lift a spear against the foe—

CALONICE: I'll get a silk gown at once.

LYSISTRATA: —or take up his shield—

CALONICE: I'll put on my sheerest gown!

LYSISTRATA: —or sword.

CALONICE: I'll buy a pair of evening slippers.

LYSISTRATA: Well then, shouldn't the women have come?

CALONICE: Come? Why, they should have *flown* here.

LYSISTRATA: Well, my dear, just watch: they'll act in true Athenian fashion—everything too late! And now there's not a woman here from the shore or from Salamis.

CALONICE: They're coming, I'm sure; at daybreak they were laying—to their oars to cross the straits.

LYSISTRATA: And those I expected would be the first to come—the women of Acharnae—they haven't arrived.

CALONICE: Yet the wife of Theagenes means to come: she consulted Hecate about it. (*Seeing a group of women approaching*) But look! Here come a few. And there are some more over here. Hurrah! Where do they come from?

LYSISTRATA: From Anagyra.

CALONICE: Yes indeed! We've raised up quite a stink from Anagyra anyway.

(*Enter* MYRRHINE *in haste, followed by several other women.*)

MYRRHINE (*breathlessly*): Have we come in time, Lysistrata? What do you say? Why so quiet?

LYSISTRATA: I can't say much for you, Myrrhine, coming at this hour on such important business.

MYRRHINE: Why, I had trouble finding my girdle in the dark. But if it's so important, we're here now; tell us.

LYSISTRATA: No. Let's wait a little for the women from Boeotia and the Peloponnesus.

MYRRHINE: That's a much better suggestion. Look! Here comes Lampito now.

(*Enter* LAMPITO *with two other women.*)

LYSISTRATA: Greetings, my dear Spartan friend. How pretty you look, my dear. What a smooth complexion and well-developed figure! You could throttle an ox.

LAMPITO: Faith, yes, I think I could. I take exercises and kick my heels against my bum. (*She demonstrates with a few steps of the Spartan "bottom-kicking" dance.*)

LYSISTRATA: And what splendid breasts you have.

LAMPITO: La! You handle me like a prize steer.

LYSISTRATA: And who is this young lady with you?

LAMPITO: Faith, she's an Ambassadress from Boeotia.

LYSISTRATA: Oh yes, a Boeotian, and blooming like a garden too.

CALONICE (*lifting up her skirt*): My word! How neatly her garden's weeded!

LYSISTRATA: And who is the other girl?

LAMPITO: Oh, she's a Corinthian swell.

MYRRHINE (*after a rapid examination*): Yes indeed. She swells very nicely (*pointing*) here and here.

LAMPITO: Who has gathered together this company of women?

LYSISTRATA: I have.

LAMPITO: Speak up, then. What do you want?

MYRRHINE: Yes, my dear, tell us what this important matter is.

LYSISTRATA: Very well, I'll tell you. But before I speak, let me ask you a little question.

MYRRHINE: Anything you like.

LYSISTRATA (*earnestly*): Tell me: don't you yearn for the fathers of your children, who are away at the wars? I know you all have husbands abroad.

CALONICE: Why, yes; mercy me! my husband's been away for five months in Thrace keeping guard on—Eucrates.

MYRRHINE: And mine for seven whole months in Pylus.

LAMPITO: And mine, as soon as ever he returns from the fray, readjusts his shield and flies out of the house again.

LYSISTRATA: And as for lovers, there's not even a ghost of one left. Since the Milesians revolted from us, I've not even seen an eight-inch dingus to be a leather consolation for us widows. Are you willing, if I can find a way, to help me end the war?

MYRRHINE: Goodness, yes! I'd do it, even if I had to pawn my dress and—get drunk on the spot!

CALONICE: And I, even if I had to let myself be split in two like a flounder

LAMPITO: I'd climb up Mt. Taygetus if I could catch a glimpse of peace.

LYSISTRATA: I'll tell you, then, in plain and simple words. My friends, if we are going to force our men to make peace, we must do without—

MYRRHINE: Without what? Tell us.

LYSISTRATA: Will you do it?

MYRRHINE: We'll do it, if it kills us.

LYSISTRATA: Well then, we must do without sex altogether. (*General consternation.*) Why do you turn away? Where go you? Why turn so pale? Why those tears? Will you do it or not? What means this hesitation?

MYRRHINE: I won't do it! Let the war go on.

CALONICE: Nor I! Let the war go on.

LYSISTRATA: So, my little flounder? Didn't you say just now you'd split yourself in half?

CALONICE: Anything else you like. I'm willing, even if I have to walk through fire. Anything rather than sex. There's nothing like it, my dear.

LYSISTRATA (*to* MYRRHINE): What about you?

MYRRHINE (*sullenly*): I'm willing to walk through fire, too.

LYSISTRATA: Oh vile and cursed breed! No wonder they make tragedies about us: we're naught but "love-affairs and bassinets." But you, my dear Spartan friend, if you alone are

with me, our enterprise might yet succeed. Will you vote with
me?

LAMPITO: 'Tis cruel hard, by my faith, for a woman to
sleep alone without her nooky; but for all that, we certainly
do need peace. *Good translation - captures owl*

LYSISTRATA: O my dearest friend! You're the only real
woman here. *sexual terms —*

CALONICE (*wavering*): Well, if we do refrain from—
(*shuddering*) what you say (God forbid!), would that bring
peace?

LYSISTRATA: My goodness, yes! If we sit at home all
rouged and powdered, dressed in our sheerest gowns, and
neatly depilated, our men will get excited and want to take
us; but if you don't come to them and keep away, they'll
soon make a truce.

LAMPITO: Aye; Menelaus caught sight of Helen's naked
breast and dropped his sword, they say.

CALONICE: What if the men give us up?

LYSISTRATA: "Flay a skinned dog," as Pherecrates says.

CALONICE: Rubbish! These make-shifts are no good. But
suppose they grab us and drag us into the bedroom?

LYSISTRATA: Hold on to the door.

CALONICE: And if they beat us?

LYSISTRATA: Give in with a bad grace. There's no pleasure
in it for them when they have to use violence. And you must
torment them in every possible way. They'll give up soon
enough; a man gets no joy if he doesn't get along with his
wife.

MYRRHINE: If this is your opinion, we agree.

LAMPITO: As for our own men, we can persuade them to
make a just and fair peace; but what about the Athenian rabble? Who will persuade them not to start any more monkey-
shines?

LYSISTRATA: Don't worry. We guarantee to convince them.

LAMPITO: Not while their ships are rigged so well and they
have that mighty treasure in the temple of Athene.

LYSISTRATA: We've taken good care for that too: we shall
seize the Acropolis today. The older women have orders to
do this, and while we are making our arrangements, they are
to pretend to make a sacrifice and occupy the Acropolis.

LAMPITO: All will be well then. That's a very fine idea.

LYSISTRATA: Let's ratify this, Lampito, with the most solemn oath.

LAMPITO: Tell us what oath we shall swear.

LYSISTRATA: Well said. Where's our Policewoman? (*to a*

Pokes fun at his contemporary artists.

Scythian slave) What are you gaping at? Set a shield upside-down here in front of me, and give me the sacred meats.

CALONICE: Lysistrata, what sort of an oath are we to take?

LYSISTRATA: What oath? I'm going to slaughter a sheep over the shield, as they do in Aeschylus.

CALONICE: Don't, Lysistrata! No oaths about peace over a shield.

LYSISTRATA: What shall the oath be, then?

CALONICE: How about getting a white horse somewhere and cutting out its entrails for the sacrifice?

LYSISTRATA: White horse indeed!

CALONICE: Well then, how shall we swear?

MYRRHINE: I'll tell you: let's place a large black bowl upside-down and then slaughter—a flask of Thasian wine. And then let's swear—not to pour in a single drop of water.

LAMPITO: Lôrd! How I like that oath!

LYSISTRATA: Someone bring out a bowl and a flask.

(*A slave brings the utensils for the sacrifice.*)

CALONICE: Look, my friends! What a big jar! Here's a cup that 'twould give me joy to handle. (*She picks up the bowl.*)

LYSISTRATA: Set it down and put your hands on our victim. (*As* CALONICE *places her hands on the flask*) O Lady of Persuasion and dear Loving Cup, graciously vouchsafe to receive this sacrifice from us women. (*She pours the wine into the bowl.*)

CALONICE: The blood has a good colour and spurts out nicely.

LAMPITO: Faith, it has a pleasant smell, too.

MYRRHINE: Oh, let me be the first to swear, ladies!

CALONICE: No, by our Lady! Not unless you're allotted the first turn.

LYSISTRATA: Place all your hands on the cup, and one of you repeat on behalf of all what I say. Then all will swear and ratify the oath. *I will suffer no man, be he husband or lover,*

CALONICE: *I will remain at home unmated,*

LYSISTRATA: *To approach me all hot and horny.* (*As* CALONICE *hesitates*) Say it!

CALONICE (*slowly and painfully*): *To approach me all hot and horny.* O Lysistrata, I feel so weak in the knees!

LYSISTRATA: *I will remain at home unmated,*

CALONICE: *I will remain at home unmated,*

LYSISTRATA: *Wearing my sheerest gown and carefully adorned,*

CALONICE: *Wearing my sheerest gown and carefully adorned,*

LYSISTRATA: *That my husband may burn with desire for me.*

CALONICE: *That my husband may burn with desire for me.*

LYSISTRATA: *And if he takes me by force against my will,*

CALONICE: *And if he takes me by force against my will,*

LYSISTRATA: *I shall do it badly and keep from moving.*

CALONICE: *I shall do it badly and keep from moving.*

LYSISTRATA: *I will not stretch my slippers toward the ceiling,*

CALONICE: *I will not stretch my slippers toward the ceiling,*

LYSISTRATA: *Nor will I take the posture of the lioness on the knife-handle.*

CALONICE: *Nor will I take the posture of the lioness on the knife-handle.*

LYSISTRATA: *If I keep this oath, may I be permitted to drink from this cup,*

CALONICE: *If I keep this oath, may I be permitted to drink from this cup,*

LYSISTRATA: *But if I break it, may the cup be filled with water.*

CALONICE: *But if I break it, may the cup be filled with water.*

LYSISTRATA: Do you all swear to this?

ALL: I do, so help me!

LYSISTRATA: Come then, I'll just consummate this offering.

(She takes a long drink from the cup.)

CALONICE *(snatching the cup away)*: Shares, my dear! Let's drink to our continued friendship.

(A shout is heard from off-stage.)

LAMPITO: What's that shouting?

LYSISTRATA: That's what I was telling you: the women have just seized the Acropolis. Now, Lampito, go home and arrange matters in Sparta; and leave these two ladies here as hostages. We'll enter the Acropolis to join our friends and help them lock the gates.

CALONICE: Don't you suppose the men will come to attack us?

LYSISTRATA: Don't worry about them. Neither threats nor fire will suffice to open the gates, except on the terms we've stated.

CALONICE: I should say not! Else we'd belie our reputation as unmanageable pests.

But it does articulate the reputation —

(LAMPITO *leaves the stage. The other women retire and enter the Acropolis through the Propylaea.*)

(*Enter the* CHORUS OF OLD MEN, *carrying fire-pots and a load of heavy sticks.*)

LEADER OF MEN: Onward, Draces, step by step, though your shoulder's aching.
Cursèd logs of olive-wood, what a load you're making!

FIRST SEMI-CHORUS OF OLD MEN (*singing*):

Aye, many surprises await a man who lives to a ripe old age;
For who could suppose, Strymodorus my lad, that the women we've nourished (alas!),
  Who sat at home to vex our days,
  Would seize the holy image here,
  And occupy this sacred shrine,
  With bolts and bars, with fell design,
  To lock the Propylaea?

LEADER OF MEN: Come with speed, Philourgus, come! to the temple hast'ning.
There we'll heap these logs about in a circle round them,
And whoever has conspired, raising this rebellion,
Shall be roasted, scorched, and burnt, all without exception,
Doomed by one unanimous vote—but first the wife of Lycon.

SECOND SEMI-CHORUS (*singing*):

No, no! by Demeter, while I'm alive, no woman shall mock at me.
Not even the Spartan Cleomenes, our citadel first to seize,
  Got off unscathed; for all his pride
  And haughty Spartan arrogance,
  He left his arms and sneaked away,
  Stripped to his shirt, unkempt, unshav'd,
  With six years' filth still on him.

LEADER OF MEN: I besieged that hero bold, sleeping at my station,
Marshalled at these holy gates sixteen deep against him.
Shall I not these cursèd pests punish for their daring,
Burning these Euripides-and-God-detested women?
Aye! or else may Marathon overturn my trophy.

FIRST SEMI-CHORUS (*singing*): There remains of my road
  Just this brow of the hill;
  There I speed on my way.
Drag the logs up the hill, though we've got no ass to help.
  (God! my shoulder's bruised and sore!)
  Onward still must we go.
  Blow the fire! Don't let it go out
  Now we're near the end of our road.

ALL (*blowing on the fire-pots*): Whew! Whew! Drat the smoke!

SECOND SEMI-CHORUS (*singing*): Lord, what smoke rushing forth
From the pot, like a dog
Running mad, bites my eyes!
This must be Lemnos-fire. What a sharp and stinging smoke!
Rushing onward to the shrine
Aid the gods. Once for all
Show your mettle, Laches my boy!
To the rescue hastening all!

ALL (*blowing on the fire-pots*): Whew! Whew! Drat the smoke!

(*The chorus has now reached the edge of the Orchestra nearest the stage, in front of the Propylaea. They begin laying their logs and fire-pots on the ground.*)

LEADER OF MEN: Thank heaven, this fire is still alive. Now let's first put down these logs here and place our torches in the pots to catch: then let's make a rush for the gates with a battering-ram. If the women don't unbar the gate at our summons, we'll have to smoke them out.

Let me put down my load. Ouch! That hurts! (*to the audience*) Would any of the generals in Samos like to lend a hand with this log? (*Throwing down a log*) Well, *that* won't break my back any more, at any rate. (*Turning to his fire-pot*) Your job, my little pot, is to keep those coals alive and furnish me shortly with a red-hot torch.

O mistress Victory, be my ally and grant me to rout these audacious women in the Acropolis.

(*While the men are busy with their logs and fires, the* CHORUS OF OLD WOMEN *enters, carrying pitchers of water.*)

LEADER OF WOMEN: What's this I see? Smoke and flames?
      Is that a fire ablazing?
Let's rush upon them. Hurry up! They'll find us women ready.

FIRST SEMI-CHORUS OF OLD WOMEN (*singing*):
With wingèd foot onward I fly,
Ere the flames consume Neodice;
Lest Critylla be overwhelmed
By a lawless, accurst herd of old men.
I shudder with fear. Am I too late to aid them?
At break of the day filled we our jars with water

Fresh from the spring, pushing our way straight through the
      crowds.
        Oh, what a din!
  Mid crockery crashing, jostled by slave-girls,
  Sped we to save them, aiding our neighbours,
  Bearing this water to put out the flames.
SECOND SEMI-CHORUS OF OLD WOMEN (*singing*):
    Such news I've heard; doddering fools
    Come with logs, like furnace-attendants,
    Loaded down with three hundred pounds,
  Breathing many a vain, blustering threat,
  That all these abhorred sluts will be burnt to charcoal.
  O goddess, I pray never may they be kindled;
Grant them to save Greece and our men, madness and war
      held them to end.
  With this as our purpose, golden-plumed Maiden,
  Guardian of Athens, seized we thy precinct.
  Be my ally, Warrior-maiden,
  'Gainst these old men, bearing water with me.

(*The women have now reached their position in the Orchestra, and their* LEADER *advances toward the* LEADER OF THE
MEN.)

LEADER OF WOMEN: Hold on there! What's this, you utter
scoundrels? No decent, God-fearing citizens would act like
this.

LEADER OF MEN: Oho! Here's something unexpected: a
swarm of women have come out to attack us.

LEADER OF WOMEN: What, do we frighten you? Surely you
don't think we're too many for you. And yet there are ten
thousand times more of us whom you haven't even seen.

LEADER OF MEN: What say, Phaedria? Shall we let these
women wag their tongues? Shan't we take our sticks and
break them over their backs?

LEADER OF WOMEN: Let's set our pitchers on the ground;
then if anyone lays a hand on us, they won't get in our way.

LEADER OF MEN: By God! If someone gave them two or
three smacks on the jaw, like Bupalus, they wouldn't talk so
much!

LEADER OF WOMEN: Go on, hit me, somebody! Here's my
jaw! But no other bitch will bite a piece out of you before
me.

LEADER OF MEN: Silence! or I'll knock out your—senility!

LEADER OF WOMEN: Just lay one finger on Stratyllis, I dare
you!

LEADER OF MEN: Suppose I dust you off with this fist? What will you do?

LEADER OF WOMEN: I'll tear the living guts out of you with my teeth.

LEADER OF MEN: No poet is more clever than Euripides: "There is no beast so shameless as a woman."

LEADER OF WOMEN: Let's pick up our jars of water, Rhodippe.

LEADER OF MEN: Why have you come here with water, you detestable slut?

LEADER OF WOMEN: And why have you come with fire, you funeral vault? To cremate yourself?

LEADER OF MEN: To light a fire and singe your friends.

LEADER OF WOMEN: And I've brought water to put out your fire.

LEADER OF MEN: What? You'll put out my fire?

LEADER OF WOMEN: Just try and see!

LEADER OF MEN: I wonder: shall I scorch you with this torch of mine?

LEADER OF WOMEN: If you've got any soap, I'll give you a bath.

LEADER OF MEN: Give *me* a bath, you stinking hag?

LEADER OF WOMEN: Yes—a bridal bath!

LEADER OF MEN: Just listen to her! What crust!

LEADER OF WOMEN: Well, I'm a free citizen.

LEADER OF MEN: I'll put an end to your bawling.

(*The men pick up their torches.*)

LEADER OF WOMEN: You'll never do jury-duty again.

(*The women pick up their pitchers.*)

LEADER OF MEN: Singe her hair for her!

LEADER OF WOMEN: Do your duty, water!

(*The women empty their pitchers on the men.*)

LEADER OF MEN: Ow! Ow! For heaven's sake!

LEADER OF WOMEN: Is it too hot?

LEADER OF MEN: What do you mean "hot"? Stop! What are you doing?

LEADER OF WOMEN: I'm watering you, so you'll be fresh and green.

LEADER OF MEN: But I'm all withered up with shaking.

LEADER OF WOMEN: Well, you've got a fire; why don't you dry yourself?

(*Enter an Athenian* MAGISTRATE, *accompanied by four Scythian policemen.*)

MAGISTRATE: Have these wanton women flared up again with their timbrels and their continual worship of Sabazius? Is this another Adonis-dirge upon the roof-tops—which we heard not long ago in the Assembly? That confounded Demostratus was urging us to sail to Sicily, and the whirling women shouted, "Woe for Adonis!" And then Demostratus said we'd best enroll the infantry from Zacynthus, and a tipsy woman on the roof shrieked, "Beat your breasts for Adonis!" And that vile and filthy lunatic forced his measure through. Such license do our women take.

LEADER OF MEN: What if you heard of the insolence of these women here? Besides their over violent acts, they threw water all over us, and we have to shake out our clothes just as if we'd leaked in them.

MAGISTRATE: And rightly, too, by God! For we ourselves lead the women astray and teach them to play the wanton; from these roots such notions blossom forth. A man goes into the jeweler's shop and says, "About that necklace you made for my wife, goldsmith: last night, while she was dancing, the fastening-bolt slipped out of the hole. I have to sail over to Salamis today; if you're free, do come around tonight and fit in a new bolt for her." Another goes to the shoe-maker, a strapping young fellow with manly parts, and says, "See here, cobbler, the sandal-strap chafes my wife's little—toe; it's so tender. Come around during the siesta and stretch it a little, so she'll be more comfortable." Now we see the results of such treatment: here I'm a special Councillor and need money to procure oars for the galleys; and I'm locked out of the Treasury by these women.

But this is no time to stand around. Bring up crow-bars there! I'll put an end to their insolence (*To one of the policemen*) What are you gasping at, you wretch? What are you staring at? Got an eye out for a tavern, eh? Set your crow-bars here to the gates and force them open. (*Retiring to a safe distance*) I'll help from over here.

(*The gates are thrown open and* LYSISTRATA *comes out followed by several other women.*)

LYSISTRATA: Don't force the gates; I'm coming out of my own accord. We don't need crow-bars here; what we need is good sound common-sense.

MAGISTRATE: Is that so, you strumpet? Where's my policeman? Officer, arrest her and tie her arms behind her back.

LYSISTRATA: By Artemis, if he lays a finger on me, he'll pay for it, even if he is a public servant.

(*The policeman retires in terror.*)

MAGISTRATE: You there, are you afraid? Seize her round the waist—and you, too. Tie her up, both of you!

FIRST WOMAN (*as the second policeman approaches* LYSISTRATA): By Pandrosus, if you but touch her with your hand, I'll kick the stuffings out of you.

(*The second policeman retires in terror.*)

MAGISTRATE: Just listen to that: "kick the stuffings out." Where's another policeman? Tie *her* up first, for her chatter.

SECOND WOMAN: By the Goddess of the Light, if you lay the tip of your finger on her, you'll soon need a doctor.

(*The third policeman retires in terror.*)

MAGISTRATE: What's this? Where's my policeman? Seize *her* too. I'll soon stop your sallies.

THIRD WOMAN: By the Goddess of Tauros, if you go near her, I'll tear out your hair until it shrieks with pain.

(*The fourth policeman retires in terror.*)

MAGISTRATE: Oh, damn it all! I've run out of policemen. But women must never defeat us. Officers, let's charge them all together. Close up your ranks!

(*The policemen rally for a mass attack.*)

LYSISTRATA: By heaven, you'll soon find out that we have four companies of warrior-women, all fully equipped within!

MAGISTRATE (*advancing*): Twist their arms off, men!

LYSISTRATA (*shouting*): To the rescue, my valiant women!
O sellers-of-barley-green-stuffs-and-eggs,
O sellers-of-garlic, ye keepers-of-taverns, and vendors-of-bread,
Grapple! Smite! Smash!
Won't you heap filth on them? Give them a tongue-lashing!

[handwritten:] always a resource for women —

Is this very different from Euripides

(*The women beat off the policemen.*)

Halt! Withdraw! No looting on the field.

MAGISTRATE: Damn it! My police-force has put up a very poor show.

LYSISTRATA: What did you expect? Did you think you were attacking slaves? Didn't you know that women are filled with passion?

MAGISTRATE: Aye, passion enough—for a good strong drink!

LEADER OF MEN: O chief and leader of this land, why spend your words in vain?
Don't argue with these shameless beasts. You know not how we've fared:
A soapless bath they've given us; our clothes are soundly soaked.

LEADER OF WOMEN: Poor fool! You never should attack or strike a peaceful girl.
But if you do, your eyes must swell. For I am quite content
To sit unmoved, like modest maids, in peace and cause no pain;
But let a man stir up my hive, he'll find me like a wasp.

CHORUS OF MEN (*singing*):
O God, whatever shall we do with creatures like Womankind?
This can't be endured by any man alive. Question them!
Let us try to find out what this means.
To what end have they seized on this shrine,
This steep and rugged, high and holy,
Undefiled Acropolis?

LEADER OF MEN: Come, put your questions; don't give in, and probe her every statement.
For base and shameful it would be to leave this plot untested.

MAGISTRATE: Well then, first of all I wish to ask her this: for what purpose have you barred us from the Acropolis?

LYSISTRATA: To keep the treasure safe, so you won't make war on account of it.

MAGISTRATE: What? Do we make war on account of the treasure?

LYSISTRATA: Yes, and you cause all our other troubles for it, too. Peisander and those greedy office-seekers keep things stirred up so they can find occasions to steal. Now let them do what they like: they'll never again make off with any of this money.

MAGISTRATE: What will you do?

LYSISTRATA: What a question! We'll administer it ourselves.

MAGISTRATE: *You* will administer the treasure?

LYSISTRATA: What's so strange in that? Don't we administer the household money for you?

MAGISTRATE: That's different.

LYSISTRATA: How is it different?

MAGISTRATE: We've got to make war with this money.

LYSISTRATA: But that's the very first thing: you mustn't make war.

MAGISTRATE: How else can we be saved?

LYSISTRATA: We'll save you.

MAGISTRATE: *You?*

LYSISTRATA: Yes, we!

MAGISTRATE: God forbid!

LYSISTRATA: We'll save you, whether you want it or not.

MAGISTRATE: Oh! This is terrible!

LYSISTRATA: You don't like it, but we're going to do it none the less.

MAGISTRATE: Good God! it's illegal!

LYSISTRATA: We *will* save you, my little man!

MAGISTRATE: Suppose I don't want you to?

LYSISTRATA: That's all the more reason.

MAGISTRATE: What business have you with war and peace?

LYSISTRATA: I'll explain.

MAGISTRATE (*shaking his fist*): Speak up, or you'll smart for it.

LYSISTRATA: Just listen, and try to keep your hands still.

MAGISTRATE: I can't. I'm so mad I can't stop them.

FIRST WOMAN: Then you'll be the one to smart for it.

MAGISTRATE: Croak to yourself, old hag! (*To* LYSISTRATA) Now then, speak up.

LYSISTRATA: Very well. Formerly we endured the war for a good long time with our usual restraint, no matter what you men did. You wouldn't let us say "boo," although nothing you did suited us. But we watched you well, and though we stayed at home we'd often hear of some terribly stupid measure you'd proposed. Then, though grieving at heart, we'd smile sweetly and say, "What was passed in the Assembly today about writing on the treaty-stone?" "What's that to you?" my husband would say. "Hold your tongue!" And I held my tongue.

FIRST WOMAN: But I wouldn't have—not I!

MAGISTRATE: You'd have been soundly smacked, if you hadn't kept still.

LYSISTRATA: So I kept still at home. Then we'd hear of some plan still worse than the first; we'd say, "Husband, how could you pass such a stupid proposal?" He'd scowl at me and say, "If you don't mind your spinning, your head will be sore for weeks. *War shall be the concern of men.*"

MAGISTRATE: And he was right, upon my word!

LYSISTRATA: Why right, you confounded fool, when your proposals were so stupid and we weren't allowed to make suggestions?

"There's not a *man* left in the country," says one. "No, not one," says another. Therefore all we women have decided in council to make a common effort to save Greece. How long should we have waited? Now, if you're willing to listen to our excellent proposals and keep silence for us in your turn, we still may save you.

MAGISTRATE: We men keep silence for you? That's terrible; I won't endure it!

LYSISTRATA: Silence!

MAGISTRATE: Silence for *you*, you wench, when you're wearing a snood? I'd rather die!

LYSISTRATA: Well, if that's all that bothers you—here! take my snood and tie it round your head. (*During the following words the women dress up the* MAGISTRATE *in women's garments.*) And *now* keep quiet! Here, take this spinning-basket, too, and card your wool with robes tucked up, munching on beans. *War shall be the concern of Women!*

LEADER OF WOMEN: Arise and leave your pitchers, girls; no time is this to falter.

We too must aid our loyal friends; our turn has come for action.

CHORUS OF WOMEN (*singing*):

I'll never tire of aiding them with song and dance; never may Faintness keep my legs from moving to and fro endlessly.

For I yearn to do all for my friends;
They have charm, they have wit, they have grace,
  With courage, brains, and best of virtues—
    Patriotic sapience.

LEADER OF WOMEN: Come, child of manliest ancient dames, offspring of stinging nettles,

Advance with rage unsoftened; for fair breezes speed you onward.

LYSISTRATA: If only sweet Eros and the Cyprian Queen of Love shed charm over our breasts and limbs and inspire our men with amorous longing and priapic spasms, I think we may soon be called Peacemakers among the Greeks.

MAGISTRATE: What will you do?

LYSISTRATA: First of all, we'll stop those fellows who run madly about the Marketplace in arms.

FIRST WOMAN: Indeed we shall, by the Queen of Paphos.

LYSISTRATA: For now they roam about the market, amid the pots and greenstuffs, armed to the teeth like Corybantes.

MAGISTRATE: That's what manly fellows ought to do!

LYSISTRATA: But it's so silly: a chap with a Gorgon-emblazoned shield buying pickled herring.

FIRST WOMAN: Why, just the other day I saw one of those long-haired dandies who command our calvary ride up on horseback and pour into his bronze helmet the egg-broth he'd bought from an old dame. And there was a Thracian slinger too, shaking his lance like Tereus; he'd scared the life out of the poor fig-peddler and was gulping down all her ripest fruit.

MAGISTRATE: How can you stop all the confusion in the various states and bring them together?

LYSISTRATA: Very easily.

MAGISTRATE: Tell me how.

LYSISTRATA: Just like a ball of wool, when it's confused and snarled: we take it thus, and draw out a thread here and a thread there with our spindles; thus we'll unsnarl this war, if no one prevents us, and draw together the various states and embassies here and embassies there.

MAGISTRATE: Do you suppose you can stop this dreadful business with balls of wool and spindles, you nit-wits?

LYSISTRATA: Why, if *you* had any wits, you'd manage all affairs of state like our wool-working.

MAGISTRATE: How so?

LYSISTRATA: First you ought to treat the city as we do when we wash the dirt out of a fleece: stretch it out and pluck and thrash out of the city all those prickly scoundrels; aye, and card out those who conspire and stick together to gain office, pulling off their heads. Then card the wool, all of it, into one fair basket of goodwill, mingling in the aliens residing here, any loyal foreigners, and anyone who's in debt to the Treasury; and consider that all our colonies lie scattered round about like remnants; from all of these collect the wool and gather it together here, wind up a great ball, and then weave a good stout cloak for the democracy.

MAGISTRATE: Dreadful! Talking about thrashing and winding balls of wool, when you haven't the slightest share in the war!

LYSISTRATA: Why, you dirty scoundrel, we bear more than twice as much as you. First, we bear children and send off our sons as soldiers.

MAGISTRATE: Hush! Let bygones be bygones!

LYSISTRATA: Then, when we ought to be happy and enjoy our youth, we sleep alone because of your expeditions

→ a correct recounting of fact.
But consider what it says —
Consider May - December marriages:

abroad. But never mind us married women; I grieve most
for the maids who grow old at home unwed.

MAGISTRATE: Don't men grow old, too? *then in reverse*

LYSISTRATA: For heaven's sake! That's not the same thing.
When a man comes home, no matter how grey he is, he soon
finds a girl to marry. But woman's bloom is short and fleet-
ing; if she doesn't grasp her chance, no man is willing to
marry her and she sits at home a prey to every fortune-teller.

MAGISTRATE (*coarsely*): But if a man can still get it up—

LYSISTRATA: See here, you: what's the matter? Aren't you
dead yet? There's plenty of room for you. Buy yourself a
shroud and I'll bake you a honey-cake. (*Handing him a copper coin for his passage across the Styx*) Here's your fare!
Now get yourself a wreath.

(*During the following dialogue the women dress up the*
MAGISTRATE *as a corpse.*)

FIRST WOMAN: Here, take this fillets.

SECOND WOMAN: Here, take this wreath.

LYSISTRATA: What do you want? What's lacking? Get moving; off to the ferry! Charon is calling you; don't keep him
from sailing.

MAGISTRATE: Am I to endure these insults? By God! I'm
going straight to the magistrates to show them how I've been
treated.

LYSISTRATA: Are you grumbling that you haven't been
properly laid out? Well, the day after tomorrow we'll send
around all the usual offerings early in the morning.

(*The* MAGISTRATE *goes out still wearing his funeral decorations.* LYSISTRATA *and the women retire into the Acropolis.*)

LEADER OF MEN: Wake, ye sons of freedom, wake! 'Tis no
time for sleeping. Up and at them, like a man! Let us strip
for action.

(*The* CHORUS OF MEN *remove their outer cloaks.*)

CHORUS OF MEN (*singing*):
Surely there is something here greater than meets the eye;
For without a doubt I smell Hippias' tyranny.
Dreadful fear assails me lest certain bands of Spartan men,
Meeting here with Cleisthenes, have inspired through treach-
      ery
All those god-detested women secretly to seize

Athens' treasure in the temple, and to stop that pay

Whence I live at my ease.

LEADER OF MEN: Now isn't it terrible for them to advise the state and chatter about shields, being mere women?

And they think to reconcile us with the Spartans—men who hold nothing sacred any more than hungry wolves. Surely this is a web of deceit, my friends, to conceal an attempt at tyranny. But they'll never lord it over me; I'll be on my guard and from now on,

"The blade I bear
A myrtle spray shall wear."

I'll occupy the market under arms and stand next to Aristogeiton.

Thus I'll stand beside him. (*He strikes the pose of the famous statue of the tyrannicides, with one arm raised.*) And here's my chance to take this accurst old hag and— (*striking the* LEADER OF WOMEN) smack her on the jaw!

LEADER OF WOMEN: You'll go home in such a state your

Ma won't recognize you!

Ladies all, upon the ground let us place these garments.

(*The* CHORUS OF WOMEN *remove their outer garments.*)

CHORUS OF WOMEN (*singing*):

Citizens of Athens, hear useful words for the state.
Rightly; for it nurtured me in my youth royally.
As a child of seven years carried I the sacred box;
Then I was a Miller-maid, grinding at Athene's shrine;
Next I wore the saffron robe and played Brauronia's Bear;
And I walked as a Basket-bearer, wearing chains of figs,

As a sweet maiden fair.

LEADER OF WOMEN: Therefore, am I not bound to give good advice to the city?

Don't take it ill that I was born a woman, if I contribute something better than our present troubles. I pay my share: for I contribute MEN. But you miserable old fools contribute nothing, and after squandering our ancestral treasure, the fruit of the Persian Wars, you make no contribution in return. And now, all on account of you, we're facing ruin.

What, muttering, are you? If you annoy me, I'll take this hard, rough slipper and— (*striking the* LEADER OF MEN) smack you on the jaw!

CHORUS OF MEN (*singing*):

This is outright insolence! Things go from bad to worse.
If you're men with any guts, prepare to meet the foe.

Let us strip our tunics off! We need the smell of male
Vigour. And we cannot fight all swaddled up in clothes.

(They strip off their tunics.)

Come then, my comrades, on to the battle, ye once to
     Leipsydrion came:
Then ye were MEN. Now call back your youthful vigour.
  With light, wingèd footstep advance,
Shaking old age from your frame.
    LEADER OF MEN: If any of us give these wenches the
slightest hold, they'll stop at nothing; such is their cunning.

    They will even build ships and sail against us, like Ar-
temisia. Or if they turn to mounting, I count our Knights as
done for: a woman's such a tricky jockey when she gets
astraddle, with a good firm seat for trotting. Just look at those
Amazons that Micon painted, fighting on horseback against
men!

    But we must throw them all in the pillory—*(seizing and
choking the LEADER OF WOMEN)* grabbing hold of yonder
neck!

    CHORUS OF WOMEN *(singing)*:
'Ware my anger! Like a boar 'twill rush upon you men.
Soon you'll bawl aloud for help, you'll be so soundly trimmed!
Come, my friends, let's strip with speed, and lay aside these
     robes;
Catch the scent of women's rage. Attack with tooth and nail!

    (They strip off their tunics.)

Now then, come near me, you miserable man! you'll never
     eat garlic or black beans again.
And if you utter a single hard word, in rage I will "nurse"
     you as once
  The beetle requited her foe.
    LEADER OF WOMEN: For you don't worry me; no, not so
long as my Lampito lives and our Theban friend, the noble
Ismenia.

    You can't do anything, not even if you pass a dozen—de-
crees! You miserable fool, all our neighbours hate you. Why,
just the other day when I was holding a festival for Hecate, I
invited as playmate from our neighbours the Boeotians a
charming, wellbred Copaic—eel. But they refused to send me
one on account of your decrees.

    And you'll never stop passing decrees until I grab your

foot and——(*tripping up the* LEADER OF MEN) toss you down and break your neck!

(*Here an interval of five days is supposed to elapse.* LYSISTRATA *comes out from the Acropolis.*)

LEADER OF WOMEN (*dramatically*): Empress of this great emprise and undertaking,
Why come you forth, I pray, with frowning brow?
LYSISTRATA: Ah, these cursèd women! Their deeds and female notions make me pace up and down in utter despair.
LEADER OF WOMEN: Ah, what sayest thou?
LYSISTRATA: The truth, alas! the truth.
LEADER OF WOMEN: What dreadful tale hast thou to tell thy friends?
LYSISTRATA: 'Tis shame to speak, and not to speak is hard.
LEADER OF WOMEN: Hide not from me whatever woes we suffer.
LYSISTRATA: Well then, to put it briefly, we want——laying!
LEADER OF WOMEN: O Zeus, Zeus!
LYSISTRATA: Why call on Zeus? That's the way things are. I can no longer keep them away from the men, and they're all deserting. I caught one wriggling through a hole near the grotto of Pan, another sliding down a rope, another deserting her post; and yesterday I found one getting on a sparrow's back to fly off to Orsilochus, and had to pull her back by the hair. They're digging up all sorts of excuses to get home. Look, here comes one of them now.

(*A woman comes hastily out of the Acropolis.*)

Here you! Where are you off to in such a hurry?
FIRST WOMAN: I want to go home. My very best wool is being devoured by moths.
LYSISTRATA: Moths? Nonsense! Go back inside.
FIRST WOMAN: I'll come right back; I swear it. I just want to lay it out on the bed.
LYSISTRATA: Well, you won't lay it out, and you won't go home, either.
FIRST WOMAN: Shall I let my wool be ruined?
LYSISTRATA: If necessary, yes.

(*Another woman comes out.*)

SECOND WOMAN: Oh dear! Oh dear! My precious flax! I left it at home all unpeeled.

LYSISTRATA: Here's another one, going home for her "flax." Come back here!

SECOND WOMAN: But I just want to work it up a little and then I'll be right back.

LYSISTRATA: No indeed! If you start this, all the other women will want to do the same.

(*A third woman comes out.*)

THIRD WOMAN: O Eilithyia, goddess of travail, stop my labour till I come to a lawful spot!

LYSISTRATA: What's this nonsense?

THIRD WOMAN: I'm going to have a baby—right now!

LYSISTRATA: But you weren't even pregnant yesterday.

THIRD WOMAN: Well, I am today. O Lysistrata, do send me home to see a midwife, right away.

LYSISTRATA: What are you talking about? (*Putting her hand on her stomach*) What's this hard lump here?

THIRD WOMAN: A little boy.

LYSISTRATA: My goodness, what have you got there? It seems hollow; I'll just find out. (*Pulling aside her robe*) Why, you silly goose, you've got Athene's sacred helmet there. And you said you were having a baby!

THIRD WOMAN: Well, I *am* having one, I swear!

LYSISTRATA: Then what's this helmet for?

THIRD WOMAN: If the baby starts coming while I'm still in the Acropolis, I'll creep into this like a pigeon and give birth to it there.

LYSISTRATA: Stuff and nonsense! It's plian enough what you're up to. You just wait here for the christening of this—helmet.

THIRD WOMAN: But I can't sleep in the Acropolis since I saw the sacred snake.

FIRST WOMAN: And I'm dying for lack of sleep: the hooting of the owls keep me awake.

LYSISTRATA: Enough of these shams, you wretched creatures. You want your husbands, I suppose. Well, don't you think they want us? I'm sure they're spending miserable nights. Hold out, my friends, and endure for just a little while. There's an oracle that we shall conquer, if we don't split up. (*Producing a roll of paper*) Here it is.

FIRST WOMAN: Tell us what it says.

LYSISTRATA: Listen.

"When in the length of time the Swallows shall gather together, Fleeing the Hoopoe's amorous flight and the Cockatoo shunning, Then shall your woes be ended and Zeus who thunders in heaven Set what's below on top—"

FIRST WOMAN: What? Are we going to be on top?

LYSISTRATA: "But if the Swallows rebel and flutter away from the temple,

Never a bird in the world shall seem more wanton and worthless.

FIRST WOMAN: That's clear enough, upon my word!

LYSISTRATA: By all that's holy, let's not give up the struggle now. Let's go back inside. It would be a shame, my dear friends, to disobey the oracle.

(The women all retire to the Acropolis again.)

CHORUS OF MEN *(singing)*:
    I have a tale to tell,
    Which I know full well.
      It was told me
      In the nursery.

    Once there was a likely lad,
      Melanion they name him;
    The thought of marriage made him mad,
      For which I cannot blame him.

    So off he went to mountains fair;
      (No women to upbraid him!)
    A mighty hunter of the hare,
      He had a dog to aid him.

    He never came back home to see
      Detested women's faces.
    He showed a shrewd mentality.
      With him I'd fain change places!

ONE OF THE MEN *(to one of the women)*: Come here, old dame; give me a kiss.

WOMAN: You'll ne'er eat garlic, if you dare!

MAN: I want to kick you—just like this!

WOMAN: Oh, there's a leg with bushy hair!

MAN: Myronides and Phormio
Were hairy—and they thrashed the foe.

CHORUS OF WOMEN *(singing)*:
    I have another tale,
    With which to assail

Your contention
'Bout Melanion.

Once upon a time a man
  Named Timon left our city,
To live in some deserted land.
  (We thought him rather witty.)

He dwelt alone amidst the thorn;
  In solitude he brooded.
From some grim Fury he was born:
  Such hatred he exuded.

He cursed you men, as scoundrels through
  And through, till life he ended.
He couldn't stand the sight of YOU!
  But women he befriended.

WOMAN (*to one of the men*): I'll smash your face in, if
you like.
MAN: Oh no, please don't! You frighten me.
WOMAN: I'll lift my foot—and thus I'll strike.
MAN: Aha! Look there! What's that I see?
WOMAN: Whate'er you see, you cannot say
That I'm not neatly trimmed today.

(LYSISTRATA *appears on the wall of the Acropolis.*)

LYSISTRATA: Hello! Hello! Girls, come here quick!

(*Several women appear beside her.*)

WOMAN: What is it? Why are you calling?
LYSISTRATA: I see a man coming: he's in a dreadful state.
He's mad with passion. O Queen of Cyprus, Cythera, and Pa-
phos, just keep on this way!
WOMAN: Where is the fellow?
LYSISTRATA: There, beside the shrine of Demeter.
WOMAN: Oh yes, so he is. Who is he?
LYSISTRATA: Let's see. Do any of you know him?
MYRRHINE: Yes indeed. That's my husband, Cinesias.
LYSISTRATA: It's up to you, now: roast him, rack him, fool
him, love him—and leave him! Do everything, except what
our oath forbids.
MYRRHINE: Don't worry; I'll do it.
LYSISTRATA: I'll stay here to tease him and warm him up
a bit. Off with you.

(The other women retire from the wall. Enter CINESIAS *followed by a slave carrying a baby.* CINESIAS *is obviously in great pain and distress.)*

CINESIAS *(groaning)*: Oh-h! Oh-h-h! This is killing me! O God, what tortures I'm suffering!

LYSISTRATA *(from the wall)*: Who's that within our lines?

CINESIAS: Me.

LYSISTRATA: A *man*?

CINESIAS *(pointing)*: A *man*, indeed!

LYSISTRATA: Well, go away!

CINESIAS: Who are you to send me away?

LYSISTRATA: The captain of the guard.

CINESIAS: Oh, for heaven's sake, call out Myrrhine for me.

LYSISTRATA: Call Myrrhine? Nonsense! Who are you?

CINESIAS: Her husband, Cinesias of Paionidai.

LYSISTRATA *(appearing much impressed)*: Oh, greetings, friend. Your name is not without honour here among us. Your wife is always talking about you, and whenever she takes an egg or an apple, she says, "Here's to my dear Cinesias!"

CINESIAS *(quivering with excitement)*: Oh, ye gods in heaven!

LYSISTRATA: Indeed she does! And whenever our conversations turn to men, your wife immediately says, "All others are mere rubbish compared with Cinesias."

CINESIAS *(groaning)*: Oh! Do call her for me.

LYSISTRATA: Why should I? What will you give me?

CINESIAS: Whatever you want. All I have is yours—and you see what I've got.

LYSISTRATA: Well then, I'll go down and call her. *(She descends.)*

CINESIAS: And hurry up! I've had no joy of life ever since she left home. When I go in the house, I feel awful: everything seems so empty and I can't enjoy my dinner. I'm in such a state all the time!

MYRRHINE *(from behind the wall)*: I *do* love him so. But he won't let me love him. No, no! Don't ask me to see him!

CINESIAS: O my darling, O Myrrhine honey, why do you do this to me?

*(*MYRRHINE *appears on the wall.)*

Come down here!

MYRRHINE: No, I won't come down.

CINESIAS: Won't you come, Myrrhine, when *I* call you?

MYRRHINE: No; you don't want me.

CINESIAS: *Don't want you?* I'm in agony!

MYRRHINE: I'm going now.

CINESIAS: Please don't. At least, listen to your baby. (*To the baby*) Here you, call your mamma! (*Pinching the baby*)

BABY: Ma-ma! Ma-ma! Ma-ma!

CINESIAS (*to* MYRRHINE): What's the matter with you? Have you no pity for your child, who hasn't been washed or fed for five whole days?

MYRRHINE: Oh, poor child; your father pays no attention to you.

CINESIAS: Come down then, you heartless wretch, for the baby's sake.

MYRRHINE: Oh, what it is to be a mother! I've got to come down, I suppose.

(*She leaves the wall and shortly reappears at the gate.*)

CINESIAS (*to himself*): She seems much younger, and she has such a sweet look about her. Oh, the way she teases me! And her pretty, provoking ways make me burn with longing.

MYRRHINE (*coming out of the gate and taking the baby*): O my sweet little angel. Naughty papa! Here, let Mummy kiss you, Mamma's little sweetheart!

(*She fondles the baby lovingly.*)

CINESIAS (*in despair*): You heartless creature, why do you do this? Why follow these other women and make us suffer so?

(*He tries to embrace her.*)

MYRRHINE: Don't touch me!

CINESIAS: You're letting all our things at home go to wrack and ruin.

MYRRHINE: I don't care.

CINESIAS: You don't care that your wool is being plucked to pieces by the chickens?

MYRRHINE: Not in the least.

CINESIAS: And you haven't celebrated the rites of Aphrodite for ever so long. Won't you come home?

MYRRHINE: Not on your life, unless you men make a truce and stop the war.

CINESIAS: Well then, if that pleases you, we'll do it.

MYRRHINE: Well then, if that pleases *you*, I'll come home—afterwards! Right now I'm on oath not to.

CINESIAS: Then just lie down here with me for a moment.

MYRRHINE: No—(*in a teasing voice*) and yet, I won't say I don't love you.

CINESIAS: You love me? Oh, do lie down here, Myrrhine dear!

MYRRHINE: What, you silly fool! in front of the baby?

CINESIAS (*hastily thrusting the baby at the slave*): Of course not. Here—home! Take him, Manes! (*The slave goes off with the baby.*) See, the baby's out of the way. Now won't you lie down?

MYRRHINE: But where, my dear?

CINESIAS: Where? The grotto of Pan's a lovely spot.

MYRRHINE: How could I purify myself before returning to the shrine?

CINESIAS: Easily: just wash here in the Clepsydra.

MYRRHINE: And then, shall I go back on my oath?

CINESIAS: On my head be it! Don't worry about the oath.

MYRRHINE: All right, then. Just let me bring out a bed.

CINESIAS: No, don't. The ground's all right.

MYRRHINE: Heavens, no! Bad as you are, I won't let you lie on the bare ground.

(*She goes into the Acropolis.*)

CINESIAS: Why, she really loves me; it's plain to see.

MYRRHINE (*returning with a bed*): There! Now hurry up and lie down. I'll just slip off this dress. But—let's see: oh yes, I must fetch a mattress.

CINESIAS: Nonsense! No mattress for me.

MYRRHINE: Yes indeed! It's not nice on the bare springs.

CINESIAS: Give me a kiss.

MYRRHINE (*giving him a hasty kiss*): There!

(*She goes.*)

CINESIAS (*in mingled distress and delight*): Oh-h! Hurry back!

MYRRHINE (*returning with a mattress*): Here's the mattress; lie down on it. I'm taking my things off now—but—let's see: you have no pillow.

CINESIAS: I don't *want* a pillow!

MYRRHINE: But I do.

(*She goes.*)

CINESIAS: Cheated again, just like Heracles and his dinner!

MYRRHINE (*returning with a pillow*): Here, lift your head. (*to herself, wondering how else to tease him*) Is that all?

CINESIAS: Surely that's all! Do come here, precious!

MYRRHINE: I'm taking off my girdle. But remember: don't go back on your promise about the truce.

CINESIAS: Hope to die, if I do.

MYRRHINE: You don't have a blanket.

CINESIAS (*shouting in exasperation*): *I don't want one!* I WANT TO—

MYRRHINE: Sh-h! There, there, I'll be back in a minute.

(*She goes.*)

CINESIAS: She'll be the death of me with these bed-clothes.

MYRRHINE (*returning with a blanket*): Here, get up.

CINESIAS: I've got *this* up!

MYRRHINE: Would you like some perfume?

CINESIAS: Good heavens, no! I won't have it!

MYRRHINE: Yes, you shall, whether you want it or not.

(*She goes.*)

CINESIAS: O lord! Confound all perfumes anyway!

MYRRHINE (*returning with a flask*): Stretch out your hand and put some on.

CINESIAS (*suspiciously*): By God, I don't much like this perfume. It smacks of shilly-shallying, and has no scent of the marriage-bed.

MYRRHINE: Oh dear! This is Rhodian perfume I've brought.

CINESIAS: It's quite all right, dear. Never mind.

MYRRHINE: Don't be silly!

(*She goes out with the flask.*)

CINESIAS: Damn the man who first concocted perfumes!

MYRRHINE (*returning with another flask*): Here, try this flask.

CINESIAS: I've got another one all ready for you. Come, you wretch, lie down and stop bringing me things.

MYRRHINE: All right; I'm taking off my shoes. But, my dear, see that you vote for peace.

CINESIAS (*absently*): I'll consider it.

(MYRRHINE *runs away to the Acropolis.*)

I'm ruined! The wench has skinned me and run away! (*chanting, in tragic style*) Alas! Alas! Deceived, deserted by this fairest of women, whom shall I—lay? Ah, my poor little child, how shall I nurture thee? Where's Cynalopex? I needs must hire a nurse!

LEADER OF MEN (*chanting*): Ah, wretched man, in dreadful wise beguiled, bewrayed, thy soul is sore distressed. I pity thee, alas! alas! What soul, what loins, what liver could stand this strain? How firm and unyielding he stands, with naught to aid him of a morning.

CINESIAS: O lord! O Zeus! What tortures I endure!

LEADER OF MEN: This is the way she's treated you, that vile and cursèd wanton.

LEADER OF WOMEN: Nay, not vile and cursèd, but sweet and dear.

LEADER OF MEN: Sweet, you say? Nay, hateful, hateful!

CINESIAS: Hateful indeed! O Zeus, Zeus!
Seize her and snatch her away,
Like a handful of dust, in a mighty,
Fiery tempest! Whirl her aloft, then let her drop
Down to the earth, with a crash, as she falls—
On the point of this waiting
Thingummybob!

(*He goes out.*)
(*Enter a Spartan* HERALD, *in an obvious state of excitement which he is doing his best to conceal.*)

HERALD: Where can I find the Senate or the Prytanes? I've got an important message.

(*The Athenian* MAGISTRATE *enters.*)

MAGISTRATE: Say there, are you a man or Priapus?

HERALD (*in annoyance*): I'm a herald, you lout! I've come from Sparta about the truce.

MAGISTRATE: Is that a spear you've got under your cloak?

HERALD: No, of course not!

MAGISTRATE: Why do you twist and turn so? Why hold your cloak in front of you? Did you rupture yourself on the trip?

HERALD: By gum, the fellow's an old fool.

MAGISTRATE (*pointing*): Why, you dirty rascal, you're all excited.

HERALD: Not at all. Stop this tom-foolery.

MAGISTRATE: Well, what's that I see?

HERALD: A Spartan message-staff.

MAGISTRATE: Oh, certainly! That's just the kind of message-staff I've got. But tell me the honest truth: how are things going in Sparta?

HERALD: All the land of Sparta is up in arms—and our allies are up, too. We need Pellene.

MAGISTRATE: What brought this trouble on you? A sudden Panic?

HERALD: No, Lampito started it and then all the women in Sparta with one accord chased their husbands out of their beds.

MAGISTRATE: How do you feel?

HERALD: Terrible. We walk around the city bent over like men lighting matches in a wind. For our women won't let us touch them until we all agree and make peace throughout Greece.

MAGISTRATE: This is a general conspiracy of the women; I see it now. Well, hurry back and tell the Spartans to send ambassadors here with full powers to arrange a truce. And I'll go tell the Council to choose ambassadors from here; I've got a little something here that will soon persuade them!

HERALD: I'll fly there; for you've made an excellent suggestion.

(*The* HERALD *and the* MAGISTRATE *depart on opposite sides of the stage.*)

LEADER OF MEN: No beast or fire is harder than womankind to tame, Nor is the spotted leopard so devoid of shame.

LEADER OF WOMEN: Knowing this, you dare provoke us to attack?

I'd be your steady friend, if you'd but take us back.

LEADER OF MEN: I'll never cease my hatred keen of womankind.

LEADER OF WOMEN: Just as you will. But now just let me help you find

That cloak you threw aside. You look so silly there

Without your clothes. Here, put it on and don't go bare.

LEADER OF MEN: That's very kind, and shows you're not entirely bad.

But I threw off my things when I was good and mad.

LEADER OF WOMEN: At last you seem a man, and won't be mocked, my lad.

If you'd been nice to me, I'd take this little gnat

That's in your eye and pluck it out for you, like that.

she is kind to him, mothering him

LEADER OF MEN: So that's what's bothered me and bit my eye so long!
Please dig it out for me. I own that I've been wrong.
    LEADER OF WOMEN: I'll do so, though you've been a most ill-natured brat.
Ye gods! See here! A huge and monstrous little gnat!
    LEADER OF MEN: Oh, how that helps! For it was digging wells in me.
And now it's out, my tears can roll down hard and free.
    LEADER OF WOMEN: Here, let me wipe them off, although you're such a knave,
And kiss me.
    LEADER OF MEN: No!
    LEADER OF WOMEN: Whate'er you say, a kiss I'll have.

(She kisses him.)

LEADER OF MEN: Oh, confound these women! They've a coaxing way about them.
He was wise and never spoke a truer word, who said,
"We can't live with women, but we cannot live without them."
Now I'll make a truce with you. We'll fight no more; instead,
    I will not injure you if you do me no wrong.
And now let's join our ranks and then begin a song.
COMBINED CHORUS *(singing)*:
    Athenians, we're not prepared,
      To say a single ugly word
    About our fellow-citizens.
Quite the contrary: we desire but to say and to do
Naught but good. Quite enough are the ills now on hand.

        Men and women, be advised:
           If anyone requires
        Money—minae two or three—
           We've got what he desires.

        My purse is yours, on easy terms:
           When Peace shall reappear,
        Whate'er you've borrowed will be due.
           So speak up without fear.

        You needn't pay me back, you see,
        If you can get a cent from me!

        We're about to entertain
           Some foreign gentlemen;

We've soup and tender, fresh-killed pork,
    Come round to dine at ten.

Come early; wash and dress with care,
    And bring the children, too.
Then step right in, no "by your leave."
    We'll be expecting you.

Walk in as if you owned the place.
You'll find the door—shut in your face!

(*Enter a group of* SPARTAN AMBASSADORS; *they are in the
same desperate condition as the Herald in the previous scene.*)

LEADER OF CHORUS: Here come the envoys from Sparta,
sprouting long beards and looking for the world as if they
were carrying pig-pens in front of them.
    Greetings, gentlemen of Sparta. Tell me, in what state
have you come?
SPARTAN: Why waste words? You can plainly see what
state we've come in!
    LEADER OF CHORUS: Wow! You're in a pretty high-strung
condition, and it seems to be getting worse.
    SPARTAN: It's indescribable. Won't someone please arrange
a peace for us—in any way you like.
    LEADER OF CHORUS: Here come our own, native ambassa-
dors, crouching like wrestlers and holding their clothes in
front of them; this seems an athletic kind of malady.

(*Enter several* ATHENIAN AMBASSADORS.)

ATHENIAN: Can anyone tell us where Lysistrata is? You see
our condition.
    LEADER OF CHORUS: Here's another case of the same com-
plaint. Tell me, are the attacks worse in the morning?
    ATHENIAN: No, we're always afflicted this way. If someone
doesn't soon arrange this truce, you'd better not let me get
my hands on—Cleisthenes!
    LEADER OF CHORUS: If you're smart, you'll arrange your
cloaks so none of these fellows who smashed the Hermae can
see you.
    ATHENIAN: Right you are; a very good suggestion.
    SPARTAN: Aye, by all means. Here, let's hitch up our
clothes.
    ATHENIAN: Greetings, Spartan. We've suffered dreadful
things.

SPARTAN: My dear fellow, we'd have suffered still worse if one of those fellows had seen us in this condition.

ATHENIAN: Well, gentlemen, we must get down to business. What's your errand here?

SPARTAN: We're ambassadors about peace.

ATHENIAN: Excellent; so are we. Only Lysistrata can arrange things for us; shall we summon her?

SPARTAN: Aye, and Lysistratus too, if you like.

LEADER OF CHORUS: No need to summon her, it seems. She's coming out of her own accord.

(*Enter* LYSISTRATA *accompanied by a statue of a nude female figure, which represents Reconciliation.*)

Hail, noblest of women; now must thou be
A judge shrewd and subtle, mild and severe,
Be sweet yet majestic: all manners employ.
The leaders of Hellas, caught by thy love-charms,
Have come to thy judgment, their charges submitting.

LYSISTRATA: This is no difficult task, if one catch them still in amorous passion, before they've resorted to each other. But I'll soon find out. Where's Reconciliation? Go, first bring the Spartans here, and don't seize them rudely and violently, as our tactless husbands used to do, but as befits a woman, like an old, familiar friend; if they won't give you their hands, take them however you can. Then go fetch these Athenians here, taking hold of whatever they offer you. Now then, men of Sparta, stand here beside me, and you Athenians on the other side, and listen to my words.

I am a woman, it is true, but I have a mind; I'm not badly off in native wit, and by listening to my father and my elders, I've had a decent schooling.

Now I intend to give you a scolding which you both deserve. With one common font you worship at the same altars, just like brothers, at Olympia, at Thermopylae, at Delphi—how many more might I name, if time permitted;—and the Barbarians stand by waiting with their armies; yet you are destroying the men and towns of Greece.

ATHENIAN: Oh, this tension is killing me!

LYSISTRATA: And now, men of Sparta,—to turn to you— don't you remember how the Spartan Pericleidas came here once as a suppliant, and sitting at our altar, all pale with fear in his crimson cloak, begged us for an army? For all Messene had attacked you and the god sent an earthquake too? Then Cimon went forth with four thousand hoplites and saved all Lacedaemon. Such was the aid you received from Athens,

and now you lay waste the country which once treated you
so well.

ATHENIAN (*hotly*): They're in the wrong, Lysistrata, upon
my word, they are!

SPARTAN (*absently, looking at the statue of Reconciliation*): We're in the wrong. What hips! How lovely they are!

LYSISTRATA: Don't think I'm going to let you Athenians
off. Don't you remember how the Spartans came in arms
when you were wearing the rough, sheepskin cloak of slaves
and slew the host of Thessalians, the comrades and allies of
Hippias? Fighting with you on that day, alone of all the
Greeks, they set you free and instead of a sheepskin gave
your folk a handsome robe to wear.

SPARTAN (*looking at* LYSISTRATA): I've never seen a more
distinguished woman.

ATHENIAN (*looking at Reconciliation*): I've never seen a
more voluptuous body!

LYSISTRATA: Why then, with these many noble deeds to
think of, do you fight each other? Why don't you stop this
villainy? Why not make peace? Tell me, what prevents it?

SPARTAN (*waving vaguely at Reconciliation*): We're willing,
if you're willing to give up your position on yonder flank.

LYSISTRATA: What position, my good man?

SPARTAN: Pylus; we've been panting for it for ever so long.

ATHENIAN: No, by God! You shan't have it!

LYSISTRATA: Let them have it, my friend.

ATHENIAN: Then what shall we have to rouse things up?

LYSISTRATA: Ask for another place in exchange.

ATHENIAN: Well, let's see: first of all (*Pointing to various
parts of Reconciliation's anatomy*) give us Echinus here, this
Maliac Inlet in back there, and these two Megarian legs.

SPARTAN: No, by heavens! You can't have *everything*, you
crazy fool!

LYSISTRATA: Let it go. Don't fight over a pair of legs.

ATHENIAN (*taking off his cloak*): I think I'll strip and do a
little planting now.

SPARTAN (*following suit*): And I'll just do a little fertiliz-
ing, by gosh!

LYSISTRATA: Wait until the truce is concluded. Now if
you've decided on this course, hold a conference and discuss
the matter with your allies.

ATHENIAN: Allies? Don't be ridiculous! They're in the same
state we are. Won't all our allies want the same thing we
do—to jump in bed with their women?

SPARTAN: Ours will, I know.

ATHENIAN: Especially the Carystians, by God!

LYSISTRATA: Very well. Now purify yourselves, that your wives may feast and entertain you in the Acropolis; we've provisions by the basketfull. Exchange your oaths and pledges there, and then each of you may take his wife and go home.

ATHENIAN: Let's go at once.

SPARTAN: Come on, where you will.

ATHENIAN: For God's sake, let's hurry!

(*They all go into the Acropolis.*)

CHORUS (*singing*):

> Whate'er I have of coverlets
>   And robes of varied hue
> And golden trinkets,—without stint
>   I offer them to you.

> Take what you will and bear it home,
>   Your children to delight,
> Or if your girl's a Basket-maid;
>   Just choose whate'er's in sight.

> There's naught within so well secured
>   You cannot break the seal
> And bear it off; just help yourselves;
>   No hesitation feel.

> But you'll see nothing, though you try,
> Unless you've sharper eyes than I!

> If anyone needs bread to feed
>   A growing family,
> I've lots of wheat and full-grown loaves;
>   So just apply to me.

> Let every poor man who desires
>   Come round and bring a sack
> To fetch the grain; my slave is there
>   To load it on his back.

> But don't come near my door, I say:
> Beware the dog, and stay away!

[handwritten marginal note: why this switch]

(*An* ATHENIAN *enters carrying a torch; he knocks at the gate.*)

ATHENIAN: Open the door! (*To the* CHORUS, *which is clustered around the gate*) Make way, won't you! What are you hanging around for? Want me to singe you with this torch? (*To himself*) No; it's a stale trick, I won't do it! (*To the audience*) Still if I've got to do it to please *you*, I suppose I'll have to take the trouble.

(*A* SECOND ATHENIAN *comes out of the gate.*)

SECOND ATHENIAN: And I'll help you.

FIRST ATHENIAN (*waving his torch at the* CHORUS): Get out! Go bawl your heads off! Move on there, so the Spartans can leave in peace when the banquet's over.

(*They brandish their torches until the* CHORUS *leaves the Orchestra.*)

SECOND ATHENIAN: I've never seen such a pleasant banquet: The Spartans are charming fellows, indeed they are! And we Athenians are very witty in our cups.

FIRST ATHENIAN: Naturally: for when we're sober we're never at our best. If the Athenians would listen to me, we'd always get a little tipsy on our embassies. As things are now, we go to Sparta when we're sober and look around to stir up trouble. And then we don't hear what they say—and as for what they *don't* say, we have all sorts of suspicions. And then we bring back varying reports about the mission. But this time everything is pleasant; even if a man should sing the Telamon-song when he ought to sing "Cleitagorus," we'd praise him and swear it was excellent.

(*The two* CHORUSES *return, as a* CHORUS OF ATHENIANS *and a* CHORUS OF SPARTANS.)

Here they come back again. Go to the devil, you scoundrels!

SECOND ATHENIAN: Get out, I say! They're coming out from the feast.

(*Enter the Spartan and Athenian envoys, followed by* LYSISTRATA *and all the women.*)

SPARTAN (*to one of his fellow-envoys*): My good fellow, take up your pipes; I want to do a fancy two-step and sing a jolly song for the Athenians.

ATHENIAN: Yes, do take your pipes, by all means. I'd love
to see you dance.

SPARTAN (*singing and dancing with the* CHORUS OF SPAR-
TANS):

These youths inspire
To song and dance, O Memory;
Stir up my Muse, to tell how we
And Athens' men, in our galleys clashing
At Artemisium, 'gainst foemen dashing
   In godlike ire
Conquered the Persian and set Greece free.

   Leonidas
Led on his valiant warriors
Whetting their teeth like angry boars.
Abundant foam on their lips was flow'ring,
A stream of sweat from their limbs was show'ring.
   The Persian was
Numberless as the sand on the shores.

O Huntress who slayest the beasts in the glade,
O Virgin divine, hither come to our truce,
Unite us in bonds which all time will not loose.
Grant us to find in this treaty, we pray,
An unfailing source of true friendship, today,
And all of our days, helping us to refrain
From weaseling tricks which bring war in their train.
   Then hither, come hither! O huntress maid.

LYSISTRATA: Come then, since all is fairly done, men of
Sparta, lead away your wives, and you, Athenians, take
yours. Let every man stand beside his wife, and every wife
beside her man, and then, to celebrate our fortune, let's
dance. And in the future, let's take care to avoid these misun-
derstandings. *The peaceful res election*

CHORUS OF ATHENIANS (*singing and dancing*):
Lead on the dances, your graces revealing,
Call Artemis hither, call Artemis' twin,
Leader of dances, Apollo the Healing,
Kindly God—hither! let's summon him in!

   Nysian Bacchus call,
Who with his Maenads, his eyes flashing fire,
   Dances, and last of all
Zeus of the thunderbolt flaming, the Sire,

And Hera in majesty,
Queen of prosperity.

Come, ye Powers who dwell above
Unforgetting, our witnesses be
Of Peace with bonds of harmonious love—
The Peace which Cypris has wrought for me.
Alleluia! Io Paean!
Leap in joy—hurrah! hurrah!
'Tis victory—hurrah! hurrah!
Euoi! Euoi! Euai! Euai!

LYSISTRATA (*to the Spartans*): Come now, sing a new song
to cap ours.

CHORUS OF SPARTANS (*singing and dancing*):
Leaving Taygetus fair and renown'd,
Muse of Laconia, hither come:
Amyclae's god in hymns resound,
Athene of the Brazen Home,
And Castor and Pollux, Tyndareus' sons,
Who sport where Eurotas murmuring runs.

On with the dance! Heia! Ho!
    All leaping along,
Mantles a-swinging as we go!
    Of Sparta our song.
There the holy chorus ever gladdens,
There the beat of stamping feet,
As our winsome fillies, lovely maidens,
Dance, beside Eurotas' banks a-skipping,—
    Nimbly go to and fro
Hast'ning, leaping feet in measures tripping,
Like the Bacchae's revels, hair a-streaming.
Leda's child, divine and mild,
Leads the holy dance, her fair face beaming.
    On with the dance! as your hand
        Presses the hair
    Streaming away unconfined.
        Leap in the air
    Light as the deer; footsteps resound
    Aiding our dance, beating the ground.
Praise Athene, Maid divine, unrivalled in her might,
Dweller in the Brazen Home, unconquered in the fight.

(*All go out singing and dancing.*)

WOMEN BEWARE WOMEN

Thomas Middleton

UPON THE TRAGEDY OF
MY FAMILIAR ACQUAINTANCE,
THO. MIDDLETON

Women beware Women; 'tis a true text
Never to be forgot; drabs of state vext
Have plots, poisons, mischiefs that seldom miss,
To murder virtue with a venom-kiss.
Witness this worthy tragedy, exprest
By him that well deserv'd among the best
Of poets in his time: he knew the rage,
Madness of women cross'd, and for the stage
Fitted their humours; hell-bred malice, strife
Acted in state, presented to the life.
I that have seen't can say, having just cause,
Never came tragedy off with more applause.

NATH. RICHARDS.

[Dramatis Personae]

DUKE OF FLORENCE
LORD CARDINAL, *brother to the Duke*
TWO CARDINALS MORE
A LORD
FABRITIO, *father to Isabella*
HIPPOLITO, *brother to Fabritio*
GUARDIANO, *uncle to the foolish ward*
THE WARD, *a rich young heir*
LEANTIO, *a factor, husband to Bianca*
SORDIDO, *the Ward's man*

LIVIA, *sister to Fabritio*
ISABELLA, *niece to Livia*
BIANCA, *Leantio's wife*
WIDOW, *his mother*

STATES OF FLORENCE
CITIZENS
A PRENTICE
BOYS
MESSENGERS
SERVANTS
[LADIES]

The Scene FLORENCE

NOTE: Since it was a tendency of Jacobean and Elizabethan authors to omit essential exits and entrances from their texts, stage directions that are clearly implied but do not appear in the original texts have been added here in brackets.

ACT. 1. Scene. 1

(*Enter* LEANTIO *with* BIANCA, *and* MOTHER.)

MOTHER: Thy sight was never yet more precious to me;
Welcome with all the affection of a mother,
That comfort can express from natural love:
Since thy birth-joy, a mother's chiefest gladness
After sh'as undergone her curse of sorrows,
Thou wast not more dear to me, than this hour
Presents thee to my heart. Welcome again.
LEANTIO [*Aside*]: 'Las poor affectionate soul, how her joys
        speak to me!
I have observ'd it often, and I know it is
The fortune commonly of knavish children
To have the loving'st mothers.
MOTHER: What's this gentlewoman?
LEANTIO: Oh you have nam'd the most unvaluedst pur-
        chase,
That youth of man had ever knowledge of.
As often as I look upon that treasure,
And know it to be mine, (there lies the blessing)
It joys me that I ever was ordain'd
To have a being, and to live 'mongst men;
Which is a fearful living, and a poor one;
Let a man truly think on't.
To have the toil and griefs of fourscore years
Put up in a white sheet, ti'd with two knots;
Methinks it should strike earthquakes in adulterers,
When ev'n the very sheets they commit sin in
May prove, for aught they know, all their last garments.
Oh what a mark were there for women then!
But beauty able to content a conqueror,
Whom earth could scarce content, keeps me in compass;
I find no wish in me bent sinfully
To this man's sister, or to that man's wife:
In love's name let 'em keep their honesties,
And cleave to their own husbands, 'tis their duties.

Now when I go to church, I can pray handsomely;
Not come like gallants only to see faces,
As if lust went to market still on Sundays.
I must confess I am guilty of one sin, Mother,
More than I brought into the world with me;
But that I glory in: 'tis theft, but noble
As ever greatness yet shot up withal.
    MOTHER: How's that?
    LEANTIO: Never to be repented (Mother,)
Though sin be death; I had di'd, if I had not sinn'd,
And here's my masterpiece: do you now behold her!
Look on her well, she's mine, look on her better:
Now say, if't be not the best piece of theft
That ever was committed; and I have my pardon for't:
'Tis seal'd from heaven by marriage.
    MOTHER: Married to her!
    LEANTIO: You must keep counsel, Mother, I am undone
        else;
If it be known, I have lost her; do but think now
What that loss is, life's but a triffle to't.
From Venice, her consent and I have brought her
From parents great in wealth, more now in rage;
But let storms spend their furies, now we have got
A shelter o'er our quiet innocent loves,
We are contented; little money sh'as brought me.
View but her face, you may see all her dowry,
Save that which lies lockt up in hidden virtues,
Like jewels kept in cabinets.
    MOTHER: Y'are to blame,
If your obedience will give way to a check,
To wrong such a perfection.
    LEANTIO: How?
    MOTHER: Such a creature,
To draw her from her fortune, which no doubt,
At the full time, might have prov'd rich and noble:
You know not what you have done; my life can give you
But little helps, and my death lesser hopes.
And hitherto your own means has but made shift
To keep you single, and that hardly too.
What ableness have you to do her right then
In maintenance fitting her birth and virtues?
Which ev'ry woman of necessity looks for,
And most to go above it, not confin'd
By their conditions, virtues, bloods, or births,
But flowing to affections, wills, and humours.

LEANTIO: Speak low, sweet Mother; you are able to spoil
    as many
As come within the hearing: if it be not
Your fortune to mar all, I have much marvel.
I pray do not you teach her to rebel,
When she's in a good way to obedience,
To rise with other women in commotion
Against their husbands, for six gowns a year,
And so maintain their cause, when they're once up,
In all things else that require cost enough.
They are all of 'em a kind of spirits soon rais'd,
But not so soon laid (Mother). As for example,
A woman's belly is got up in a trice,
A simple charge ere it be laid down again:
So even in all their quarrels, and their courses,
And I'm a proud man I hear nothing of 'em,
They're very still, I thank my happiness,
And sound asleep; pray let not your tongue wake 'em.
If you can but rest quiet, she's contented
With all conditions that my fortunes bring her to;
To keep close as a wife that loves her husband;
To go after the rate of my ability,
Not the licentious swing of her own will,
Like some of her old school-fellows; she intends,
To take out other works in a new sampler,
And frame the fashion of an honest love,
Which knows no wants, but, mocking poverty,
Brings forth more children, to make rich men wonder
At divine Providence, that feeds mouths of infants,
And sends them none to feed, but stuffs their rooms
With fruitful bags, their beds with barren wombs.
Good Mother, make not you things worse than they are,
Out of your too much openness; pray take heed on't;
Nor imitate the envy of old people,
That strive to mar good sport, because they are perfit.
I would have you more pitiful to youth,
Especially to your own flesh and blood.
I'll prove an excellent husband, here's my hand,
Lay in provision, follow my business roundly,
And make you a grandmother in forty weeks.
Go, pray salute her, bid her welcome cheerfully.
    MOTHER: Gentlewoman, thus much is a debt of courtesy
    [*greeting her*]
Which fashionable strangers pay each other
At a kind meeting; then there's more than one
Due to the knowledge I have of your nearness.

I am bold to come again, and now salute you
By th' name of daughter, which may challenge more
Than ordinary respect.
    LEANTIO [*Aside*]:   Why, this is well now,
And I think few mothers of threescore will mend it.
    MOTHER: What I can bid you welcome to, is mean;
But make it all your own; we are full of wants,
And cannot welcome worth.
    LEANTIO [*Aside*]:   Now this is scurvy,
And spake as if a woman lack'd her teeth.
These old folks talk of nothing but defects,
Because they grow so full of 'em themselves.
    BIANCA: Kind Mother, there is nothing can be wanting
To her that does enjoy all her desires.
Heaven send a quiet peace with this man's love,
And I am as rich, as virtue can be poor;
Which were enough after the rate of mind,
To erect temples for content plac'd here;
I have forsook friends, fortunes, and my country,
And hourly I rejoice in't. Here's my friends,
And few is the good number; thy successes,
How e'er they look, I will still name my fortunes,
Hopeful or spiteful, they shall all be welcome:
Who invites many guests has of all sorts,
As he that traffics much drinks of all fortunes,
Yet they must all be welcome, and us'd well.
I'll call this place the place of my birth now,
And rightly too; for here my love was born,
And that's the birth-day of a woman's joys.
You have not bid me welcome since I came.
    LEANTIO: That I did questionless.
    BIANCA: No sure, how was't?
I have quite forgot it.
    LEANTIO: Thus. [*Kisses her.*]
    BIANCA: Oh Sir, 'tis true;
Now I remember well: I have done thee wrong,
Pray take't again Sir. [*Kisses him.*]
    LEANTIO: How many of these wrongs
Could I put up in an hour, and turn up
The glass for twice as many more!
    MOTHER: Wilt please
You to walk in, Daughter?
    BIANCA: Thanks, sweet Mother;
The voice of her that bare me is not more pleasing. (*Exeunt.*)
[*Manet* LEANTIO.]
    LEANTIO: Though my own care, and my rich master's trust,

Lay their commands both on my factorship,
This day and night, I'll know no other business
But her and her dear welcome. 'Tis a bitterness
To think upon tomorrow, that I must leave her
Still to the sweet hopes of the week's end,
That pleasure should be so retrain'd and curb'd
After the course of a rich work-master,
That never pays till Saturday night. Marry,
It comes together in a round sum then,
And does more good, you'll say. Oh fair-ey'd Florence!
Didst thou but know what a most matchless jewel
Thou now art mistress of, a pride would take thee,
Able to shoot destruction through the bloods
Of all thy youthful sons; but 'tis great policy
To keep choice treasures in obscurest places:
Should we show thieves our wealth, 'twould make 'em bolder;
Temptation is a devil will not stick
To fasten upon a saint; take heed of that;
The jewel is cas'd up from all men's eyes.
Who could imagine now a gem were kept,
Of that great value under this plain roof?
But how in times of absence? what assurance
Of this restraint then? Yes, yes, there's one with her.
Old mothers know the world; and such as these,
When sons lock chests, are good to look to keys. (*Exit.*)

Scene. 2

(*Enter* GUARDIANO, FABRITIO, *and* LIVIA.)

GUARDIANO: What, has your daughter seen him yet? know
    you that?
FABRITIO: No matter, she shall love him.
GUARDIANO: Nay, let's have fair
                                                          play;
He has been now my ward some fifteen year,
And 'tis my purpose (as time calls upon me)
By custom seconded, and such moral virtues,
To tender him a wife; now sir, this wife
I'd fain elect out of a daughter of yours.
You see my meaning's fair; if now this daughter
So tendered (let me come to your own phrase, sir)
Should offer to refuse him, I were hansell'd.

[Aside] Thus am I fain to calculate all my words,
For the meridian of a foolish old man,
To take his understanding.—What do you answer, sir?
 FABRITIO: I say still she shall love him.
 GUARDIANO: Yet again?
And shall she have no reason for this love?
 FABRITIO: Why, do you think that women love with rea-
  son?
 GUARDIANO *[Aside]*: I perceive fools are not at all hours
  foolish,
No more than wisemen wise.
 FABRITIO: I had a wife,
She ran mad for me; she had no reason for't,
For aught I could perceive: what think you, Lady Sister?
 GUARDIANO *[Aside]*: 'Twas a fit match that, being both out
  of their wits:
—A loving wife, it seem'd
She strove to come as near you as she could.
 FABRITIO: And if her daughter prove not mad for love too,
She takes not after her, nor after me
If she prefer reason before my pleasure.
You're an experienc'd widow, Lady Sister,
I pray let your opinion come amongst us.
 LIVIA: I must offend you then, if truth will do't,
And take my niece's part, and call't injustice
To force her love to one she never saw.
Maids should both see, and like; all little enough
If they love truly after that, 'tis well
Counting the time, she takes one man till death,
That's a hard task, I tell you; but one may
Enquire at three years' end, amongst young wives,
And mark how the game goes.
 FABRITIO: Why, is not a man
Ti'd to the same observance, Lady Sister,
And in one woman?
 LIVIA: 'Tis enough for him:
Besides he tastes of many sundry dishes
That we poor wretches never lay our lips to;
As obedience forsooth, subjection, duty, and such
Kickshaws, all of our making, but serv'd in
To them; and if we lick a finger then
Sometimes, we are not to blame: your best cooks use it.
 FABRITIO: Th'art a sweet Lady, Sister, and a witty——
 LIVIA: A witty! Oh the bud of commendation
Fit for a girl of sixteen; I am blown, man,
I should be wise by this time, and for instance,

I have buried my two husbands in good fashion,
And never mean more to marry.
    GUARDIANO: No, why so, Lady?
    LIVIA: Because the third shall never bury me:
I think I am more than witty; how think you, sir?
    FABRITIO: I have paid often fees to a counsellor
Has had a weaker brain.
    LIVIA: Then I must tell you.
Your money was soon parted.
    GUARDIANO: Like enow.
    LIVIA: Brother,
Where is my niece? let her be sent for straight,
If you have any hope 'twill prove a wedding;
'Tis fit i'faith she should have one sight of him,
And stop upon't, and not be join'd in haste,
As if they went to stock a new found land.
    FABRITIO: Look out her uncle, and y'are sure of her,
Those two are nev'r asunder, they've been heard
In argument at midnight, moon-shine nights
Are noondays with them; they walk out their sleeps;
Or rather at those hours appear like those
That walk in 'em, for so they did to me.
Look you, I told you truth; they're like a chain,
Draw but one link, all follows.

    (*Enter* HIPPOLITO, *and* ISABELLA *the niece.*)
    GUARDIANO: Oh affinity,
What piece of excellent workmanship art thou!
'Tis work clean wrought, for there's no lust, but love in't,
And that abundantly: when in stranger things,
There is no love at all, but what lust brings.
    FABRITIO: On with your mask; for 'tis your part to see
           now,
And not be seen: go to, make use of your time;
See what you mean to like; nay, and I charge you,
Like what you see: do you hear me? there's no dallying:
The gentleman's almost twenty, and 'tis time
He were getting lawful heirs, and you a-breeding on 'em.
    ISABELLA: Good Father!
    FABRITIO: Tell me not of tongues and ru-
                                 mours.
You'll say the gentleman is somewhat simple—
The better for a husband, were you wise;
For those that marry fools, live ladies' lives.
On with the mask, I'll hear no more, he's rich;
The fool's hid under bushels.

LIVIA: Not so hid neither
But here's a foul great piece of him methinks;
What will he be, when he comes altogether?

(*Enter the* WARD *with a trap-stick, and* SORDIDO *his man.*)
WARD: Beat him?
I beat him out o'th'field with his own cat-stick,
Yet gave him the first hand.
SORDIDO: Oh strange!
WARD: I did it,
Then he set jacks on me.
SORDIDO: What, my lady's tailor?
WARD: Ay, and I beat him too.
SORDIDO: Nay, that's no wonder,
He's used to beating.
WARD: Nay, I tickl'd him
When I came once to my tippings.
SORDIDO: Now you talk on 'em, there was a poulterer's wife
made a great complaint of you last night to your guardianer,
that you struck a bump in her child's head, as big as an egg.
WARD: An egg may prove a chicken, then in time the poul-
terer's wife will get by't. When I am in game, I am furious;
came my mother's eyes in my way, I would not lose a fair
end: no, were she alive, but with one tooth in her head, I
should venture the striking out of that. I think of no body,
when I am in play, I am so earnest. Coads me, my guardi-
aner!
   Prethee lay up my cat and cat-stick safe.
SORDIDO: Where, sir, i'th'chimney-corner?
WARD: Chimney-corner!
SORDIDO: Yes sir, your cats are always safe i'th'chimney-
corner, unless they burn their coats.
WARD: Marry, that I am afraid on!
SORDIDO: Why, then I will bestow your cat i'th'gutter,
And there she's safe I am sure.
WARD: If I but live
To keep a house, I'll make thee a great man,
If meat and drink can do't. I can stoop gallantly,
And pitch out when I list: I'm dog at a hole.
I mar'l my guardianer does not seek a wife for me: I protest
I'll have a bout with the maids else, or contract my self at
midnight to the larder-woman, in presence of a fool, or a
sack-posset.
GUARDIANO: Ward.
WARD: I feel my self after any exercise.

Horribly prone: let me but ride, I'm lusty,
A cock-horse straight i'faith.
GUARDIANO: Why, Ward, I say.
    WARD: I'll forswear eating eggs in moon-shine nights;
There's never a one I eat, but turns into a cock
In four and twenty hours; if my hot blood
Be not took down in time, sure 'twill crow shortly.
    GUARDIANO: Do you hear, sir? follow me, I must now
school you.
    WARD: School me? I scorn that now, I am past schooling.
I am not so base to learn to write and read;
I was born to better fortunes in my cradle.

(*Exit* [*with* SORDIDO *and* GUARDIANO].)

    FABRITIO: How do you like him, girl? this is your husband.
Like him, or like him not, wench, you shall have him,
And you shall love him.
    LIVIA: Oh soft there, Brother! though you be a justice,
Your warrant cannot be serv'd out of your liberty;
You may compel, out of the power of a father,
Things merely harsh to a maid's flesh and blood;
But when you come to love, there the soil alters;
Y'are in an other country, where your laws
Are no more set by, than the cacklings
Of geese in Rome's great Capitol.
    FABRITIO: Marry him she shall then,
Let her agree upon love afterwards. (*Exit.*)
    LIVIA: You speak now, Brother, like an honest mortal
That walks upon th'earth with a staff; you were
Up i'th'clouds before, you'd command love,
And so do most old folks that go without it.
My best and dearest Brother, I could dwell here;
There is not such another seat on earth,
Where all good parts better express themselves.
    HIPPOLITO: You'll make me blush anon.
    LIVIA: 'Tis but like saying grace before a feast then,
And that's most comely; thou art all a feast,
And she that has thee, a most happy guest,
Prethee cheer up thy niece with special counsel. (*Exit.*)
    HIPPOLITO [*Aside*]: I would 'twere fit to speak to her what
        I would; but
'Twas not a thing ordain'd, Heaven has forbid it,
And 'tis most meet, that I should rather perish
Than the decree divine receive least blemish:

Feed inward, you my sorrows, make no noise,
Consume me silent, let me be stark dead
Ere the world know I'm sick. You see my honesty;
If you befriend me, so.
    ISABELLA [*Aside*]:   Marry a fool!
Can there be greater misery to a woman
That means to keep her days true to her husband,
And know no other man! so virtue wills it.
Why; how can I obey and honour him,
But I must needs commit idolatry?
A fool is but the image of a man,
And that but ill-made neither: oh the heart-breakings
Of miserable maids, where love's enforc'd!
The best condition is but bad enough;
When women have their choices, commonly
They do but buy their thraldoms, and bring great portions
To men to keep 'em in subjection,
As if a fearful prisoner should bribe
The keeper to be good to him, yet lies in still,
And glad of a good usage, a good look sometimes.
By'r Lady, no misery surmounts a woman's.
Men buy their slaves, but women buy their masters;
Yet honesty and love makes all this happy,
And next to angels', the most blest estate.
That Providence, that has made ev'ry poison
Good for some use, and sets four warring elements
At peace in man, can make a harmony
In things that are most strange to human reason.
Oh but this marriage!—What, are you sad too, Uncle?
Faith, then there's a whole household down together:
Where shall I go to seek my comfort now
When my best friend's distress'd? what is't afflicts you, sir?
    HIPPOLITO: Faith, nothing but one grief that will not leave
      me,
And now 'tis welcome; ev'ry man has something
To bring him to his end, and this will serve
Join'd with your father's cruelty to you,
That helps it forward.
    ISABELLA: Oh be cheer'd, sweet Uncle!
How long has't been upon you? I never spi'd it:
What a dull sight have I, how long I pray, sir?
    HIPPOLITO: Since I first saw you, Niece, and left Bologna.
    ISABELLA: And could you deal so unkindly with my heart,
To keep it up so long hid from my pity?

Alas, how shall I trust your love hereafter?
Have we past through so many arguments,
And miss'd of that still, the most needful one?
Walk'd out whole nights together in discourses,
And the main point forgot? We are to blame both;
This is an obstinate wilful forgetfulness,
And faulty on both parts: let's lose no time now,
Begin, good Uncle, you that feel't; what is it?
   HIPPOLITO: You of all creatures, Niece, must never hear
      on't,
'Tis not a thing ordain'd for you to know.
   ISABELLA: Not I, sir! all my joys that word cuts off;
You made profession once you lov'd me best;
'Twas but profession!
   HIPPOLITO: Yes, I do't too truly,
And fear I shall be chid for't. Know the worst then:
I love thee dearlier than an uncle can.
   ISABELLA: Why, so you ever said, and I believ'd it.
   HIPPOLITO [*Aside*]: So simple is the goodness of her
      thoughts,
They understand not yet th'unhallowed language
Of a near sinner: I must yet be forced
(Though blushes be my venture) to come nearer.
—As a man loves his wife, so love I thee.
   ISABELLA: What's that?
Methought I heard ill news come toward me,
Which commonly we understand too soon,
Then over-quick at hearing. I'll prevent it,
Though my joys fare the harder; welcome it:
It shall nev'r come so near mine ear again.
Farewell all friendly solaces and discourses,
I'll learn to live without ye, for your dangers
Are greater than your comforts; what's become
Of truth in love, if such we cannot trust,
When blood that should be love, is mix'd with lust? (*Exit.*)
   HIPPOLITO: The worst can be but death, and let it come,
He that lives joyless, ev'ry day's his doom. (*Exit.*)

Scene. 3

(*Enter* LEANTIO *alone.*)
   LEANTIO: Methinks I'm ev'n as dull now at departure,
As men observe great gallants the next day

After a revels; you shall see 'em look
Much of my fashion, if you mark 'em well.
'Tis ev'n a second hell to part from pleasure,
When man has got a smack on't: as many holidays,
Coming together, makes your poor heads idle
A great while after, and are said to stick
Fast in their fingers' ends, ev'n so does game
In a new-married couple; for the time
It spoils all thrift, and indeed lies abed
To invent all the new ways for great expenses.
    (BIANCA *and* MOTHER *above.*)
See, and she be not got on purpose now
Into the window to look after me.
I have no power to go now, and I should be hang'd:
Farewell all business, I desire no more
Than I see yonder; let the goods at key
Look to themselves; why should I toil my youth out?
It is but begging two or three year sooner,
And stay with her continually; is't a match?
O fie, what a religion have I leap'd into!
Get out again for shame; the man loves best
When his care's most, that shows his zeal to love.
Fondness is but the idiot to affection,
That plays at hot-cockles with rich merchants' wives;
Good to make sport withal when the chest's full,
And the long warehouse cracks. 'Tis time of day
For us to be more wise; 'tis early with us,
And if they lose the morning of their affairs,
They commonly lose the best part of the day:
Those that are wealthy, and have got enough,
'Tis after sun-set with 'em, they may rest,
Grow fat with ease, banket, and toy and play,
When such as I enter the heat o'th'day,
And I'll do't cheerfully.
  BIANCA: I perceive sir,
Y'are not gone yet, I have good hope you'll stay now.
   LEANTIO: Farewell, I must not.
  BIANCA: Come, come, pray return;
Tomorrow, adding but a little care more,
Will dispatch all as well; believe me 'twill, sir.
   LEANTIO: I could well wish my self where you would have
      me;
But love that's wanton must be rul'd awhile
By that that's careful, or all goes to ruin;
As fitting is a government in love,

As in a kingdom; where 'tis all mere lust,
'Tis like an insurrection in the people
That, rais'd in self-will, wars against all reason:
But love that is respective for increase
Is like a good king, that keeps all in peace.
Once more farewell.

BIANCA: But this one night, I prethee.

LEANTIO: Alas I'm in for twenty, if I stay,
And then for forty more; I've such a luck to flesh,
I never bought a horse, but he bore double.
If I stay any longer, I shall turn
An everlasting spendthrift, as you love
To be maintain'd well, do not call me again,
For then I shall not care which end goes forward:
Again farewell to thee. (*Exit.*)

BIANCA: Since it must, farewell too.

MOTHER: 'Faith, Daughter, y'are to blame, you take the
        course
To make him an ill husband, troth you do,
And that disease is catching, I can tell you,
Ay, and soon taken by a youngman's blood,
And that with little urging. Nay fie, see now,
What cause have you to weep? would I had no more
That have liv'd threescore years; there were a cause
And 'twere well thought on; trust me y'are to blame,
His absence cannot last five days at utmost.
Why should those tears be fetch'd forth? cannot love
Be ev'n as well express'd in a good look,
But it must see her face still in a fountain?
It shows like a country maid dressing her head
By a dish of water: come, 'tis an old custom
To weep for love.

(*Enter two or three* BOYS, *and a* CITIZEN *or two, with an*
APPRENTICE.)

BOYS: Now they come, now they come.

2. BOY: The Duke!

3. BOY: The States!

CITIZEN: How near, boy?

1. BOY: I'th'next street sir, hard at hand.

CITIZEN: You sirrah, get a standing for your mistress,
The best in all the city.

APPRENTICE: I have't for her sir,

'Twas a thing I provided for her over night,
'Tis ready at her pleasure.
    CITIZEN: Fetch her to't then,
Away sir!
    BIANCA: What's the meaning of this hurry,
Can you tell, Mother?
    MOTHER: What a memory
Have I! I see by that years come upon me.
Why, 'tis a yearly custom and solemnity,
Religiously observ'd by th'Duke and State
To St. Mark's Temple, the fifteenth of April:
See if my dull brains had not quite forgot it.
'Twas happily question'd of thee, I had gone down else,
Sat like a drone below, and never thought on't.
I would not to be ten years younger again
That you had lost the sight; now you shall see
Our Duke, a goodly gentleman of his years.
    BIANCA: Is he old then?
    MOTHER: About some fifty-five.
    BIANCA: That's no great age in man, he's then at best
For wisdom, and for judgment.
    MOTHER: The Lord Cardinal,
His noble brother, there's a comely gentleman,
And greater in devotion than in blood.
    BIANCA: He's worthy to be mark'd.
    MOTHER: You shall behold
All our chief states of Florence, you came fortunately
Against this solemn day.
    BIANCA: I hope so always. (*Music.*)
    MOTHER: I hear 'em near us now, do you stand easily?
    BIANCA: Exceeding well, good Mother.
    MOTHER: Take this stool.
    BIANCA: I need it not, I thank you.
    MOTHER: Use your will then.

(*Enter in great solemnity six* KNIGHTS *bare-headed, then two* CARDINALS, *and then the* LORD CARDINAL, *then the* DUKE; *after him the* STATES OF FLORENCE *by two and two, with variety of music and song. Exeunt.*)

    MOTHER: How like you, Daughter?
    BIANCA: 'Tis a noble state.
Methinks my soul could dwell upon the reverence
Of such a solemn and most worthy custom.

Did not the Duke look up? me-thought he saw us.
   MOTHER: That's ev'ry one's conceit that sees a duke:
If he looks steadfastly, he looks straight at them,
When he perhaps, good careful gentleman,
Never minds any; but the look he casts
Is at his own intentions, and his object
Only the public good.
   BIANCA: Most likely so.
   MOTHER: Come, come, we'll end this argument below.
   (*Exeunt.*)

ACT. 2. Scene. 1

(*Enter* HIPPOLITO, *and Lady* LIVIA *the Widow.*)

   LIVIA: A strange affection (Brother) when I think on't!
I wonder how thou cam'st by't.
Ev'n as easily   HIPPOLITO:
As man comes by destruction, which oft-times
He wears in his own bosom.
   LIVIA: Is the world
So populous in women, and creation
So prodigal in beauty and so various,
Yet does love turn thy point to thine won blood?
'Tis somewhat too unkindly; must thy eye
Dwell evilly on the fairness of thy kinred,
And seek not where it should? it is confin'd
Now in a narrower prison than was made for't:
It is allow'd a stranger, and where bounty
Is made the great man's honour, 'tis ill husbandry
To spare, and servants shall have small thanks for't.
So he heaven's bounty seems to scorn and mock,
That spares free means, and spends of his own stock.
   HIPPOLITO: Never was man's misery so soon sew'd up,
Counting how truly.
   LIVIA: Nay, I love you so,
That I shall venture much to keep a change from you
So fearful as this grief will bring upon you.
'Faith it even kills me, when I see you faint
Under a reprehension, and I'll leave it,
Though I know nothing can be better for you:
Prethee (sweet Brother) let not passion waste

The goodness of thy time, and of thy fortune:
Thou keep'st the treasure of that life I love
As dearly as mine own; and if you think
My former words too bitter, which were minist'red
By truth and zeal, 'tis but a hazarding
Of grace and virtue, and I can bring forth
As pleasant fruits as sensuality wishes
In all her teeming longings: this I can do.
   HIPPOLITO: Oh nothing that can make my wishes perfect!
   LIVIA: I would that love of yours were pawn'd to't, Brother,
And as soon lost that way as I could win.
Sir, I could give as shrewd a lift to chastity
As any she that wears a tongue in Florence.
Sh'ad need be a good horse-woman, and sit fast,
Whom my strong argument could not fling at last.
Prethee take courage, man; though I should counsel
Another to despair, yet I am pitiful
To thy afflictions, and will venture hard;
I will not name for what, 'tis not handsome;
Find you the proof, and praise me.
   HIPPOLITO: Then I fear me
I shall not praise you in haste.
   LIVIA: This is the comfort,
You are not the first (Brother) has attempted
Things more forbidden than this seems to be:
I'll minister all cordials now to you,
Because I'll cheer you up sir.
   HIPPOLITO: I am past hope.
   LIVIA: Love, thou shalt see me do a strange cure then,
As e'er was wrought on a disease so mortal,
And near akin to shame; when shall you see her?
   HIPPOLITO: Never in comfort more.
   LIVIA: Y'are so impatient too.
   HIPPOLITO: Will you believe? death, sh'has forsworn my
         company,
And seal'd it with a blush.
   LIVIA: So, I perceive
All lies upon my hands then; well, the more glory
When the work's finish'd.—How now sir, the news!

(*Enter* SERVANT.)

   SERVANT: Madam, your niece, the virtuous Isabella,
Is lighted now to see you.
   LIVIA: That's great fortune;

Your stars bless you.—Simple, lead her in. (*Exit* SERVANT.)
HIPPOLITO: What's this to me?
  LIVIA: Your absence, gentle brother;
I must bestir my wits for you.
  HIPPOLITO: Ay, to great purpose. (*Exit*
                 HIPPOLITO.)
  LIVIA: Beshrew you, would I lov'd you not so well:
I'll go to bed, and leave this deed undone:
I am the fondest where I once affect;
The careful'st of their healths, and of their ease forsooth,
That I look still but slenderly to mine own.
I take a course to pity him so much now,
That I have none left for modesty and my self.
This 'tis to grow so liberal; y'have few sisters
That love their brothers' ease 'bove their own honesties:
But if you question my affections,
That will be found my fault.

  (*Enter* ISABELLA *the Niece.*)

           Niece, your love's welcome.
Alas, what draws that paleness to thy cheeks?
This enforc'd marriage towards?
  ISABELLA: It helps, good Aunt,
Amongst some other griefs; but those I'll keep
Lock'd up in modest silence; for they're sorrows
Would shame the tongue more than they grieve the thought.
  LIVIA: Indeed, the Ward is simple.
  ISABELLA: Simple! that were well:
Why, one might make good shift with such a husband.
But he's a fool entail'd, he halts downright in't.
  LIVIA: And knowing this, I hope 'tis at your choice
To take or refuse, Niece.
  ISABELLA: You see it is not.
I loathe him more than beauty can hate death
Or age her spiteful neighbour.
  LIVIA: Let't appear then.
  ISABELLA: How can I, being born with that obedience,
That must submit unto a father's will?
If he command, I must of force consent.
  LIVIA: Alas poor soul! Be not offended prethee,
If I set by the name of niece awhile,
And bring in pity in a stranger fashion:
It lies here in this breast would cross this match.
  ISABELLA: How, cross it, Aunt?
  LIVIA: Ay, and give thee more liberty

Than thou hast reason yet to apprehend.

ISABELLA: Sweet Aunt, in goodness keep not hid from me
What may befriend my life.

LIVIA:　　　　　　　　　　Yes, yes, I must,
When I return to reputation,
And think upon the solemn vow I made
To your dead mother, my most loving sister;
As long as I have her memory 'twixt mine eye-lids,
Look for no pity now.

ISABELLA:　　　　　Kind, sweet, dear Aunt——

LIVIA: No, 'twas a secret I have took special care of,
Delivered by your mother on her death-bed,
That's nine years now, and I'll not part from't yet,
Though nev'r was fitter time, nor greater cause for't.

ISABELLA: As you desire the praises of a virgin——

LIVIA: Good sorrow! I would do thee any kindness,
Not wronging secrecy, or reputation.

ISABELLA: Neither of which (as I have hope of fruitness)
Shall receive wrong from me.

LIVIA:　　　　　　　Nay 'twould be your own wrong,
As much as any's, should it come to that once.

ISABELLA: I need no better means to work persuasion then.

LIVIA: Let it suffice, you may refuse this fool,
Or you may take him, as you see occasion
For your advantage; the best wits will do't;
Y'have liberty enough in your own will,
You cannot be enforc'd; there grows the flow'r,
If you could pick it out, makes whole life sweet to you.
That which you call your father's command's nothing;
Then your obedience must needs be as little.
If you can make shift here to taste your happiness,
Or pick out aught that likes you, much good do you:
You see your cheer, I'll make you no set dinner.

ISABELLA: And trust me, I may starve for all the good
I can find yet in this: sweet Aunt, deal plainlier.

LIVIA: Say I should trust you now upon an oath,
And give you in a secret that would start you,
How am I sure of you, in faith and silence?

ISABELLA: Equal assurance may I find in mercy,
As you for that in me.

LIVIA:　　　　　　It shall suffice.
Then know, however custom has made good,
For reputation's sake, the names of niece
And aunt 'twixt you and I, w'are nothing less.

ISABELLA: How's that?

LIVIA:　　　　　　I told you I should start your blood.

You are no more alli'd to any of us,
Save what the courtesy of opinion casts
Upon your mother's memory and your name,
Than the mer'st stranger is, or one begot
At Naples, when the husband lies at Rome;
There's so much odds betwixt us. Since your knowledge
Wish'd more instruction, and I have your oath
In pledge for silence, it makes me talk the freelier.
Did never the report of that fam'd Spaniard,
Marquess of Coria, since your time was ripe
For understanding, fill your ear with wonder?
   ISABELLA: Yes, what of him? I have heard his deeds of
      honour
Often related when we liv'd in Naples.
   LIVIA: You heard the praises of your father then.
   ISABELLA: My father!
   LIVIA: That was he: but all the business
So carefully and so discreetly carried,
That fame receiv'd no spot by't, not a blemish;
Your mother was so wary to her end,
None knew it, but her conscience, and her friend,
Till penitent confession made it mine,
And now my pity yours: it had been long else,
And I hope care and love alike in you,
Made good by oath, will see it take no wrong now:
How weak his commands now, whom you call father!
How vain all his enforcements, your obedience,
And what a largeness in your will and liberty,
To take, or to reject, or to do both!
For fools will serve to father wise men's children:
All this y'have time to think on. O my wench!
Nothing o'erthrows our sex but indiscretion,
We might do well else of a brittle people,
As any under the great canopy:
I pray forgot not but to call me aunt still;
Take heed of that, it may be mark'd in time else,
But keep your thoughts to your self, from all the world,
Kinred, or dearest friend, nay, I entreat you,
From him that all this while you have call'd uncle;
And though you love him dearly, as I know
His deserts claim as much ev'n from a stranger,
Yet let not him know this, I prethee do not;
As ever thou hast hope of second pity
If thou should'st stand in need on't, do not do't.
   ISABELLA: Believe my oath, I will not.
   LIVIA: Why, well said.

[*Aside*] Who shows more craft t'undo a maidenhead,
I'll resign my part to her.

(*Enter* HIPPOLITO.)

                            —She's thine own, go. (*Exit.*)
HIPPOLITO: Alas, fair flattery cannot cure my sorrows!
ISABELLA [*Aside*]: Have I past so much time in ignorance,
And never had the means to know my self
Till this blest hour? Thanks to her virtuous pity
That brought it now to light; would I had known it
But one day sooner, he had then receiv'd
In favours what (poor gentleman) he took
In bitter words; a slight and harsh reward
For one of his deserts.
HIPPOLITO [*Aside*]:   There seems to me now
More anger and distraction in her looks.
I'm gone, I'll not endure a second storm;
The memory of the first is not past yet.
ISABELLA [*Aside*]: Are you return'd, you comforts of my
                            life,
In this man's presence? I will keep you fast now,
And sooner part eternally from the world,
Than my good joys in you.—Prethee forgive me,
I did but chide in jest; the best loves use it
Sometimes, it sets an edge upon affection:
When we invite our best friends to a feast,
'Tis not all sweet-meats that we set before them,
There's somewhat sharp and salt, both to whet appetite,
And make 'em taste their wine well: so me thinks,
After a friendly, sharp and savoury chiding,
A kiss tastes wondrous well, and full o'th'grape. [*Kisses
            him.*]
How think'st thou, does't not?
HIPPOLITO: 'Tis so excellent,
I know now how to praise it, what to say to't.
ISABELLA: This marriage shall go forward.
HIPPOLITO: With the ward?
Are you in earnest?
ISABELLA: 'Twould be ill for us else.
HIPPOLITO [*Aside*]: For us? how means she that?
ISABELLA: Troth I
                                            begin
To be so well methinks, within this hour,
For all this match able to kill one's heart.
Nothing can pull me down now; should my father

Provide a worse fool yet (which I should think
Were a hard thing to compass) I'd have him either;
The worse the better, none can come amiss now,
If he want wit enough: so discretion love me,
Desert and judgment, I have content sufficient.
She that comes once to be a house-keeper
Must not look every day to fare well, sir,
Like a young waiting gentlewoman in service,
For she feeds commonly as her lady does;
No good bit passes her, but she gets a taste on't;
But when she comes to keep house for her self,
She's glad of some choice cates then once a week,
Or twice at most, and glad if she can get 'em:
So must affection learn to fare with thankfulness.
Pray make your love no stranger, sir, that's all,
[*Aside*] Though you be one your self, and know not on't,
And I have sworn you must not. (*Exit.*)
   HIPPOLITO: This is beyond me!
Never came joys so unexpectedly
To meet desires in man; how came she thus?
What has she done to her, can any tell?
'Tis beyond sorcery this, drugs, or love-powders;
Some art that has no name sure, strange to me
Of all the wonders I e'er met withal
Throughout my ten years' travels; but I'm thankful for't.
This marriage now must of necessity forward;
It is the only veil wit can devise
To keep our acts hid from sin-piercing eyes. (*Exit.*)

Scene. 2

(*Enter* GUARDIANO *and* LIVIA.)

   LIVIA: How sir? a gentlewoman, so young, so fair
As you set forth, spi'd from the widow's window?
   GUARDIANO: She!
   LIVIA: Our Sunday-dinner woman?
   GUARDIANO: And Thursday-supper woman, the same still.
I know not how she came by her, but I'll swear
She's the prime gallant for a face in Florence;
And no doubt other parts follow their leader:
The Duke himself first spi'd her at the window,
Then in a rapture, as if admiration

Were poor when it were single, beck'ned me,
And pointed to the wonder warily,
As one that fear'd she would draw in her splendour
Too soon, if too much gaz'd at: I nev'r knew him
So infinitely taken with a woman,
Nor can I blame his appetite, or tax
His raptures of slight folly, she's a creature
Able to draw a state from serious business,
And make it their best piece to do her service:
What course shall we devise? h'as spoke twice now.

LIVIA: Twice?

GUARDIANO: 'Tis beyond your apprehension
How strangely that one look has catch'd his heart:
'Twould prove but too much worth in wealth and favour
To those should work his peace.

LIVIA: And if I do't not,
Or at least come as near it (if your art
Will take a little pains, and second me)
As any wench in Florence of my standing,
I'll quite give o'er, and shut up shop in cunning.

GUARDIANO: 'Tis for the Duke, and if I fail your purpose,
All means to come, by riches or advancement,
Miss me, and skip me over.

LIVIA: Let the old woman then
Be sent for with all speed, then I'll begin.

GUARDIANO: A good conclusion follow, and a sweet one
After this stale beginning with old ware!
Within there!

(*Enter* SERVANT.)

SERVANT: Sir, do you call?

GUARDIANO: Come near, list hither. [*Whispers.*]

LIVIA: I long my self to see this absolute creature,
That wins the heart of love and praise so much.

GUARDIANO: Go sir, make haste.

LIVIA: Say I entreat her company;
Do you hear, sir?

SERVANT: Yes, Madam. (*Exit.*)

LIVIA: That brings her quickly.

GUARDIANO: I would 'twere done, the Duke waits the good
    hour,
And I wait the good fortune that may spring from't.
I have had a lucky hand these fifteen year
At such court passage with three dice in a dish.
Signor Fabritio!

(*Enter* FABRITIO.)

FABRITIO: Oh sir, I bring
An alteration in my mouth now.
   GUARDIANO [*Aside*]: An alteration! no wise speech I hope;
He means not to talk wisely, does he, trow?
—Good! what's the change, I pray, sir?
   FABRITIO: A new change.
   GUARDIANO: Another yet! 'faith, there's enough already.
   FABRITIO: My daughter loves him now.
   GUARDIANO: What, does she, sir?
   FABRITIO: Affects him beyond thought, who but the Ward
      forsooth!
No talk but of the Ward; she would have him
To choose 'bove all the men she ever saw.
My will goes not so fast, as her consent now;
Her duty gets before my command still.
   GUARDIANO: Why then sir, if you'll have me speak my
      thoughts,
I smell 'twill be a match.
   FABRITIO: Ay, and a sweet young couple,
If I have any judgment.
   GUARDIANO [*Aside*]:   'Faith, that's little.
—Let her be sent tomorrow before noon,
And handsomely trick'd up; for 'bout that time
I mean to bring her in, and tender her to him.
   FABRITIO: I warrant you for handsome, I will see
Her things laid ready, every one in order,
And have some part of her trick'd up tonight.
   GUARDIANO: Why, well said.
   FABRITIO: 'Twas a use her mother had,
When she was invited to an early wedding;
She'd dress her head o'ernight, sponge up her self,
And give her neck three lathers.
   GUARDIANO [*Aside*]:   Ne'er a halter?
   FABRITIO: On with her chain of pearl, her ruby bracelets,
Lay ready for her tricks and jiggam-bobs.
   GUARDIANO: So must your daughter.
   FABRITIO: I'll about it straight, sir.

(*Exit* FABRITIO.)

   LIVIA: How he sweats in the foolish zeal of fatherhood,
After six ounces an hour, and seems
To toil as much as if his cares were wise ones!

GUARDIANO: Y'have let his folly blood in the right vein,
Lady.

LIVIA: And here comes his sweet son-in-law that shall be;
They're both ally'd in wit before the marriage;
What will they be hereafter, when they are nearer?
Yet they can go no further than the fool:
There's the world's end in both of 'em.

(*Enter* WARD *and* SORDIDO, *one with a shittlecock, the
other a battledore.*)

GUARDIANO: Now, young heir.

WARD: What's the next business after shittlecock now?

GUARDIANO: Tomorrow you shall see the gentlewoman
Must be your wife.

WARD: There's even another thing too
Must be kept up with a pair of battledores.
My wife! what can she do?

GUARDIANO: Nay, that's a question you should ask your
self, Ward,
When y'are alone together.

WARD: That's as I list.
A wife's to be ask anywhere, I hope;
I'll ask her in a congregation,
If I have a mind to't, and so save a license:

[GUARDIANO *and* LIVIA *talk apart.*]

My guardiner has no more wit than an herb-woman,
That sells away all her sweet herbs and nosegays,
And keeps a stinking breath for her own pottage.

SORDIDO: Let me be at the choosing of your beloved,
If you desire a woman of good parts.

WARD: Thou shalt, sweet Sordido.

SORDIDO: I have a plaguy guess; let me alone to see what
she is; if I but look
upon her—'way, I know all the faults to a hair, that you may
refuse her for.

WARD: Dost thou! I prethee let me hear 'em, Sordido.

SORDIDO: Well, mark 'em then; I have 'em all in rhyme.
The wife your guardiner ought to tender
Should be pretty, straight and slender;
Her hair not short, her foot not long,
Her hand not huge, nor too too loud her tongue:
No pearl in eye, nor ruby in her nose,
No burn or cut, but what the catalogue shows.

She must have teeth, and that no black ones,
And kiss most sweet when she does smack once:
Her skin must be both white and plumpt,
Her body straight, not hopper-rumpt,
Or wriggle sideways like a crab;
She must be neither slut nor drab,
Nor go too splay-foot with her shoes,
To make her smock lick up the dews.
And two things more, which I forgot to tell ye,
She neither must have bump in back, nor belly.
These are the faults that will not make her pass.
   WARD: And if I spy not these, I am a rank ass.
   SORDIDO: Nay more; by right, sir, you should see her naked,
For that's the ancient order.
   WARD: See her naked?
That were good sport i'faith: I'll have the books turn'd over;
And if I find her naked on record,
She shall not have a rag on: but stay, stay,
How if she should desire to see me so too?
I were in a sweet case then—such a foul skin!
   SORDIDO: But y'have a clean shirt, and that makes amends,
      sir.
   WARD: I will not see her naked for that trick, though. (*Exit.*)
   SORDIDO: Then take her with all faults, with her clothes on!
And they may hide a number with a bum-roll.
'Faith, choosing of a wench in a huge farthingale is like the
burying of ware under a great pent-house. What with the de-
ceit of one, and the false light of th'other, mark my speeches,
he may have a diseas'd wench in's bed, and rotten stuff in's
breeches. (*Exit.*)
   GUARDIANO: It may take handsomely.
   LIVIA: I see small hindrance.
How now, so soon return'd?

(*Enter* MOTHER.)

   GUARDIANO: She's come.
   LIVIA: That's well.
Widow, come, come, I have a great quarrel to you,
'Faith I must chide you, that you must be sent for!
You make your self so strange, never come at us;
And yet so near a neighbour, and so unkind;
Troth y'are to blame, you cannot be more welcome
To any house in Florence, that I'll tell you.
   MOTHER: My thanks must needs acknowledge so much,
      Madam.

LIVIA: How can you be so strange then! I sit here
Sometimes whole days together without company,
When business draws this gentleman from home,
And should be happy in society,
Which I so well affect as that of yours.
I know y'are alone too; why should not we,
Like two kind neighbours, then, supply the wants
Of one another, having tongue discourse,
Experience in the world, and such kind helps
To laugh down time, and meet age merrily?
    MOTHER: Age (Madam): you speak mirth; 'tis at my door,
But a long journey from your Ladyship yet.
    LIVIA: My faith I'm nine and thirty, ev'ry stroke, wench,
And 'tis a general observation
'Mongst knights' wives or widows, we accompt our selves
Then old, when young men's eyes leave looking at's:
'Tis a true rule amongst us, and ne'er fail'd yet
In any but in one, that I remember;
Indeed she had a friend at nine and forty;
Marry, she paid well for him, and in th'end
He kept a quean or two with her own money,
That robb'd her of her plate, and cut her throat.
    MOTHER: She had her punishment in this world (Madam)
And a fair warning to all other women,
That they live chaste at fifty.
    LIVIA: Ay, or never, wench:
Come, now I have thy company I'll not part with't
Till after supper.
    MOTHER: Yes, I must crave pardon (Madam).
    LIVIA: I swear you shall stay supper; we have no strangers,
        woman,
None but my sojourners and I; this gentleman
And the young heir his ward; you know our company.
    MOTHER: Some other time, I will make bold with you,
    Madam.
    GUARDIANO: Nay, pray stay, widow.
    LIVIA: 'Faith, she shall not go.
Do you think I'll be forsworn?

(*Table and Chess.*)

    MOTHER: 'Tis a great while
Till supper time; I'll take my leave then now (Madam)
And come again i'th'evening, since your Ladyship
Will have it so.
    LIVIA: I'th'evening? by my troth, wench,

I'll keep you while I have you; you have great business, sure,
To sit alone at home; I wonder strangely
What pleasure you take in't! were't to me now,
I should be ever at one neighbour's house
Or other all day long; having no charge,
Or none to chide you, if you go, or stay,
Who may live merrier, ay, or more at heart's-ease?
Come, we'll to chess, or draughts; there are an hundred tricks
To drive out time till supper, never fear't, wench.
    MOTHER: I'll but make one step home, and return straight
      (Madam).
    LIVIA: Come, I'll not trust you; you use more excuses
To your kind friends than ever I knew any.
What business can you have, if you be sure
Y'have lock'd the doors? and that being all you have,
I know y'are careful on't: one afternoon
So much to spend here! say I should entreat you now
To lie a night or two, or a week with me,
Or leave your own house for a month together,
It were a kindness that long neighbourhood
And friendship might well hope to prevail in:
Would you deny such a request i'faith?
Speak truth, and freely.
    MOTHER: I were then uncivil, Madam.
    LIVIA: Go to then, set your men; we'll have whole nights
Of mirth together, ere we be much older, wench.
    MOTHER [*Aside*]: As good now tell her then, for she will
      know't;
I have always found her a most friendly lady.
    LIVIA: Why widow, where's your mind?
    MOTHER: Troth, ev'n at home, Madam.
To tell you truth, I left a gentlewoman
Ev'n sitting all alone, which is uncomfortable,
Especially to young bloods.
    LIVIA: Another excuse!
    MOTHER: No, as I hope for health, Madam, that's a truth;
Please you to send and see.
    LIVIA: What gentlewoman? pish.
    MOTHER: Wife to my son indeed, but not known (Madam)
To any but your self.
    LIVIA: Now I beshrew you,
Could you be so unkind to her and me,
To come and not bring her? 'Faith, 'tis not friendly.
    MOTHER: I fear'd to be too bold.
    LIVIA: Too bold? Oh what's become

Of the true hearty love was wont to be
'Mongst neighbours in old time?
    MOTHER: And she's a stranger (Madam).
    LIVIA: The more should be her welcome; when is courtesy
In better practice than when 'tis employ'd
In entertaining strangers? I could chide i'faith.
Leave her behind, poor gentlewoman, alone too!
Make some amends, and send for her betimes, go.
    MOTHER: Please you command one of your servants,
    Madam.
    LIVIA: Within there.

(*Enter* SERVANT.)

    SERVANT: Madam.
    LIVIA: Attend the gentlewoman.
    MOTHER: It must be carried wondrous privately
From my son's knowledge, he'll break out in storms else.
Hark you, sir. [*Whispers to* SERVANT, *who goes out.*]
    LIVIA: [*To* GUAR.]: Now comes in the heat of your part.
    GUARDIANO: True, I know it (Lady) and if I be out,
May the Duke banish me from all employments,
Wanton or serious.
    LIVIA: So, have you sent, widow?
    MOTHER: Yes (Madam) he's almost at home by this.
    LIVIA: And 'faith let me entreat you, that henceforward
All such unkind faults may be swept from friendship,
Which does but dim the lustre; and think thus much
It is a wrong to me, that have ability
To bid friends welcome, when you keep 'em from me,
You cannot set greater dishonour near me;
For bounty is the credit and the glory
Of those that have enough: I see y'are sorry,
And the good mends is made by't.
    MOTHER: Here she's, Madam.

(*Enter* BIANCA, *and* SERVANT.)
[*Exit* SERVANT.]

    BIANCA [*Aside*]: I wonder how she comes to send for me
        now?
    LIVIA: Gentlewoman, y'are most welcome, trust me y'are,
As courtesy can make one, or respect
Due to the presence of you.
    BIANCA: I give you thanks, Lady.
    LIVIA: I heard you were alone, and 't had appear'd

An ill condition in me, though I knew you not,
Nor ever saw you, (yet humanity
Thinks ev'ry case her own) to have kept your company
Here from you, and left you all solitary:
I rather ventur'd upon boldness then
As the least fault, and wish'd your presence here;
A thing most happily motion'd of that gentleman,
Whom I request you, for his care and pity,
To honour and reward with your acquaintance,
A gentleman that ladies' rights stands for,
That's his profession.

BIANCA: 'Tis a noble one,
And honours my acquaintance.

GUARDIANO: All my intentions
Are servants to such mistresses.

BIANCA: 'Tis your modesty,
It seems, that makes your deserts speak so low, sir.

LIVIA: Come widow: look you, Lady, here's our business;

[LIVIA *and* MOTHER *sit down to chess.*]

Are we not well employ'd, think you! an old quarrel
Between us, that will never be at an end.

BIANCA: No, and methinks there's men enough to part you
    (Lady).

LIVIA: Ho! but they set us on, let us come off
As well as we can, poor souls, men care no farther.
I pray sit down forsooth, if you have the patience
To look upon two weak and tedious gamesters.

GUARDIANO: 'Faith Madam, set these by till evening,
You'll have enough on't then; the gentlewoman,
Being a stranger, would take more delight
To see your rooms and pictures.

LIVIA: Marry, good sir,
And well rememb'red, I beseech you show 'em her;
That will beguile time well; pray heartily do, sir,
I'll do as much for you; here take these keys,
Show her the monument too, and that's a thing
Every one sees not; you can witness that, widow.

MOTHER: And that's worth sight indeed, Madam.

BIANCA: Kind lady,
I fear I came to be a trouble to you.

LIVIA: Oh nothing less forsooth.

BIANCA: And to this courteous gentleman,
That wears a kindness in his breast so noble
And bounteous to the welcome of a stranger.

GUARDIANO: If you but give acceptance to my service,
You do the greatest grace and honour to me
That courtesy can merit.
BIANCA: I were to blame else,
And out of fashion much. I pray you lead, sir.
LIVIA: After a game or two, w'are for you, gentlefolks.
GUARDIANO: We wish no better seconds in society
Than your discourses, Madam, and your partner's there.
MOTHER: I thank your praise, I listen'd to you, sir;
Though when you spoke, there came a paltry rook
Full in my way, and chokes up all my game.

(*Exit* GUARDIANO & BIANCA.)

LIVIA: Alas poor widow, I shall be too hard for thee.
MOTHER: Y'are cunning at the game, I'll be sworn (Madam).
LIVIA: It will be found so, ere I give you over:
She that can place her man well——
MOTHER: As you do (Madam).
LIVIA: As I shall (wench) can never lose her game;
Nay, nay, the black king's mine.
MOTHER: Cry you mercy (Madam).
LIVIA: And this my queen.
MOTHER: I see't now.
LIVIA: Here's a duke
Will strike a sure stroke for the game anon;
Your pawn cannot come back to relieve it self.
MOTHER: I know that (Madam).
LIVIA: You play well the whilst;
How she belies her skill! I hold two ducats,
I give you check and mate to your white king:
Simplicity it self, you saintish king there.
MOTHER: Well, ere now, Lady,
I have seen the fall of subtilty: jest on.
LIVIA: Ay, but simplicities receives two for one.
MOTHER: What remedy but patience!

(*Enter above* GUARDIANO *and* BIANCA.)

BIANCA: Trust me, sir,
Mine eye nev'r met with fairer ornaments.
GUARDIANO: Nay, livelier, I'm persuaded, neither Florence
Nor Venice can produce.
BIANCA: Sir, my opinion
Takes your part highly.
GUARDIANO: There's a better piece

Yet than all these (—*The* DUKE *above*.)
BIANCA: Not possible, sir!
GUARDIANO: Believe it,
You'll say so when you see't: turn but your eye now,
Y'are upon't presently. (*Exit*.)
BIANCA: Oh sir.
DUKE: He's gone, beauty!
Pish, look not after him: he's but a vapour,
That, when the sun appears, is seen no more.
BIANCA: Oh treachery to honour!
DUKE: Prethee tremble not;
I feel thy breast shake like a turtle panting
Under a loving hand that makes much on't;
Why art so fearful? as I'm a friend to brightness,
There's nothing but respect and honour near thee:
You know me, you have seen me; here's a heart
Can witness I have seen thee.
BIANCA: The more's my danger.
DUKE: The more's thy happiness. Pish, strive not, sweet;
This strength were excellent employ'd in love now,
But here 'tis spent amiss; strive not to seek
Thy liberty, and keep me still in prison.
I'faith you shall not out, till I'm releast now;
We'll be both freed together, or stay still by't;
So is captivity pleasant.
BIANCA: Oh my Lord.
DUKE: I am not here in vain; have but the leisure
To think on that, and thou'lt be soon resolv'd:
The lifting of thy voice is but like one
That does exalt his enemy, who proving high,
Lays all the plots to confound him that rais'd him.
Take warning, I beseech three; thou seem'st to me
A creature so compos'd of gentleness,
And delicate meekness; such as bless the faces
Of figures that are drawn for goddesses,
And makes art proud to look upon her work:
I should be sorry the least force should lay
An unkind touch upon thee.
BIANCA: Oh my extremity!
My Lord, what seek you?
DUKE: Love.
BIANCA: 'Tis gone already,
I have a husband.
DUKE: That's a single comfort,
Take a friend to him.

BIANCA: That's a double mischief,
Or else there's no religion.
DUKE: Do not tremble
At fears of thine own making.
BIANCA: Nor, great Lord,
Make me not bold with death and deeds of ruin,
Because they fear not you; me they must fright,
Then am I best in health. Should thunder speak,
And none regard it, it had lost the name,
And were as good be still. I'm not like those
That take their soundest sleeps in greatest tempests,
Then wake I most, the weather fearfullest,
And call for strength to virtue.
DUKE: Sure I think
Thou know'st the way to please me. I affect
A passionate pleading, 'bove an easy yielding,
But never pitied any, (they deserve none)
That will not pity me: I can command,
Think upon that; yet if thou truly knewest
The infinite pleasure my affection takes
In gentle, fair entreatings, when love's businesses
Are carried courteously 'twixt heart and heart,
You'd make more haste to please me.
BIANCA: Why should you seek, sir,
To take away that you can never give?
DUKE: But I give better in exchange: wealth, honour;
She that is fortunate in a duke's favour
Lights on a tree that bears all women's wishes:
If your own mother saw you pluck fruit there,
She would commend your wit, and praise the time
Of your nativity. Take hold of glory:
Do not I know y'have cast away your life
Upon necessities, means merely doubtful
To keep you in indifferent health and fashion,
(A thing I heard too lately, and soon pitied)
And can you be so much your beauty's enemy,
To kiss away a month or two in wedlock,
And weep whole years in wants for ever after?
Come play the wise wench, and provide for ever;
Let storms come when they list, they find thee shelter'd:
Should any doubt arise, let nothing trouble thee;
Put trust in our love for the managing
Of all to thy heart's peace. We'll walk together,
And show a thankful joy for both our fortunes. (*Exeunt above.*)
LIVIA: Did not I say my duke would fetch you over (widow)?

MOTHER: I think you spoke in earnest when you said it
  (Madam).

LIVIA: And my black king makes all the haste he can too.

MOTHER: Well (Madam) we may meet with him in time
  yet.

LIVIA: I have given thee blind mate twice.

MOTHER: You may see
                           (Madam)

My eyes begin to fail.

  LIVIA: I'll swear they do, wench.

(*Enter* GUARDIANO.)

GUARDIANO [*Aside*]: I can but smile as often as I think on't,
How prettily the poor fool was beguil'd:
How unexpectedly; it's a witty age,
Never were finer snares for women's honesties
Than are devis'd in these days; no spider's web
Made of a daintier thread than are now practis'd
To catch love's flesh-fly by the silver wing:
Yet to prepare her stomach by degrees
To Cupid's feast, because I saw 'twas queasy,
I show'd her naked pictures by the way;
A bit to stay the appetite. Well, advancement!
I venture hard to find thee; if thou com'st
With a greater title set upon thy crest,
I'll take that first cross patiently, and wait
Until some other comes greater than that.
I'll endure all.

  LIVIA: The game's ev'n at the best now;
You may see, widow, how all things draw to
An end.

MOTHER: Ev'n so do I, Madam.

  LIVIA: I pray
Take some of your neighbours along with you.

  MOTHER: They must be those are almost twice your years
  then,
If they be chose fit matches for my time, Madam.

LIVIA: Has not my duke bestirr'd himself?

MOTHER: Yes 'faith, Madam;
H'as done me all the mischief in this game.

LIVIA: H'as show'd himself in's kind.

MOTHER: In's kind, call you it?
I may swear that.

  LIVIA: Yes 'faith, and keep your oath.

GUARDIANO [*To* LIVIA]: Hark, list, there's somebody coming down; 'tis she.

(*Enter* BIANCA.)

  BIANCA [*Aside*]: Now bless me from a blasting; I saw that
      now,
Fearful for any woman's eye to look on;
Infectious mists and mildews hang at's eyes:
The weather of a doomsday dwells upon him.
Yet since mine honour's leprous, why should I
Preserve that fair that caus'd the leprosy?
Come poison all at once.—[*To* GUARDIANO] Thou in whose
      baseness
The bane of virtue broods, I'm bound in soul
Eternally to curse thy smooth-brow'd treachery,
That wore the fair veil of a friendly welcome,
And I a stranger; think upon't, 'tis worth it.
Murders pil'd up upon a guilty spirit
At his last breath will not lie heavier
Than this betraying act upon thy conscience:
Beware of off'ring the first-fruits to sin;
His weight is deadly who commits with strumpets,
After they have been abas'd, and made for use;
If they offend to th'death, as wise men know,
How much more they then that first make 'em so!
I give thee that to feed on; I'm made bold now,
I thank thy treachery; sin and I'm acquainted,
No couple greater; and I'm like that great one,
Who, making politic use of a base villain,
He likes the treason well, but hates the traitor;
So hate I thee, slave.
  GUARDIANO: Well, so the Duke love me,
I fare not much amiss then; two great feasts
Do seldom come together in one day;
We must not look for 'em.
  BIANCA: What, at it still, Mother?
  MOTHER: You see we sit by't; are you so soon return'd?
  LIVIA [*Aside*]: So lively, and so cheerful, a good sign that.
  MOTHER: You have not seen all since, sure?
BIANCA: That have I, Mother,
The monument and all: I'm so beholding
To this kind, honest, courteous gentleman,
You'd little think it (Mother) show'd me all,
Had me from place to place, so fashionably;
The kindness of some people, how't exceeds!
'Faith, I have seen that I little thought to see,
I'th'morning when I rose.

MOTHER: Nay, so I told you
Before you saw't, it would prove worth your sight.
I give you great thanks for my daughter, sir,
And all your kindness towards her.
GUARDIANO: O good widow!
Much good may't do her; [*Aside*] forty weeks hence, i'faith.

(*Enter* SERVANT.)

LIVIA: Now sir.
SERVANT: May't please you, Madam, to walk in?
Supper's upon the table.
LIVIA: Yes, we come; [*Exit* SERVANT.]
Will't please you gentlewoman?
BIANCA: Thanks virtuous lady,
(Y'are a damn'd bawd) I'll follow you forsooth,
Pray take my mother in, [*Aside*] an old ass go with you;
This gentleman and I vow not to part.
LIVIA: Then get you both before.
BIANCA: There lies his art.

(*Exeunt* [BIANCA & GUARDIANO].)

LIVIA: Widow, I'll follow you. [*Exit* MOTHER.] Is't so,
        damn'd bawd?
Are you so bitter? 'Tis but want of use;
Her tender modesty is sea-sick a little,
Being not accustom'd to the breaking billow
Of woman's wavering faith, blown with temptations.
'Tis but a qualm of honour, 'twill away,
A little bitter for the time, but lasts not.
Sin tastes at the first draught like wormwood water,
But drunk again, 'tis nectar ever after. (*Exit.*)

ACT. 3. Scene. 1

(*Enter* MOTHER.)

MOTHER: I would my son would either keep at home,
Or I were in my grave;
She was but one day abroad, but ever since,
She's grown so cutted, there's no speaking to her:
Whether the sight of great cheer at my Lady's,

And such mean fare at home, work discontent in her,
I know not; but I'm sure she's strangely alter'd.
I'll nev'r keep daughter-in-law i'th'house with me
Again, if I had an hundred: when read I of any
That agreed long together, but she and her mother
Fell out in the first quarter! nay, sometime
A grudging of a scolding the first week, by'r Lady;
So takes the new disease, methinks, in my house;
I'm weary of my part, there's nothing likes her;
I know not how to please her, here a-late;
And here she comes.

(*Enter* BIANCA.)

BIANCA: This is the strangest house
For all defects, as ever gentlewoman
Made shift withal, to pass away her love in:
Why is there not a cushion-cloth of drawn work,
Or some fair cut-work pinn'd up in my bedchamber?
A silver and gilt casting-bottle hung by't?
Nay, since I am content to be so kind to you,
To spare you for a silver basin and ew'r,
Which one of my fashion looks for of duty;
She's never offered under, where she sleeps.
  MOTHER: She talks of things here my whole state's not
     worth.
  BIANCA: Never a green silk quilt is there i'th'house, Mother,
To cast upon my bed?
  MOTHER: No by troth is there,
Nor orange tawny neither.
  BIANCA: Here's a house
For a young gentlewoman to be got with child in.
  MOTHER: Yes, simple though you make it, there has been
     three
Got in a year in't, since you move me to't;
And all as sweet-fac'd children, and as lovely,
As you'll be mother of; I will not spare you:
What, cannot children be begot, think you,
Without gilt casting-bottles? Yes, and as sweet ones.
The miller's daughter brings forth as white boys,
And she that bathes her self with milk and bean-flour.
'Tis an old saying, one may keep good cheer
In a mean house; so may true love affect
After the rate of princes in a cottage.
  BIANCA: Troth you speak wondrous well for your old
     house here;

'Twill shortly fall down at your feet to thank you,
Or stoop when you go to bed, like a good child
To ask you blessing. Must I live in want,
Because my fortune matcht me with your son?
Wives do not give away themselves to husbands,
To the end to be quite cast away; they look
To be the better us'd and tender'd rather,
Highlier respected, and maintain'd the richer;
They're well rewarded else for the free gift
Of their whole life to a husband. I ask less now
Than what I had at home when I was a maid,
And at my father's house, kept short of that
Which a wife knows she must have, nay, and will;
Will, Mother, if she be not a fool born;
And report went of me, that I could wrangle
For what I wanted when I was two hours old,
And by that copy, this land still I hold.
You hear me, Mother. (*Exit.*)
MOTHER: Ay, too plain methinks;
And were I somewhat deafer when you spake,
'Twere nev'r a whit the worse for my quietness:
'Tis the most sudden'st, strangest alteration,
And the most subtilest that ev'r wit at threescore
Was puzzled to find out: I know no cause for't; but
She's no more like the gentlewoman at first,
Than I am like her that nev'r lay with man yet,
And she's a very young thing where'er she be;
When she first lighted here, I told her then
How mean she should find all things; she was pleas'd for-
          sooth,
None better: I laid open all defects to her,
She was contented still; but the devil's in her,
Nothing contents her now. Tonight my son
Promis'd to be at home, would he were come once,
For I'm weary of my charge, and life too:
She'd be serv'd all in silver by her good will,
By night and day; she hates the name of pewterer,
More than sick men the noise, or diseas'd bones
That quake at fall o'th'hammer, seeming to have
A fellow-feeling with't at every blow:
What course shall I think on? she frets me so. (*Exit.*)

(*Enter* LEANTIO.)

LEANTIO: How near am I now to a happiness,
The earth exceeds not! not another like it;

The treasures of the deep are not so precious.
As are the conceal'd comforts of a man,
Lockt up in woman's love. I scent the air
Of blessings when I come but near the house;
What a delicious breath marriage sends forth!
The violet-bed's not sweeter. Honest wedlock
Is like a banqueting-house built in a garden,
On which the spring's chaste flowers take delight
To cast their modest odours; when base lust,
With all her powders, paintings, and best pride,
Is but a fair house built by a ditch-side.
When I behold a glorious dangerous strumpet,
Sparkling in beauty and destruction too,
Both at a twinkling, I do liken straight
Her beautifi'd body to a goodly temple
That's built on vaults where carcasses lie rotting,
And so by little and little I shrink back again,
And quench desire with a cool meditation,
And I'm as well methinks. Now for a welcome
Able to draw men's envies upon man:
A kiss now that will hang upon my lip,
As sweet as morning dew upon a rose,
And full as long; after a five days' fast
She'll be so greedy now, and cling about me,
I take care how I shall be rid of her;
And here't begins.

[*Enter* BIANCA *and* MOTHER.]

    BIANCA: Oh sir, y'are welcome home.
    MOTHER: Oh is he come? I am glad on't.
    LEANTIO: Is that all?
Why, this is as dreadful now as sudden death
To some rich man, that flatters all his sins
With promise of repentance when he's old,
And dies in the midway before he comes to't.
Sure y'are not well, Bianca. How dost, prethee?
    BIANCA: I have been better than I am at this time.
    LEANTIO: Alas, I thought so.
    BIANCA: Nay, I have been worse too,
Than now you see me, sir.
    LEANTIO: I'm glad thou mend'st yet,
I feel my heart mend too: how came it to thee?
Has any thing dislik'd thee in my absence?
    BIANCA: No certain, I have had the best content
That Florence can afford.

LEANTIO: Thou makest the best on't.
Speak Mother, what's the cause? you must needs know.
    MOTHER: Troth I know none, son, let her speak her self;
Unless it be the same gave Lucifer
A tumbling cast; that's pride.
    BIANCA: Methinks this house
Stands nothing to my mind; I'd have
Some pleasant lodging i'th'high street, sir,
Or if 'twere near the court, sir, that were much better;
'Tis a sweet recreation for a gentlewoman,
To stand in a bay-window, and see gallants.
    LEANTIO: Now I have another temper, a mere stranger
To that of yours, it seems; I should delight
To see none but your self.
    BIANCA: I praise not that:
Too fond is as unseemly as too churlish;
I would not have a husband of that proneness,
To kiss me before company, for a world:
Beside, 'tis tedious to see one thing still (sir),
Be it the best that ever heart affected;
Nay, were't your self, whose love had power, you know,
To bring me from my friends, I would not stand thus,
And gaze upon you always: troth I could not, sir;
As good be blind, and have no use of sight,
As look on one thing still: what's the eye's treasure,
But change of objects? You are learned, sir,
And know I speak not ill; 'tis full as virtuous
For woman's eye to look on several men,
As for her heart (sir) to be fix'd on one.
    LEANTIO: Now thou com'st home to me, a kiss for that
                    word.
    BIANCA: No matter for a kiss, sir, let it pass,
'Tis but a toy, we'll not so much as mind it,
Let's talk of other business, and forget it.
What news now of the pirates, any stirring?
Prethee discourse a little.
    MOTHER [*Aside*]:   I am glad he's here yet
To see her tricks himself; I had lied monstrously,
If I had told 'em first.
    LEANTIO: Speak, what's the humour (sweet)
You make your lip so strange? this was not wont.
    BIANCA: Is there no kindness betwix man and wife,
Unless they make a pigeon-house of friendship,
And be still billing? 'tis the idlest fondness
That ever was invented, and 'tis pity
It's grown a fashion for poor gentlewomen;

There's many a disease kiss'd in a year by't,
And a French curtsy made to't. Alas, sir,
Think of the world, how we shall live, grow serious;
We have been married a whole fortnight now.
    LEANTIO: How? a whole fortnight! why, is that so long?
    BIANCA: 'Tis time to leave off dalliance; 'tis a doctrine
Of your own teaching, if you be rememb'red,
And I was bound to obey it.
    MOTHER [*Aside*]:   Here's one fits him;
This was well catch'd i'faith, son, like a fellow
That rids another country of a plague,
And brings it home with him to his own house. (*Knock within.*)
—Who knocks?
    LEANTIO: Who's there now? withdraw you Bianca,
Thous art a gem no stranger's eye must see,
Howev'r thou pleas'd now to look dull on me.

    (*Exit* [BIANCA, *with* MOTHER].)

    (*Enter* MESSENGER.)

Y'are welcome, sir; to whom your business, pray?
    MESSENGER: To one I see not here now.
    LEANTIO: Who should that be, sir?
    MESSENGER: A young gentlewoman, I was sent to.
    LEANTIO: A young gentlewoman?
    MESSENGER: Ay sir, about sixteen; why look you wildly, sir?
    LEANTIO: At your strange error: y'have mistook the house, sir.
There's none such here, I assure you.
    MESSENGER: I assure you too,
The man that sent me cannot be mistook.
    LEANTIO: Why, who is't sent you, sir?
    MESSENGER: The Duke.
    LEANTIO: The Duke?
    MESSENGER: Yes, he entreats her company at a banquet
At Lady Livia's house.
    LEANTIO: Troth, shall I tell you, sir,
It is the most erroneous business
That e'er your honest pains was abus'd with;
I pray forgive me, if I smile a little
(I cannot choose i'faith, sir) at an error

So comical as this (I mean no harm though).
His grace has been most wondrous ill inform'd,
Pray so return it (sir). What should her name be?
   MESSENGER: That I shall tell you straight too: Bianca
      Capella.
   LEANTIO: How sir, Bianca? What do you call th'other?
   MESSENGER: Capella; sir, it seems you know no such then?
   LEANTIO: Who should this be? I never heard o'th'name.
   MESSENGER: Then 'tis a sure mistake.
   LEANTIO: What if you enquir'd
In the next street, sir? I saw gallants there
In the new houses that are built of late.
Ten to one, there you find her.
   MESSENGER: Nay, no matter,
I will return the mistake, and seek no further.
   LEANTIO: Use your own will and pleasure, sir, y'are wel-
      come.

(Exit MESSENGER.*)*

What shall I think of first? Come forth Bianca,
Thou art betray'd, I fear me.

(Enter BIANCA *[and* MOTHER].*)*

   BIANCA: Betray'd, how sir?
   LEANTIO: The Duke knows thee.
   BIANCA: Knows me! how know you
                            that, sir?
   LEANTIO: H'as got thy name.
   BIANCA *[Aside]*:   Ay, and my good name too,
That's worse o'th'twain.
   LEANTIO: How comes this work about?
   BIANCA: How should the Duke know me? can you guess,
      Mother?
   MOTHER: Not I with all my wits, sure we kept house close.
   LEANTIO: Kept close! not all the locks in Italy
Can keep you women so; you have been gadding,
And ventur'd out at twilight, to th'court-green yonder,
And met the gallant bowlers coming home;
Without your masks too, both of you, I'll be hang'd else;
Thou hast been seen, Bianca, by some stranger;
Never excuse it.
   BIANCA: I'll not seek the way, sir;
Do you think y'have married me to mew me up
Not to be seen? what would you make of me?

LEANTIO: A good wife, nothing else.

BIANCA: Why, so are some
That are seen ev'ry day, else the devil take 'em.

LEANTIO: No more then; I believe all virtuous in thee,
Without an argument; 'twas but thy hard chance
To be seen somewhere, there lies all the mischief;
But I have devis'd a riddance.

MOTHER: Now I can tell you, son,
The time and place.

LEANTIO: When, where?

MOTHER: What wits have I!
When you last took your leave, if you remember,
You left us both at window.

LEANTIO: Right, I know that.

MOTHER: And not the third part of an hour after,
The Duke pass'd by in a great solemnity, .
To St. Mark's temple, and to my apprehension
He look'd up twice to th'window.

LEANTIO: Oh, there quick'ned
The mischief of this hour!

BIANCA [*Aside*]:   If you call't mischief,
It is a thing I fear I am conceiv'd with.

LEANTIO: Look'd he up twice, and could you take no warning?

MOTHER: Why, once may do as much harm, son, as a
   thousand;
Do not you know one spark has fir'd an house,
As well as a whole furnace?

LEANTIO: My heart flames for't:
Yet let's be wise, and keep all smother'd closely;
I have bethought a means; is the door fast?

MOTHER: I lockt it my self after him.

LEANTIO: You know, Mother,
At the end of the dark parlour there's a place
So artificially contriv'd for a conveyance,
No search could ever find it: when my father
Kept in for man-slaughter, it was his sanctuary;
There will I lock my life's best treasure up.
Bianca!

BIANCA: Would you keep me closer yet?
Have you the conscience? y'are best ev'n choke me up, sir!
You make me fearful of your health and wits,
You cleave to such wild courses; what's the matter?

LEANTIO: Why, are you so insensible of your danger
To ask that now? the Duke himself has sent for you
To Lady Livia's, to a banquet forsooth.

BIANCA: Now I beshrew you heartily, has he so!
And you the man would never yet vouchsafe
To tell me on't till now: you show your loyalty
And honesty at once; and so farewell, sir.
  LEANTIO: Bianca, whether now?
  BIANCA: Why, to the Duke, sir.
You say he sent for me.
  LEANTIO: But thou dost not mean
To go, I hope.
  BIANCA: No? I shall prove unmannerly,
Rude, and uncivil, mad, and imitate you.
Come Mother, come, follow his humour no longer,
We shall be all executed for treason shortly.
  MOTHER: Not I, i'faith; I'll first obey the Duke,
And taste of a good banquet, I'm of thy mind.
I'll step but up, and fetch two handkerchiefs
To pocket up some sweet-meats, and o'ertake thee. (*Exit.*)
  BIANCA [*Aside*]: Why, here's an old wench would trot into
          a bawd now,
For some dry sucket, or a colt in march-pane. (*Exit.*)
  LEANTIO: Oh thou the ripe time of man's misery, wedlock;
When all his thoughts, like overladen trees,
Crack with the fruits they bear, in cares, in jealousies.
Oh that's a fruit that ripens hastily,
After 'tis knit to marriage; it begins,
As soon as the sun shines upon the bride,
A little to show colour. Blessed powers!
Whence comes this alteration? the distractions,
The fears and doubts it brings are numberless,
And yet the cause I know not. What a peace
Has he that never marries! if he knew
The benefit he enjoy'd, or had the fortune
To come and speak with me, he should know then
The infinite wealth he had, and discern rightly
The greatness of his treasure by my loss:
Nay, what a quietness has he 'bove mine,
That wears his youth out in a strumpet's arms,
And never spends more care upon a woman
Than at the time of lust; but walks away,
And if he find her dead at his return,
His pity is soon done, he breaks a sigh
In many parts, and gives her but a piece on't!
But all the fears, shames, jealousies, costs and troubles,
And still renew'd cares of a marriage-bed,
Live in the issue, when the wife is dead.

(*Enter* MESSENGER.)

MESSENGER: A good perfection to your thoughts.
LEANTIO: The news,
sir?

MESSENGER: Though you were pleas'd of late to pin an er-
ror on me,
You must not shift another in your stead too:
The Duke has sent me for you.
LEANTIO: How, for me, sir?
[*Aside*] I see then 'tis my theft; w'are both betray'd:
Well, I'm not the first has stol'n away a maid,
My countrymen have us'd it.—I'll along with you, sir.

(*Exeunt.*)

Scene. 2

(*A banquet prepared: enter* GUARDIANO *and* WARD.)

GUARDIANO: Take you especial note of such a gentle-
woman,
She's here on purpose, I have invited her,
Her father, and her uncle, to this banquet;
Mark her behaviour well, it does concern you;
And what her good parts are, as far as time
And place can modestly require a knowledge of,
Shall be laid open to your understanding.
You know I'm both your guardian and your uncle,
My care of you is double, ward and nephew,
And I'll express it here.
WARD: 'Faith, I should know her
Now by her mark among a thousand women:
A lettle pretty deft and tidy thing, you say?
GUARDIANO: Right.
WARD: With a lusty sprouting sprig in her hair.
GUARDIANO: Thou goest the right way still; take one mark
more,
Thou shalt nev'r find her hand out of her uncle's,
Or else his out of hers, if she be near him:
The love of kinred never yet stuck closer
Than theirs to one another; he that weds her
Marries her uncle's heart too.

WARD: Say you so, sir?
Then I'll be ask'd i'th'church to both of them. (*Cornets*
    [*within*].)
GUARDIANO: Fall back, here comes the Duke.
WARD: He brings a
                                          gentlewoman,
I should fall forward rather.

(*Enter* DUKE, BIANCA, FABRITIO, HIPPOLITO, LIVIA, MOTHER,
ISABELLA, *and* ATTENDANTS.)

DUKE: Come Bianca,
Of purpose sent into the world to show
Perfection once in woman; I'll believe
Hence forward they have ev'ry one a soul too
'Gainst all the uncourteous opinions
That man's uncivil rudeness ever held of 'em.
Glory of Florence, light into mine arms!

(*Enter* LEANTIO.)

BIANCA: Yon comes a grudging man will chide you, sir;
The storm is now in's heart, and would get nearer,
And fall here if it durst, it pours down yonder.
DUKE: If that be he, the weather shall soon clear.
 List, and I'll tell thee how. [*Whispers* BIANCA.]
LEANTIO [*Aside*]:   A-kissing too?
I see 'tis plain lust now; adultery bold'ned;
What will it prove anon, when 'tis stufft full
Of wine and sweetmeats, being so impudent fasting?
DUKE: We have heard of your good parts, sir, which we
    honour
With our embrace and love; is not the captainship
Of Rouans citadel, since the late deceas'd,
Suppli'd by any yet?
GENTLEMAN: By none, my Lord.
DUKE: Take it, the place is yours then, and as faithfulness
And desert grows, our favour shall grow with't: [LEANTIO
    kneels.]
Rise now the captain of our fort at Rouans.
LEANTIO: The service of whole life give your Grace thanks.
DUKE: Come sit, Bianca.
LEANTIO [*Aside*]:   This is some good yet,
And more than ev'r I look'd for, a fine bit
To stay a cuckold's stomach: all preferment

That springs from sin and lust, it shoots up quickly,
As gardeners' crops do in the rotten'st grounds;
So is all means rais'd from base prostitution,
Ev'n like a sallet growing upon a dunghill:
I'm like a thing that never was yet heard of,
Half merry, and half mad, much like a fellow
That eats his meat with a good appetite,
And wears a plague-sore that would fright a country;
Or rather like the barren hard'ned ass,
That feeds on thistles till he bleeds again;
And such is the condition of my misery.

    LIVIA: Is that your son, widow?
    MOTHER: Yes, did your Ladyship
Never know that till now?
    LIVIA: No, trust me, did I,
[Aside] Nor ever truly felt the power of love,
And pity to a man, till now I knew him;
I have enough to buy me my desires,
And yet to spare; that's one good comfort.—Hark you,
Pray let me speak with you, sir, before you go.
    LEANTIO: With me, Lady? you shall, I am at your service:
[Aside] What will she say now, trow, more goodness yet?
    WARD [Aside]: I see her now, I'm sure; the ape's so little,
I shall scarce feel her; I have seen almost
As tall as she sold in the fair for ten pence.
See how she simpers it, as if marmalade would not
Melt in her mouth; she might have the kindness i'faith
To send me a gilded bull from her own trencher,
A ram, a goat, or somewhat to be nibbling.
These women, when they come to sweet things once,
They forget all their friends, they grow so greedy;
Nay, oftentimes their husbands.
    DUKE: Here's a health now, gallants,
To the best beauty at this day in Florence.
    BIANCA: Whoe'er she be, she shall not go unpledg'd, sir.
    DUKE: Nay, you're excus'd for this.
    BIANCA: Who, I, my Lord?
    DUKE: Yes, by the law of Bacchus; plead your benefit,
You are not bound to pledge your own health, Lady.
    BIANCA: That's a good way, my Lord, to keep me dry.
    DUKE: Nay, then I will not offend Venus so much,
Let Bacchus seek his mends in another court,
Here's to thy self, Bianca.
    BIANCA: Nothing comes
More welcome to that name than your Grace.
    LEANTIO [Aside]:   So, so;

Here stands the poor thief now that stole the treasure,
And he's not thought on; ours is near kin now
To a twin-misery born into the world.
First the hard-conscienc'd worldling, he hoards wealth up,
Then comes the next, and he feasts all upon't:
One's dam'd for getting, th'other for spending on't:
Oh equal justice, thou hast met my sin
With a full weight, I'm rightly now opprest,
All her friends' heavy hearts lie in my breast.

DUKE: Methinks there is no spirit amongst us, gallants,
But what divinely sparkles from the eyes
Of bright Bianca; we sat all in darkness,
But for that splendour. Who was't told us lately
Of a match-making right, a marriage-tender?

GUARDIANO: 'Twas I, my Lord.

DUKE: 'Twas you indeed: where is she?

GUARDIANO: This is the gentlewoman.

FABRITIO: My Lord, my daughter.

DUKE [*Aside*]: Why, here's some stirring yet.

FABRITIO: She's a dear child
                                     to me.

DUKE: That must needs be; you say she is your daughter.

FABRITIO: Nay, my good Lord, dear to my purse I mean,
Beside my person, I nev'r reckon'd that.
She has the full qualities of a gentlewoman;
I have brought her up to music, dancing, what not,
That may commend her sex, and stir her husband.

DUKE: And which is he now?

GUARDIANO: This young heir, my Lord.

DUKE: What is he brought up to?

HIPPOLITO [*Aside*]:   To cat and trap.

GUARDIANO: My Lord, he's a great ward, wealthy, but simple, His parts consist in acres.

DUKE: Oh, wise-acres.

GUARDIANO: Y'have spoke him in a word, sir.

BIANCA: 'Las, poor
                                gentlewoman,
She's ill bested, unless sh'as dealt the wiselier,
And laid in more provision for her youth:
Fools will not keep in summer.

LEANTIO [*Aside*]:   No, nor such wives
From whores in winter.

DUKE: Yeah, the voice too, sir?

FABRITIO: Ay, and a sweet breast too, my Lord, I hope,
Or I have cast away my money wisely;
She took her pricksong earlier, my Lord,

Than any of her kinred ever did:
A rare child, though I say't, but I'd not have
The baggage hear so much, 'twould make her swell straight:
And maids of all things must not be puft up.

DUKE: Let's turn us to a better banquet then,
For music bids the soul of a man to a feast,
And that's indeed a noble entertainment,
Worthy Bianca's self; you shall perceive, beauty,
Our Florentine damsels are not brought up idlely.

BIANCA: They are wiser of themselves, it seems my Lord,
And can take gifts, when goodness offers 'em (*Music.*)

LEANTIO [*Aside*]: True, and damnation has taught you
        that wisdom,
You can take gifts too. Oh that music mocks me!

LIVIA [*Aside*]: I am as dumb to any language now
But love's, as one that never learn'd to speak:
I am not yet so old, but he may think of me;
My own fault, I have been idle a long time;
But I'll begin the week, and paint tomorrow,
So follow my true labour day by day:
I never thriv'd so well, as when I us'd it.

SONG [*sung by* ISABELLA]

> *What harder chance can fall to woman,*
> *Who was born to cleave to some man,*
> *Than to bestow her time, youth, beauty,*
> *Life's observance, honour, duty,*
> *On a thing for no use good*
> *But to make physic work, or blood*
> *Force fresh in an old lady's cheek?*
> *She that would be*
> *Mother of fools, let her compound with me.*

WARD [*Aside*]: Here's a tune indeed; pish, I had rather hear
        one ballad
sung i'th'nose now of the lamentable drowning of fat sheep
        and oxen,
than all these simpering tunes play'd upon cat's-guts, and
        sung by little kitlings.

FABRITIO: How like you her breast now, my Lord?

BIANCA [*To* DUKE]:   Her breast?
He talks as if his daughter had given suck
Before she were married, as her betters have;
The next he praises sure will be her nipples.

DUKE [*To* BIANCA]: Methinks now, such a voice to such a
    husband
Is like a jewel of unvalued worth
Hung at a fool's ear.
    FABRITIO: May it please your Grace
To give her leave to show another quality?
    DUKE: Marry, as many good ones as you will, sir,
The more the better welcome.
    LEANTIO [*Aside*]:   But the less
The better practis'd: that soul's black indeed
That cannot commend virtue; but who keeps it?
The extortioner will say to a sick beggar,
'Heaven comfort thee,' though he give none himself:
This good is common.
    FABRITIO: Will it please you now, sir,
To entreat your ward to take her by the hand,
And lead her in a dance before the Duke?
    GUARDIANO: That will I, sir, 'tis needful; hark you, Nephew.
    FABRITIO: Nay, you shall see, young heir, what y'have for
          your money,
Without fraud or imposture.
    WARD: Dance with her!
Not I, sweet Guardiner, do not urge my heart to't,
'Tis clean against my blood; dance with a stranger!
Let who will do't, I'll not begin first with her.
    HIPPOLITO [*Aside*]: No, fear't not, fool, sh'as took a bet-
        ter order.
    GUARDIANO: Why, who shall take her then?
    WARD: Some other
                             gentleman;
Look, there's her uncle, a fine-timber'd reveller,
Perhaps he knows the manner of her dancing too,
I'll have him do't before me, I have sworn, Guardiner,
Then may I learn the better.
    GUARDIANO: Thou'lt be an ass still.
    WARD: I? All that uncle shall not fool me out.
Pish, I stick closer to my self than so.
    GUARDIANO: I must entreat you, sir, to take your niece
And dance with her; my ward's a little wilful,
He would have you show him the way.
    HIPPOLITO: Me, sir?
He shall command it at all hours, pray tell him so.
    GUARDIANO: I thank you for him, he has not wit himself,
        sir.
    HIPPOLITO: Come, my life's peace. [*Aside*] I have a strange
        office on't here:

'Tis some man's luck to keep the joys he likes
Conceal'd for his own bosom; but my fortune
To set 'em out now, for another's liking,
Like the mad misery of necessitous man,
That parts from his good horse with many praises,
And goes on foot himself; need must be obey'd
In ev'ry action, it mars man and maid.

(*Music. A dance, making honours to the* D[UKE] *and curtsy to themselves, both before and after.*)

DUKE: Signor Fabritio, y'are a happy father,
Your cares and pains are fortunate you see,
Your cost bears noble fruits. Hippolito, thanks.
FABRITIO: Here's some amends for all my charges yet;
She wins both prick and praise, where e'er she comes.
DUKE: How lik'st, Bianca?
BIANCA: All things well, my Lord:
But this poor gentlewoman's fortune, that's the worst.
DUKE: There is no doubt, Bianca, she'll find leisure
To make that good enough; he's rich and simple.
BIANCA: She has the better hope o'th'upper hand indeed,
Which women strive for most.
GUARDIANO: Do't when I bid you, sir.
WARD: I'll venture but a hornpipe with her, Guardiner,
Or some such married man's dance.
GUARDIANO: Well, venture something, sir.
WARD: I have rhyme for what I do.
GUARDIANO: But little reason, I think.
WARD: Plain men dance the measures, the cinquepace the
          gay:
Cuckolds dance the hornpipe; and farmers dance the hay:
Your soldiers dance the round, and maidens that grow big:
Your drunkards the canaries; your whore and bawd the jig.
Here's your eight kind of dancers, he that finds
The ninth, let him pay the minstrels.
DUKE: Oh here he appears once in his own person;
I thought he would have married her by attorney,
And lain with her so too.
BIANCA: Nay, my kind Lord,
There's very seldom any found so foolish
To give away his part there.
LEANTIO [*Aside*]:   Bitter scoff!
Yet I must do't; with what a cruel pride
The glory of her sin strikes by my afflictions!

(*Music.* WARD *and* ISABELLA *dance, he ridiculously imitates* HIPPOLITO.)

DUKE: This thing will make shift (sirs) to make a husband,
For aught I see in him; how think'st, Bianca?
BIANCA: 'Faith, an ill-favoured shift, my Lord, methinks;
If he would take some voyage when he's married,
Dangerous, or long enough, and scarce be seen
Once in nine year together, a wife then
Might make indifferent shift to be content with him.
DUKE: A kiss; that wit deserves to be made much on.
Come, our caroche.
GUARDIANO: Stands ready for your Grace.
DUKE: My thanks to all your loves. Come, fair Bianca,
We have took special care of you, and provided
Your lodging near us now.
BIANCA: Your love is great, my Lord.
DUKE: Once more our thanks to all.
OMNES: All blest honours guard
                                                you.

(*Exe. all but* LEANTIO *and* LIVIA; *cornets flourish.*)

LEANTIO [*Aside*]: Oh hast thou left me then, Bianca, utterly!
Bianca! now I miss thee; oh return,
And save the faith of woman! I nev'r felt
The loss of thee till now; 'tis an affliction
Of greater weight than youth was made to bear;
As if a punishment of after-life
Were fall'n upon man here; so new it is
To flesh and blood, so strange, so insupportable,
A torment, ev'n mistook, as if a body
Whose death were drowning, must needs therefore suffer it
In scalding oil.
LIVIA: Sweet sir!
LEANTIO [*Aside*]:   As long as mine eye saw thee,
I half enjoy'd thee.
LIVIA: Sir?
LEANTIO [*Aside*]:   Canst thou forget
The dear pains my love took, how it has watcht
Whole nights together, in all weathers for thee,
Yet stood in heart more merry than the tempests
That sung about mine ears (like dangerous flatterers
That can set all their mischief to sweet tunes),
And then receiv'd thee from thy father's window,

Into these arms at midnight, when we embrac'd
As if we had been statues only made for't,
To show art's life, so silent were our comforts,
And kiss'd as if our lips had grown together?
    LIVIA [*Aside*]: This makes me madder to enjoy him now.
    LEANTIO [*Aside*]: Canst thou forget all this? and better joys
That we met after this, which then new kisses
Took pride to praise?
    LIVIA [*Aside*]:   I shall grow madder yet.—Sir!
    LEANTIO [*Aside*]: This cannot be but of some close bawd's
        working.
—Cry mercy, Lady. What would you say to me?
My sorrow makes me so unmannerly,
So comfort bless me, I had quite forgot you.
    LIVIA: Nothing but ev'n in pity to that passion
Would give your grief good counsel.
    LEANTIO: Marry, and welcome, Lady,
It never could come better.
    LIVIA: Then first, sir,
To make away all your good thoughts at once of her,
Know most assuredly, she is a strumpet.
    LEANTIO: Ha: most assuredly! Speak not a thing
So vilde so certainly, leave it more doubtful.
    LIVIA: Then I must leave all truth, and spare my knowledge,
A sin which I too lately found and wept for.
    LEANTIO: Found you it?
    LIVIA: Ay, with wet eyes.
    LEANTIO: Oh perjurious
                                  friendship!
    LIVIA: You miss'd your fortunes when you met with her, sir.
Young gentlemen, that only love for beauty,
They love not wisely; such a marriage rather
Proves the destruction of affection;
It brings on want, and want's the key of whoredom.
I think y'had small means with her.
    LEANTIO: Oh not any, Lady.
    LIVIA: Alas poor gentleman, what meant'st thou, sir,
Quite to undo thy self with thine own kind heart?
Thou art too good and pitiful to woman:
Marry, sir, thank thy stars for this blest fortune
That rids the summer of thy youth so well
From many beggars that had lain a-sunning
In thy beams only else, till thou hadst wasted
The whole days of thy life in heat and labour.
What would you say now to a creature found
As pitiful to you, and as it were

Ev'n sent on purpose from the whole sex general,
To requite all that kindness you have shown to't?
   LEANTIO: What's that, Madam?
   LIVIA: Nay, a gentlewoman, and
                                               one able
To reward good things, ay, and bears a conscience to't;
Couldst thou love such a one, that (blow all fortunes)
Would never see thee want?
Nay more, maintain thee to thine enemy's envy,
And shalt not spend a care for't, stir a thought,
Nor break a sleep, unless love's music wak'd thee;
No storm of fortune should. Look upon me,
And know that woman.
   LEANTIO: Oh my life's wealth, Bianca!
   LIVIA [*Aside*]: Still with her name? will nothing wear it out?
—That deep sigh went but for a strumpet, sir.
   LEANTIO: It can go for no other that loves me.
   LIVIA [*Aside*]: He's vext in mind; I came too soon to him;
Where's my discretion now, my skill, my judgment?
I'm cunning in all arts but my own love:
'Tis as unseasonable to tempt him now
So soon, as for a widow to be courted
Following her husband's corse, or to make bargain
By the grave-side, and take a young man there:
Her strange departure stands like a hearse yet
Before his eyes; which time will take down shortly. (*Exit.*)
   LEANTIO: Is she my wife till death? yet no more mine?
That's a hard measure; then what's marriage good for?
Me thinks by right I should not now be living,
And then 'twere all well: what a happiness
Had I been made of, had I never seen her!
For nothing makes man's loss grievous to him,
But knowledge of the worth of what he loses;
For what he never had he never misses;
She's gone for ever, utterly; there is
As much redemption of a soul from hell,
As a fair woman's body from his palace.
Why should my love last longer than her truth?
What is there good in woman to be lov'd,
When only that which makes her so has left her?
I cannot love her now, but I must like
Her sin, and my own shame too, and be guilty
Of law's breach with her, and mine own abusing;
All which were monstrous: then my safest course,
For health of mind and body, is to turn
My heart, and hate her, most extremely hate her;

I have no other way: those virtuous powers,
Which were chaste witnesses of both our troths,
Can witness she breaks first, and I'm rewarded
With captainship o'th'fort; a place of credit
I must confess, but poor; my factorship
Shall not exchange means with't; he that di'd last in't,
He was no drunkard, yet he di'd a beggar
For all his thrift; besides, the place not fits me;
It suits my resolution, not my breeding.

    (*Enter* LIVIA.)

    LIVIA [*Aside*]: I have tri'd all ways I can, and have not
        power
To keep from sight of him.—How are you now, sir?
    LEANTIO: I feel a better ease, Madam.
    LIVIA: Thanks to blessedness!
You will do well, I warrant you, fear it not, sir;
Join but your own good will to't; he's not wise
That loves his pain or sickness, or grows fond
Of a disease, whose property is to vex him,
And spitefully drink his blood up. Out upon't, sir,
Youth knows no greater loss; I pray let's walk, sir,
You never saw the beauty of my house yet,
Nor how abundantly fortune has blest me
In worldly treasure; trust me, I have enough, sir,
To make my friend a rich man in my life,
A great man at my death; your self will say so:
If you want any thing, and spare to speak,
Troth I'll condemn you for a wilful man, sir.
    LEANTIO: Why, sure
This can be but the flattery of some dream.
    LIVIA: Now by this kiss, my love, my soul and riches,
'Tis all true substance. [*Kisses him.*]
Come, you shall see my wealth, take what you list,
The gallanter you go, the more you please me:
I will allow you too your page and footman,
Your racehorses, or any various pleasure
Exercis'd youth delights in; but to me
Only, sir, wear your heart of constant stuff:
Do but you love enough, I'll give enough.
    LEANTIO: Troth then, I'll love enough, and take enough.
Then we are both pleas'd enough.

    (*Exeunt.*)

Scene. 3

(*Enter* GUARDIANO *and* ISABELLA *at one door, and the* WARD *and* SORDIDO *at another.*)

GUARDIANO: Now Nephew, here's the gentlewoman again.
WARD: Mass, here she's come again; mark her now, Sordido.
GUARDIANO: This is the maid my love and care has chose
Out for your wife, and so I tender her to you;
Your self has been eye-witness of some qualities
That speak a courtly breeding, and are costly.
I bring you both to talk together now,
'Tis time you grew familiar in your tongues;
Tomorrow you join hands, and one ring ties you,
And one bed holds you; (if you like the choice)
Her father and her friends are i'th'next room,
And stay to see the contract ere they part;
Therefore dispatch, good Ward, be sweet and short;
Like her, or like her not, there's but two ways;
And one your body, th'other your purse pays.
WARD: I warrant you, Guardiner, I'll not stand all day
   thrumming,
But quickly shoot my bolt at your next coming.
GUARDIANO: Well said: good fortune to your birding then.
   (*Exit.*)
WARD: I never miss'd mark yet.
SORDIDO: Troth I think, master, if the truth were known,
You never shot at any but the kitchen-wench,
And that was a she-woodcock, a mere innocent,
That was oft lost, and cri'd at eight-and-twenty.
WARD: No more of that meat, Sordido, here's eggs o'th'spit
   now,
We must turn gingerly: draw out the catalogue
Of all the faults of women.
SORDIDO: How, all the faults!
Have you so little reason to think so much paper will lie in
my breeches? Why, ten carts will not carry it, if you set down
but the bawds. All the faults? pray let's be content with a few
of 'em; and if they were less, you would find 'em enough, I
warrant you: look you, sir.
ISABELLA [*Aside*]: But that I have th'advantage of the fool,
As much as woman's heart can wish and joy at,

What an infernal torment 'twere to be
Thus bought and sold, and turn'd and pri'd into,
When alas
The worst bit is too good for him! and the comfort is
H'as but a cater's place on't, and provides
All for another's table; yet how curious
The ass is, like some nice professor on't,
That buys up all the daintiest food i'th'markets,
And seldom licks his lips after a taste on't!

SORDIDO: Now to her, now y'have scann'd all her parts over.

WARD: But at which end shall I begin now, Sordido?

SORDIDO: Oh ever at a woman's lip, while you live, sir; do you ask that question?

WARD: Methinks, Sordido, sh'as but a crabbed face to begin with.

SORDIDO: A crabbed face? that will save money.

WARD: How! save money, Sordido?

SORDIDO: Ay, sir: for having a crabbed face of her own, she'll eat the less verjuice with her mutton; 'twill save verjuice at year's end, sir.

WARD: Nay, and your jests begin to be saucy once, I'll make you eat your meat without mustard.

SORDIDO: And that in some kind is a punishment.

WARD: Gentlewoman, they say 'tis your pleasure to be my wife, and you shall know shortly whether it be mine or no to be your husband; and thereupon thus I first enter upon you. [Kisses her.] Oh most delicious scent! Methinks it tasted as if a man had stept into a comfit-maker's shop to let a cart go by, all the while I kiss'd her. It is reported, gentlewoman, you'll run mad for me, if you have me not.

ISABELLA: I should be in great danger of my wits, sir,
For being so forward. [Aside] Should this ass kick backward now!

WARD: Alas poor soul! And is that hair your own?

ISABELLA: Mine own, yes sure, sir, I owe nothing for't.

WARD: 'Tis a good hearing, I shall have the less to pay when I have married you. Look, does her eyes stand well?

SORDIDO: They cannot stand better than in her head, I think, where would you have them? And for her nose, 'tis of a very good last.

WARD: I have known as good as that has not lasted a year though.

SORDIDO: That's in the using of a thing; will not any strong bridge fall down in time, if we do nothing but beat at the bottom? A nose of bluff would not last always, sir, especially if it came into th'camp once.

WARD: But Sordido, how shall we do to make her laugh, that I may see what teeth she has? For I'll not bate her a tooth, nor take a black one into th'bargain.

SORDIDO: Why, do but you fall in talk with her, you cannot choose but one time or other make her laugh, sir.

WARD: It shall go hard, but I will. Pray, what qualities have you beside singing and dancing? can you play at shittlecock forsooth?

ISABELLA: Ay, and at stool-ball too, sir; I have great luck at it.

WARD: Why, can you catch a ball well?

ISABELLA: I have catcht two in my lap at one game.

WARD: What, have you woman? I must have you learn
To play at trap too, then y'are full and whole.

ISABELLA: Any thing that you please to bring me up to,
I shall take pains to practise.

WARD: 'Twill not do, Sordido, we shall never get her mouth open'd wide enough.

SORDIDO: No, sir? that's strange! then here's a trick for your learning.

*(He yawns. [*ISABELLA *likewise, but covers her face with a handkerchief].)*

Look now, look now; quick, quick there.

WARD: Pox of that scurvy mannerly trick with handkerchief! It hind'red me a little, but I am satisfied. When a fair woman gapes, and stops her mouth so, it shows like a clothstopple in a cream-pot; I have fair hope of her teeth now, Sordido.

SORDIDO: Why then, y'have all well, sir; for aught I see,
She's right and straight enough, now as she stands;
They'll commonly lie crooked, that's no matter:
Wise gamesters
Never find fault with that, let 'em lie so still.

WARD: I'd fain mark how she goes, and then I have all: for of all creatures I cannot abide a splay-footed woman, she's an unlucky thing to meet in a morning; her heels keep together so, as if she were beginning an Irish dance still, and the wriggling of her bum playing the tune to't. But I have bethought a cleanly shift to find it; dab down as you see me, and peep of one side, when her back's toward you; I'll show you the way.

SORDIDO: And you shall find me apt enough to peeping,
I have been one of them has seen mad sights
Under your scaffolds.

WARD: Will it please you walk forsooth,
A turn or two by your self? you are so pleasing to me,
I take delight to view you on both sides.
    ISABELLA: I shall be glad to fetch a walk to your love, sir;
'Twill get affection a good stomach, sir,
[*Aside*] Which I had need to have, to fall to such coarse vic-
        tuals. [*Walks.*]
    WARD: Now go thy ways for a clean-treading wench,
As ever man in modesty peept under.
    SORDIDO: I see the sweetest sight to please my master:
Never went Frenchman righter upon ropes
Than she on Florentine rushes.
    WARD: 'Tis enough forsooth.
    ISABELLA: And how do you like me now, sir?
    WARD: 'Faith, so well,
I never mean to part with thee, sweet-heart,
Under some sixteen children, and all boys.
    ISABELLA: You'll be at simple pains, if you prove kind,
And breed 'em all in your teeth.
    WARD: Nay by my faith,
What serves your belly for? 'twould make my cheeks
Look like blown bagpipes.

(*Enter* GUARDIANO.)

    GUARDIANO: How now, Ward and Nephew,
Gentlewoman and Niece! speak, is it so or not?
    WARD: 'Tis so, we are both agreed, sir.
    GUARDIANO: Into your kinred then;
There's friends, and wine, and music waits to welcome you.
    WARD: Then I'll be drunk for joy.
    SORDIDO: And I for company,
I cannot break my nose in a better action.

(*Exeunt.*)

ACT. 4. Scene. 1

(*Enter* BIANCA *attended by two* LADIES.)

BIANCA: How goes your watches, Ladies? what's a-clock
        now?
1. LADY: By mine full nine.

2. LADY: By mine a quarter past.

1. LADY: I set mine by St. Mark's.

2. LADY: St. Anthony's, they say,
Goes truer.

1. LADY: That's but your opinion, Madam,
Because you love a gentleman o'th'name.

2. LADY: He's a true gentleman then.

1. LADY: So may he be
That comes to me tonight, for aught you know.

BIANCA: I'll end this strife straight: I set mine by the sun,
I love to set by th'best, one shall not then
Be troubled to set often.

2. LADY: You do wisely in't.

BIANCA: If I should set my watch, as some girls do,
By ev'ry clock i'th'town, 'twould nev'r go true;
And too much turning of the dial's point,
Or tamp'ring with the spring, might in small time
Spoil the whole work too; here it wants of nine now.

1. LADY: It does indeed forsooth; mine's nearest truth yet.

2. LADY: Yet I have found her lying with an advocate,
Which show'd
Like two false clocks together in one parish.

BIANCA: So now I thank you, Ladies, I desire
A while to be alone.

1. LADY: And I am nobody,
Methinks, unless I have one or other with me.
[*Aside*] 'Faith, my desire and hers will nev'r be sisters.

(*Exeunt* LADIES.)

BIANCA: How strangely woman's fortune comes about!
This was the farthest way to come to me,
All would have judg'd, that knew me born in Venice
And there with many jealous eyes brought up,
That never thought they had me sure enough,
But when they were upon me; yet my hap
To meet it here, so far off from my birth-place,
My friends, or kinred; 'tis not good, in sadness,
To keep a maid so strict in her young days;
Restraint
Breeds wand'ring thoughts, as many fasting days
A great desire to see flesh stirring again:
I'll nev'r use any girl of mine so strictly;
Howev'r they're kept, their fortunes find 'em out,
I see't in me; if they be got in court,
I'll never forbid 'em the country, nor the court,

Though they be born i'th'country: they will com to't,
And fetch their falls a thousand mile about,
Where one would little think on't.

(*Enter* LEANTIO [*richly dressed*].)

LEANTIO [*Aside*]: I long to see how my despiser looks,
Now she's come here to court; these are her lodgings,
She's simply now advanc'd: I took her out
Of no such window, I remember, first;
That was a great deal lower, and less carv'd.
    BIANCA: How now! What silkworm's this, i'th'name of
        pride?
What, is it he?
    LEANTIO: A bow i'th'ham to your greatness;
You must have now three legs, I take it, must you not?
    BIANCA: Then I must take another, I shall want else
The service I should have; you have but two there.
    LEANTIO: Y'are richly plac'd.
    BIANCA: Methinks y'are wondrous brave, sir.
    LEANTIO: A sumptuous lodging.
    BIANCA: Y'ave an excellent suit there.
    LEANTIO: A chair of velvet.
    BIANCA: Is your cloak lin'd through, sir?
    LEANTIO: Y'are very stately here.
    BIANCA: 'Faith, something proud, sir.
    LEANTIO: Stay, stay, let's see your cloth-of-silver slippers.
    BIANCA: Who's your shoemaker? h'as made you a neat boot.
    LEANTIO: Will you have a pair?
The Duke will lend you spurs.
    BIANCA: Yes, when I ride.
    LEANTIO: 'Tis a brave life you lead.
    BIANCA: I could nev'r see you
In such good clothes in my time.
    LEANTIO: In your time?
    BIANCA: Sure I think, sir,
We both thrive best asunder.
    LEANTIO: Y'are a whore.
    BIANCA: Fear nothing, sir.
    LEANTIO: An impudent spiteful strumpet.
    BIANCA: Oh sir, you give me thanks for your captainship;
I thought you had forgot all your good manners.
    LEANTIO: And to spite thee as much, look there, there
        read, [*Gives letter*.]
Vex, gnaw, thou shalt find there I am not love-starv'd.
The world was never yet so cold, or pitiless,

But there was ever still more charity found out
Than at one proud fool's door; and 'twere hard, 'faith,
If I could not pass that. Read to thy shame there;
A cheerful and a beauteous benefactor too,
As ev'r erected the good works of love.
    BIANCA [*Aside*]: Lady Livia!
Is't possible? Her worship was my pandress.
She dote, and send and give, and all to him!
Why, here's a bawd plagu'd home.—Y'are simply happy, sir,
Yet I'll not envy you.
    LEANTIO: No, court-saint, not thou!
You keep some friend of a new fashion;
There's no harm in your devil, he's a suckling,
But he will breed teeth shortly, will he not?
    BIANCA: Take heed you play not then too long with him.
    LEANTIO: Yes, and the great one too: I shall find time
To play a hot religious bout with some of you,
And perhaps drive you and your course of sins
To their eternal kennels; I speak softly now,
'Tis manners in a noble woman's lodgings,
And I well know all my degrees of duty.
But come I to your everlasting parting once,
Thunder shall seem soft music to that tempest.
    BIANCA: 'Twas said last week there would be change of
        weather,
When the moon hung so, and belike you heard it.
    LEANTIO: Why, here's sin made, and nev'r a conscience put
    to't;
A monster with all forehead, and no eyes.
Why do I talk to thee of sense or virtue,
That art as dark as death? and as much madness
To set light before thee, as to lead blind folks
To see the monuments, which they may smell as soon
As they behold; marry, oft-times their heads,
For want of light, may feel the hardness of 'em.
So shall thy blind pride my revenge and anger,
That canst not see it now; and it may fall
At such an hour, when thou least seest of all;
So to an ignorance darker than thy womb
I leave thy perjur'd soul: a plague will come. (*Exit.*)
    BIANCA: Get you gone first, and then I fear no greater,
Nor thee will I fear long; I'll have this sauciness
Soon banish'd from these lodgings, and the rooms
Perfum'd well after the corrupt air it leaves:
His breath has made me almost sick in troth:

A poor base start-up! Life! because he's got
Fair clothes by foul means, comes to rail, and show 'em.

(*Enter the* DUKE.)

DUKE: Who's that?
BIANCA: Cry you mercy, sir.
DUKE: Prethee who's that?
BIANCA: The former thing, my Lord, to whom you gave
The captainship; he eats his meat with grudging still.
DUKE: Still!
BIANCA: He comes vaunting here of his new love,
And the new clothes she gave him; Lady Livia—
Who but she now his mistress?
DUKE: Lady Livia?
Be sure of what you say.
BIANCA: He show'd me her name, sir,
In perfum'd paper, her vows, her letter,
With an intent to spite me; so his heart said,
And his threats made it good; they were as spiteful
As ever malice utter'd, and as dangerous,
Should his hand follow the copy.
DUKE: But that must not:
Do not you vex your mind; prethee to bed, go,
All shall be well and quiet.
BIANCA: I love peace, sir.
DUKE: And so do all that love; take you no care for't,
It shall be still provided to your hand. (*Exit* [BIANCA].)
Who's near us there?

(*Enter* MESSENGER.)

MESSENGER: My Lord.
DUKE: Seek out Hippolito,
Brother to Lady Livia, with all speed.
MESSENGER: He was the last man I saw, my Lord.
DUKE: Make haste.

(*Exit* [MESSENGER].)

He is a blood soon stirr'd, and as he's quick
To apprehend a wrong, he's bold, and sudden
In bringing forth a ruin: I know likewise
The reputation of his sister's honour's
As dear to him as life-blood to his heart;
Beside, I'll flatter him with a goodness to her,

Which I now thought on, but nev'r meant to practise
(Because I know her base), and that wind drives him.
The ulcerous reputation feels the poise
Of lightest wrongs, as sores are vext with flies:
He comes. Hippolito, welcome.

(*Enter* HIPPOLITO.)

HIPPOLITO: My lov'd Lord.
DUKE: How does that lusty widow, thy kind sister?
Is she not sped yet of a second husband?
A bed-fellow she has, I ask not that,
I know she's sped of him.
HIPPOLITO: Of him, my Lord?
DUKE: Yes, of a bed-fellow; is the news so strange to you?
HIPPOLITO: I hope 'tis so to all.
DUKE: I wish it were, sir;
But 'tis confest too fast; her ignorant pleasures,
Only by lust instructed, have receiv'd
Into their services an impudent boaster,
One that does raise his glory from her shame,
And tells the midday sun what's done in darkness;
Yet, blinded with her appetite, wastes her wealth,
Buys her disgraces at a dearer rate,
Than bounteous housekeepers purchase their honour.
Nothing sads me so much, as that in love
To thee, and to thy blood, I had pickt out
A worthy match for her, the great Vincentio,
High in our favour, and in all men's thoughts.
HIPPOLITO: Oh thou destruction of all happy fortunes,
Unsated blood! Know you the name, my Lord,
Of her abuser?
DUKE: One Leantio.
HIPPOLITO: He's
A factor.
DUKE: He nev'r made so brave a voyage,
By his own talk.
HIPPOLITO: The poor old widow's son.
I humbly take my leave.
DUKE [*Aside*]:   I see 'tis done.
—Give her good counsel, make her see her error,
I know she'll hearken to you.
HIPPOLITO: Yes, my Lord,
I make no doubt, as I shall take the course,
Which she shall never know till it be acted;
And when she wakes to honour, then she'll thank me for't.

I'll imitate the pities of old surgeons
To this lost limb, who, ere they show their art,
Cast one asleep, then cut the diseas'd part.
So out of love to her I pity most,
She shall not feel him going till he's lost,
Then she'll commend the cure. (*Exit*.)
    DUKE: The great cure's past;
I count this done already; his wrath's sure,
And speaks an injury deep; farewell Leantio.
This place will never hear thee murmur more.
Our noble brother, welcome!

(*Enter* LORD CARDINAL *attended*.)

    CARDINAL: Set those lights down:
Depart till you be call'd. [*Exeunt* ATTENDANTS.]
    DUKE: [*Aside*]:   There's serious business
Fix'd in his look, nay, it inclines a little
To the dark colour of a discontentment.
—Brother, what is't commands your eye so powerfully?
Speak, you seem lost.
    CARDINAL: The thing I look on seems so
To my eyes, lost for ever.
    DUKE: You look on me.
    CARDINAL: What a grief 'tis to a religious feeling,
To think a man should have a friend so goodly,
So wise, so noble, nay, a duke, a brother,
And all this certainly damn'd!
    DUKE: How!
    CARDINAL: 'Tis no wonder,
If your great sin can do't; dare you look up
For thinking of a vengeance? dare you sleep
For fear of never waking but to death,
And dedicate unto a strumpet's love
The strength of your affections, zeal and health?
Here you stand now; can you assure your pleasures,
You shall once more enjoy her, but once more?
Alas you cannot; what a misery 'tis then
To be more certain of eternal death
Than of a next embrace! nay, shall I show you
How more unfortunate you stand in sin
Than the low private man? all his offences,
Like inclos'd grounds, keep but about himself,
And seldom stretch beyond his own soul's bounds;
And when a man grows miserable, 'tis some comfort

When he's no further charg'd than with himself;
'Tis a sweet ease to wretchedness: but, great man,
Ev'ry sin thou commit'st shows like a flame
Upon a mountain, 'tis seen far about,
And with a big wind made of popular breath,
The sparkles fly through cities: here one takes,
Another catches there, and in short time
Waste all to cinders: but remember still,
What burnt the valleys first came from the hill;
Ev'ry offence draws his particular pain,
But 'tis example proves the great man's bane.
The sins of mean men lie like scatter'd parcels
Of an unperfect bill; but when such fall,
Then comes example, and that sums up all:
And this your reason grants, if men of good lives,
Who by their virtuous actions stir up others
To noble and religious imitation,
Receive the greater glory after death,
As sin must needs confess, what may they feel
In height of torments, and in weight of vengeance,
Not only they themselves not doing well,
But sets a light up to show men to hell?
   DUKE: If you have done, I have; no more, sweet Brother.
   CARDINAL: I know time spent in goodness is too tedious;
This had not been a moment's space in lust now;
How dare you venture on eternal pain,
That cannot bear a minute's reprehension?
Methinks you should endure to hear that talkt of
Which you so strive to suffer. Oh my brother?
What were you, if you were taken now!
My heart weeps blood to think on't; 'tis a work
Of infinite mercy (you can never merit)
That yet you are not death-struck, no not yet:
I dare not stay you long, for fear you should not
Have time enough allow'd you to repent in.
There's but this wall betwixt you and destruction,
When y'are at strongest, and but poor thin clay.
Think upon't, Brother; can you come so near it,
For a fair strumpet's love, and fall into
A torment that knows neither end nor bottom
For beauty but the deepness of a skin,
And that not of their own neither? Is she a thing
Whom sickness dare not visit, or age look on,
Or death resist? does the worm shun her grave?
If not (as your soul knows it), why should lust
Bring man to lasting pain, for rotten dust?

DUKE: Brother of spotless honour, let me weep
The first of my repentance in thy bosom,
And show the blest fruits of a thankful spirit;
And if I e'er keep woman more unlawfully,
May I want penitence at my greatest need!
And wisemen know there is no barren place
Threatens more famine than a dearth in grace.
　　CARDINAL: Why, here's a conversion is at this time, Brother,
Sung for a hymn in heaven; and at this instant
The powers of darkness groan, makes all hell sorry.
First, I praise heaven, then in my work I glory.
Who's there attends without?

(*Enter* SERVANTS.)

　　SERVANT:　　　　　　My Lord!
　　CARDINAL: Take up those lights; there was a thicker darkness,
When they came first. The peace of a fair soul
Keep with my noble brother! (*Exit* CARDINAL, *&c.*)
　　DUKE:　　　　　　Joys be with you, sir.
She lies alone tonight for't, and must still,
Though it be hard to conquer, but I have vow'd
Never to know her as a strumpet more,
And I must save my oath; if fury fail not,
Her husband dies tonight, or at the most,
Lives not to see the morning spent tomorrow;
Then will I make her lawfully mine own,
Without this sin and horror. Now I'm chidden,
For what I shall enjoy then unforbidden,
And I'll not freeze in stoves; 'tis but a while:
Live like a hopeful bridgroom, chaste from flesh,
And pleasure then will seem new, fair and fresh. (*Exit.*)

Scene. 2

(*Enter* HIPPOLITO.)

　　HIPPOLITO: The morning so far wasted, yet his baseness
So impudent? See if the very sun
Do not blush at him!
Dare he do thus much, and know me alive!
Put case one must be vicious, and I know my self

Monstrously guilty, there's a blind time mad for't;
He might use only that, 'twere conscionable:
Art, silence, closeness, subtlety, and darkness
Are fit for such a business; but there's no pity
To be bestow'd on an apparent sinner,
An impudent daylight lecher; the great zeal
I bear to her advancement in this match
With Lord Vincentio, as the Duke has wrought it,
To the perpetual honour of our house,
Puts fire into my blood, to purge the air
Of this corrpution, fear it spread too far,
And poison the whole hopes of this fair fortune.
I love her good so dearly, that no brother
Shall venture farther for a sister's glory
Than I for her preferment.

(*Enter* LEANTIO, *and a* PAGE.)

LEANTIO [*Aside*]:   Once again
I'll see that glist'ring whore, shines like a serpent
Now the court sun's upon her.—Page!
    PAGE: Anon, sir!
    LEANTIO [*Aside*]: I'll go in state too.—See the coach be
        ready. [*Exit* PAGE.]
I'll hurry away presently.
    HIPPOLITO: Yes, you shall hurry,
And the devil after you; take that at setting forth. [*Strikes
        him.*]
Now, and you'll draw, we are upon equal terms, sir.
Thou took'st advantage of my name in honour,
Upon my sister; I nev'r saw the stroke
Come, till I found my reputation bleeding;
And therefore count it I no sin to valour
To serve thy lust so. Now we are of even hand, [LEANTIO
        draws.]
Take your best course against me. You must die.
    LEANTIO: How close sticks envy to man's happiness!
When I was poor, and little car'd for life,
I had no such means offer'd me to die,
No man's wrath minded me. Slave, I turn this to thee,
To call thee to account, for a wound lately
Of a base stamp upon me.
    HIPPOLITO: 'Twas most fit
For a base mettle. Come and fetch one now
More noble then, for I will use thee fairer
Than thou hast done thine soul, or our honour; [*Fight.*]

And there I think 'tis for thee. [LEANTIO *falls.*]
   WITHIN: Help, help! Oh part 'em.
   LEANTIO: False wife! I feel now th'hast pray'd heartily for
      me;
Rise, strumpet, by my fall, thy lust may reign now;
My heart-string, and the marriage-knot that ty'd thee,
Breaks both together. [*Dies.*]
   HIPPOLITO: There I heard the sound on't,
And never lik'd string better.

(*Enter* GUARDIANO, LIVIA, ISABELLA, WARD, *and* SORDIDO.)

   LIVIA: 'Tis my brother.
Are you hurt, sir?
   HIPPLITO: Not any thing.
   LIVIA: Bless'd fortune!
Shift for thy self; what is he thou hast kill'd?
   HIPPOLITO: Our honour's enemy.
   GUARDIANO: Know you this man, Lady?
   LIVIA: Leantio? My love's joy? Wounds stick upon thee
As deadly as thy sins; art thou not hurt
(The devil take that fortune) and he dead?
Drop plagues into thy bowels without voice,
Secret, and fearful! Run for officers,
Let him be apprehended with all speed,
For fear he scape away; lay hands on him,
We cannot be too sure, 'tis wilful murder;
You do heaven's vengeance, and the law just service.
You know him not as I do, he's a villain,
As monstrous as a prodigy, and as dreadful.
   HIPPOLITO: Will you but entertain a noble patience,
Till you but hear the reason, worthy Sister?
   LIVIA: The reason! that's a jest hell falls a-laughing at:
Is there a reason found for the destruction
Of our more lawful loves? and was there none
To kill the black lust 'twixt thy niece and thee,
That has kept close so long?
   GUARDIANO: How's that, good Madam?
   LIVIA: Too true, sir, there she stands, let her deny't;
The deed cries shortly in the midwife's arms,
Unless the parents' sin strike it still-born;
And if you be not deaf, and ignorant,
You'll hear strange notes ere long. Look upon me, wench!
'Twas I betray'd thy honour subtilly to him
Under a false tale; it lights upon me now;
His arm has paid me home upon thy breast,

My sweet belov'd Leantio!

GUARDIANO: Was my judgment,
And care in choice, so dev'lishly abus'd,
So beyond shamefully?—All the world will grin at me.

WARD: Oh Sordido, Sordido, I'm damn'd, I'm damn'd!

SORDIDO: Damn'd? why, sir?

WARD: One of the wicked; dost not see't? a cuckold, a plain reprobate cuckold.

SORDIDO: Nay, and you be damn'd for that, be of good cheer, sir! Y'have gallant company of all professions; I'll have a wife next Sunday too, because I'll along with you my self.

WARD: That will be some comfort yet.

LIVIA: You sir, that bear your load of injuries,
As I of sorrows, lend me your griev'd strength
To this sad burthen; who in life wore actions,
Flames were not nimbler: we will talk of things
May have the luck to break our hearts together.

GUARDIANO: I'll list to nothing, but revenge and anger,
Whose counsels I will follow.

(*Exeunt* LIVIA *and* GUARDIANO, [*with* LEANTIO'S *body*].)

SORDIDO: A wife quoth 'a?
Here's a sweet plum-tree of your guardiner's graffing!

WARD: Nay, there's a worse name belongs to this fruit yet,
And you could hit on't, a more open one:
for he that marries a whore looks like a fellow bound all his lifetime to a medlar-tree, and that's good stuff; 'tis no sooner ripe, but it looks rotten; and so do some queans at nineteen. A pox on't,
I thought there was some knavery abroach,
For something
Stirr'd in her belly, the first night I lay with her.

SORDIDO: What, what, sir!

WARD: This is she brought up so courtly, can sing, and dance, and tumble too, methinks! I'll never marry wife again that has so many qualities.

SORDIDO: Indeed they are seldom good, Master; for likely when they are taught so many, they will have one trick more of their own finding out. Well, give me a wench but with one good quality, to lie with none but her husband, and that's bringing up enough for any woman breathing.

WARD: This was the fault, when she was tend'red to me;
You never look'd to this.

SORDIDO: Alas, how would you have me see through a

great farthingal, sir? I cannot peep through a mill-stone, or
in the going, to see what's done i'th'bottom.
    WARD: Her father prais'd her breast, sh'ad the voice for-
        sooth;
I marvell'd she sung so small indeed, being no maid.
Now I perceive there's a young querister in her belly:
This breeds a singing in my head, I'm sure.
    SORDIDO: 'Tis but the tune of your wive's cinquapace,
Danc'd in a featherbed.
'Faith, go lie down, Master—but take heed your horns do
not make holes in the pillowbers. [*Aside*] I would not batter
brows with him for a hogshead of angels, he would prick my
skull as full of holes as a scrivener's sand-box.

    (*Exeunt* WARD *and* SORDIDO.)

    ISABELLA [*Aside*]: Was ever maid so cruelly beguil'd
To the confusion of life, soul, and honour,
All of one woman's murd'ring! I'd fain bring
Her name no nearer to my blood than woman,
And 'tis too much of that. Oh shame and horror!
In that small distance, from yon man to me,
Lies sin enough to make a whole world perish.
—'Tis time we parted, sir, and left the sight
Of one another, nothing can be worse
To hurt repentance; for our very eyes
Are far more poisonous to religion,
Than basilisks to them; if any goodness
Rest in you, hope of comforts, fear of judgments,
My request is, I nev'r may see you more;
And so I turn me from you everlastingly,
So is my hope to miss you; but for her,
That durst so dally with a sin so dangerous,
And lay a snare so spitefully for my youth,
If the least means but favour my revenge,
That I may practise the like cruel cunning
Upon her life, as she has on mine honour,
I'll act it without pity.
    HIPPOLITO [*Aside*]: Here's a care
Of reputation, and a sister's fortune,
Sweetly rewarded by her: would a silence,
As great as that which keeps among the graves,
Had everlastingly chain'd up her tongue;
My love to her has made mine miserable.

    (*Enter* GUARDIANO *and* LIVIA.)

GUARDIANO: If you can but dissemble your heart's griefs now,
Be but a woman so far.
    LIVIA: Peace! I'll strive, sir.
    GUARDIANO: As I can wear my injuries in a smile;
Here's an occasion offer'd, that gives anger
Both liberty and safety to perform
Things worth the fire it holds, without the fear
Of danger, or of law; for mischiefs acted
Under the privilege of a marriage-triumph
At the Duke's hasty nuptials, will be thought
Things merely accidental; all's by chance,
Not got of their own natures.
    LIVIA: I conceive you, sir,
Even to a longing for performance on't;
What I am now, return'd to sense and judgment,
And here behold some fruits. [*Kneels to* HIPPOLITO & ISA-
BELLA.]
                    Forgive me both:
Is not the same rage and distraction
Presented lately to you; that rude form
Is gone for ever. I am now my self,
That speaks all peace, and friendship; and these tears
Are the true springs of hearty penitent sorrow
For those foul wrongs, which my forgetful fury
Sland'red your virtues with. This gentleman
Is well resolv'd now.
    GUARDIANO: I was never otherways,
I knew (alas) 'twas but your anger spake it,
And I nev'r thought on't more.
    HIPPOLITO: Pray rise, good Sister.
    ISABELLA [*Aside*]: Here's ev'n as sweet amends made for
            a wrong now,
As one that gives a wound, and pays the surgeon;
All the smart's nothing, the great loss of blood,
Or time of hindrance: well, I had a mother,
I can dissemble too.—What wrongs have slipt
Through anger's ignorance (Aunt) my heart forgives.
    GUARDIANO: Why, this is tuneful now!
    HIPPOLITO: And what I did, Sister,
Was all for honour's cause, which time to come
Will approve to you.
    LIVIA: Being awak'd to goodness,
I understand so much, sir, and praise now
The fortune of your arm, and of your safety;
For by his death y'have rid me of a sin

As costly as ev'r woman doted on:
'T has pleas'd the Duke so well too, that (behold, sir)
Has sent you here your pardon, which I kist
With most affectionate comfort; when 'twas brought,
Then was my fit just past, it came so well, me thought,
To glad my heart.

    HIPPOLITO: I see his Grace thinks on me.

    LIVIA: There's no talk now but of the preparation
For the great marriage.

    HIPPOLITO: Does he marry her then?

    LIVIA: With all speed, suddenly, as fast as cost
Can be laid on with many thousand hands.
This gentleman and I had once a purpose
To have honour'd the first marriage of the Duke
With an invention of his own; 'twas ready,
The pains well past, most of the charge bestow'd on't;
Then came the death of your good mother (Niece)
And turn'd the glory of it all to black:
'Tis a device would fit these times so well too,
Art's treasury not better; if you'll join,
It shall be done, the cost shall all be mine.

    HIPPOLITO: Y'have my voice first, 'twill well approve my
        thankfulness
For the Duke's love and favour.

    LIVIA: What say you, Niece?

    ISABELLA: I am content to make one.

    GUARDIANO: The plot's full then;
Your pages, Madam, will make shift for Cupids.

    LIVIA: That will they, sir.

    GUARDIANO: You'll play your old part still.

    LIVIA: What is't? good troth, I have ev'n forgot it.

    GUARDIANO: Why Juno Pronuba, the marriage goddess.

    LIVIA: 'Tis right indeed.

    GUARDIANO: And you shall play the nymph,
That offers sacrifice to appease her wrath.

    ISABELLA: Sacrifice, good sir?

    LIVIA: Must I be appeased then?

    GUARDIANO: That's as you list your self, as you see cause.

    LIVIA: Methinks 'twould show the more state in her deity
To be incenst.

    ISABELLA: 'Twould, but my sacrifice
Shall take a course to appease you, [Aside] or I'll fail in't,
And teach a sinful bawd to play a goddess. [Exit.]

    GUARDIANO: For our parts, we'll not be ambitious, sir;
Please you walk in, and see the project drawn,

Then take your choice.

HIPPOLITO: I weigh not, so I have one. (*Exit.*)

LIVIA: How much ado have I to restrain fury
From breaking into curses! Oh how painful 'tis
To keep great sorrow smother'd! sure I think
'Tis harder to dissemble grief, than love:
Leantio, here the weight of thy loss lies,
Which nothing but destruction can suffice. (*Exeunt.*)

Scene. 3

(*Hoboys. Enter in great state the* DUKE *and* BIANCA, *richly attir'd, with* LORDS, CARDINALS, LADIES, *and other* ATTENDANTS. *They pass solemnly over. Enter* LORD CARDINAL *in a rage, seeming to break off the ceremony.*)

LORD CARDINAL: Cease, cease! Religious honours done to sin
Disparage virtue's reverence, and will pull
Heaven's thunder upon Florence; holy ceremonies
Were made for sacred uses, not for sinful.
Are these the fruits of your repentance, Brother?
Better it had been you had never sorrow'd,
Than to abuse the benefit, and return
To worse than where sin left you.
Vow'd you then never to keep strumpet more,
And are you now so swift in your desires,
To knit your honours, and your life fast to her?
Is not sin sure enough to wretched man,
But he must bind himself in chains to't? Worse!
Must marriage, that immaculate robe of honour,
That renders virtue glorious, fair, and fruitful
To her great Master, be now made the garment
Of leprosy and foulness? is this penitence
To sanctify hot lust? what is it otherways
Than worship done to devils? is this the best
Amends that sin can make after her riots?
As if a drunkard, to appease heaven's wrath,
Should offer up his surfeit for a sacrifice:
If that be comely, then lust's offerings are
On wedlock's sacred altar.

DUKE: Here y'are bitter
Without cause, Brother: what I vow'd I keep,
As safe as you your conscience, and this needs not;

I taste more wrath in't than I do religion;
And envy more than goodness; the path now
I tread is honest, leads to lawful love,
Which virtue in her strictness would not check:
I vow'd no more to keep a sensual woman:
'Tis done,
I mean to make a lawful wife of her.
    CARDINAL: He that taught you that craft,
Call him not master long, he will undo you:
Grow not too cunning for your soul, good Brother;
Is it enough to use adulterous thefts,
And then take sanctuary in marriage?
I grant, so long as an offender keeps
Close in a privileg'd temple, his life's safe;
But if he ever venture to come out,
And so be taken, then he surely dies for't:
So now y'are safe; but when you leave this body,
Man's only privileg'd temple upon earth,
In which the guilty soul takes sanctuary,
Then you'll perceive what wrongs chaste vows endure,
When lust usurps the bed that should be pure.
    BIANCA: Sir, I have read you over all this while
In silence, and I find great knowledge in you,
And severe learning, yet 'mongst all your virtues
I see not charity written, which some call
The first-born of religion, and I wonder
I cannot see't in yours. Believe it, sir,
There is no virtue can be sooner miss'd,
Or later welcom'd; it begins the rest,
And sets 'em all in order; heaven and angels
Take great delight in a converted sinner.
Why should you then, a servant and professor,
Differ so much from them? If ev'ry woman
That commits evil should be therefore kept
Back in desires of goodness, how should virtue
Be known and honour'd? From a man that's blind
To take a burning taper, 'tis no wrong,
He never misses it: but to take light
From one that sees, that's injury and spite.
Pray, whether is religion better serv'd,
When lives that are licentious are made honest,
Than when they still run through a sinful blood?
'Tis nothing virtue's temples to deface;
But build the ruins, there's a work of grace.
    DUKE: I kiss thee for that spirit; thou hast prais'd thy wit
A modest way. On, on there. (*Hoboys.*)

CARDINAL: Lust is bold,
And will have vengeance speak, ere't be controll'd. (*Exeunt.*)

ACT. 5. Scene. 1

(*Enter* GUARDIANO *and* WARD.)

GUARDIANO: Speak, hast thou any sense of thy abuse?
Dost thou know what wrong's done thee?
WARD: I were an ass else.
I cannot wash my face but I am feeling on't.
GUARDIANO: Here take this galtrop then, convey it secretly
Into the place I show'd you; look you sir,
This is the trap-door to't.
WARD: I know't of old, Uncle, since the last triumph; here
rose up a devil with one eye, I remember, with a company of
fireworks at's tail.
GUARDIANO: Prethee leave squibbing now, mark me, and
fail not;
But when thou hear'st me give a stamp, down with't:
The villain's caught then.
WARD: If I miss you, hang me.
I love to catch a villain, and your stamp shall go current, I
warrant you. But how shall I rise up, and let him down too,
all at one hole? that will be a horrible puzzle. You know I
have a part in't, I play Slander.
GUARDIANO: True, but never make you ready for't.
WARD: No? my clothes are bought and all, and a foul
fiend's head with a long contumelious tongue i'th'chaps on't, a
very fit shape for Slander i'th'out-parishes.
GUARDIANO: It shall not come so far, thou understand'st it
not.
WARD: Oh, oh!
GUARDIANO: He shall lie deep enough ere that time,
And stick first upon those.
WARD: Now I conceive you, Guardiner.
GUARDIANO: Away, list to the privy stamp, that's all thy
part.
WARD: Stamp my horns in a mortar if I miss you, and give
the powder in white wine to sick cuckolds, a very present
remedy for the headache.

(*Exit* WARD.)

GUARDIANO: If this should any way miscarry now,
As, if the fool be nimble enough, 'tis certain,
The pages that present the swift-wing'd Cupids
Are taught to hit him with their shafts of love,
Fitting his part, which I have cunningly poison'd;
He cannot 'scape my fury; and those ills
Will be laid all on fortune, not our wills,
That's all the sport on't; for who will imagine
That at the celebration of this night
Any mischance that haps can flow from spite? (*Exit.*)

Scene. 2

(*Flourish. Enter above,* DUKE, BIANCA, L. CARDINAL, FAB-
RITIO, *and other* CARDINALS, LORDS *and* LADIES *in State.*)

DUKE: Now, our fair Duchess, your delight shall witness
How y'are belov'd and honour'd; all the glories
Bestow'd upon the gladness of this night
Are done for your bright sake.
BIANCA: I am the more
In debt, my Lord, to loves and courtesies,
That offer up themselves so bounteously
To do me honour'd grace, without my merit.
DUKE: A goodness set in greatness; how it sparkles
Afar off like pure diamonds set in gold!
How perfect my desires were, might I witness
But a fair noble peace 'twixt your two spirits!
The reconcilement would be more sweet to me,
Than longer life to him that fears to die.
Good sir!
CARDINAL: I profess peace, and am content.
DUKE: I'll see the seal upon't, and then 'tis firm.
CARDINAL: You shall have all you wish. [*Kisses* BIANCA'S
        hand.]
DUKE: I have all indeed now.
BIANCA [*Aside*]: But I have made surer work; this shall
        not blind me;
He that begins so early to reprove,
Quickly rid him, or look for little love;
Beware a brother's envy, he's next heir too.
Cardinal, you die this night, the plot's laid surely:
In time of sports death may steal in securely;

Then 'tis least thought on:
For he that's most religious, holy friend,
Does not at all hours think upon his end;
He has his times of frailty, and his thoughts
Their transportations too, through flesh and blood,
For all his zeal, his learning, and his light,
As well as we, poor souls, that sin by night.
    DUKE: What's this, Fabritio?
    FABRITIO: Marry, my Lord, the model
Of what's presented.
    DUKE: Oh, we thank their loves;
Sweet Duchess, take your seat, list to the argument.
Reads.
There is a Nymph that haunts the woods and springs,
In love with two at once, and they with her;
Equal it runs; but to decide these things,
The cause to mighty Juno they refer,
She being the marriage-goddess; the two lovers
They offer sighs, the Nymph a sacrifice,
All to please Juno, who by signs discovers
How the event shall be, so that strife dies:
Then springs a second; for the man refus'd
Grows discontent, and, out of love abus'd.
He raises Slander up, like a black fiend,
To disgrace th'other, which pays him i'th'end.
    BIANCA: In troth, my Lord, a pretty pleasing argument,
And fits th'occasion well; envy and slander
Are things soon rais'd against two faithful lovers;
But comfort is, they are not long unrewarded. (*Music.*)
    DUKE: This music shows they're upon entrance now.
    BIANCA: Then enter all my wishes.

(*Enter* HYMEN *in yellow,* GANYMED *in a blue robe powdered with stars, and* HEBE *in a white robe with golden stars, with covered cups in their hands*: *they dance a short dance, then bowing to the* DUKE, &c. HYMEN *speaks.*)

HYMEN:*To thee fair bride Hymen offers up*
Of nuptial joys this the celestial cup.
Taste it, and thou shalt ever find
Love in thy bed, peace in thy mind.
    BIANCA: We'll taste you sure, 'twere pity to disgrace
So pretty a beginning.
    DUKE: 'Twas spoke nobly.
    GANYMED: *Two cups of Nectar have we begg'd from Jove;*
Hebe, give that to innocence, I this to love.

Take heed of stumbling more, look to your way;
Remember still the Via Lactea. [DUKE & CARDINAL *drink.*]
   HEBE: *Well, Ganymed, you have more faults, though not*
      so known;
I spill'd one cup, but you have filch'd many a one.
   HYMEN: *No more, forbear for Hymen's sake;*
In love we met, and so let's part. (*Exeunt* [MASQUERS].)
   DUKE: But soft! here's no such persons in the argument,
As these three, Hymen, Hebe, Ganymed.
The actors that this model here discovers
Are only four, Juno, a nymph, two lovers.
   BIANCA: This is some antimasque belike, my Lord,
To entertain time. [*Aside*] Now my peace is perfect:
Let sports come on apace.—Now is their time, my Lord.
      (*Music.*)
Hark you, you hear from 'em!
   DUKE: The nymph indeed.

(*Enter two drest like Nymphs, bearing two tapers lighted;*
then ISABELLA *drest with flowers and garlands, bearing a cen-*
ser with fire in it; they set the censer and tapers on Juno's al-
tar with much reverence; this ditty being sung in parts.)

   DITTY.
Juno nuptial goddess, thou that rul'st o'er coupled bodies,
Ti'st man to woman, never to forsake her, thou only power-
      ful marriage-maker,
Pity this amaz'd affection; I love both, and both love me,
Now know I where to give rejection, my heart likes so equally,
     Till thou set'st right my peace of life,
     And with thy power conclude this strife.
   ISABELLA: *Now with my thanks depart you to the springs,*
I to these wells of love. Thou sacred goddess, [*Exeunt*
     NYMPHS.]
And queen of nuptials, daughter to great Saturn,
Sister and wife to Jove, imperial Juno,
Pity this passionate conflict in my breast,
This tedious mar, 'twixt two affections;
Crown me with victory, and my heart's at peace.

(*Enter* HIPPOLITO *and* GUARDIANO, *like shepherds.*)

   HIPPOLITO: *Make me that happy man, thou mighty goddess.*
   GUARDIANO: *But I live most in hope, if truest love*
Merit the greatest comfort.
   ISABELLA: *I love both*
With such an even and fair affection,

I know not which to speak for, which to wish for,
Till thou, great arbitress, 'twixt lovers' hearts,
By thy auspicious grace, design the man;
Which pity I implore.
BOTH: *We all implore it.*
  ISABELLA: *And after sighs, contritions, truest odours,*
I offer to thy powerful deity
This precious incense, may it ascend peacefully!
[*Aside*] And if it keep true touch, my good Aunt Juno,
'Twill try your immortality ere't be long:
I fear you'll never get so nigh heaven again,
When you're once down.

  (LIVIA *descends like Juno* [*attended by* PAGES *as* CUPIDS].)

  LIVIA: *Though you and your affections*
Seem all as dark to our illustrious brightness
As night's inheritance, hell, we pity you,
And your requests are granted. You ask signs;
They shall be given you, we'll be gracious to you.
He of those twain which we determine for you
Love's arrows shall wound twice, the later wound
Betokens love in age; for so are all,
Whose love continues firmly all their lifetime,
Twice wounded at their marriage; else affection
Dies when youth ends. [*Aside*] This savour overcomes me.
—*Now for a sign of wealth and golden days,*
Bright-ey'd prosperity, which all couples love,
Ay, and makes love—take that: *our brother Jove*
Never denies us of his burning treasure,
T'express bounty. [ISABELLA *falls and dies.*]
  DUKE: She falls down upon't.
What's the conceit of that?
  FABRITIO: As overjoy'd belike:
Too much prosperity overjoys us all,
And she has her lapful, it seems, my Lord.
  DUKE: This swerves a little from the argument though:
Look you, my Lords.
  GUARDIANO [*Aside*]: All's fast; now comes my part
To toll him hither; then with a stamp given,
He's dispatch'd as cunningly.
  HIPPOLITO: Stark dead:
O treachery! cruelly made away! How's that?

[*The trap-door opens and* GUARDIANO *falls through.*]

FABRITIO: Look, there's one of the lovers dropt away too.

DUKE: Why, sure this plot's drawn false, here's no such
thing.

LIVIA: Oh I am sick to th'death, let me down quickly;
This fume is deadly: oh 't'has poison'd me!
My subtilty is sped, her art has quitted me;
My own ambition pulls me down to ruin. [Falls and dies.]

HIPPOLITO: Nay, then I kiss thy cold lips, and applaud
This thy revenge in death. [Kisses ISABELLA.]

FABRITIO: Look, Juno's down too: (CUPIDS shoot.)
What makes she there? her pride should keep aloft.
She was wont to scorn the earth in other shows:
Methinks her peacocks' feathers are much pull'd.

HIPPOLITO: Oh death runs through my blood, in a wild
        flame too:
Plague of those Cupids; some lay hold on 'em.
Let 'em not 'scape, they have spoil'd me; the shaft's
Deadly.

DUKE: I have lost my self in this quite.

HIPPOLITO: My great Lords, we are all confounded.

DUKE: How?

HIPPOLITO: Dead; and I worse.

FABRITIO: Dead? my girl dead? I hope
My sister Juno has not serv'd me so.

HIPPOLITO: Lust, and forgetfulness has been amongst us,
And we are brought to nothing. Some blest charity
Lend me the speeding pity of his sword
To quench this fire in blood. Leantio's death
Has brought all this upon us (now I taste it)
And made us lay plots to confound each other;
The event so proves it, and man's understanding
Is riper at his fall, than all his lifetime.
She, in a madness for her lover's death,
Reveal'd a fearful lust in our near bloods,
For which I am punish'd dreadfully and unlook'd for;
Prov'd her own ruin too, vengeance met vengeance,
Like a set match; as if the plagues of sin
Had been agreed to meet here altogether.
But how her fawning partner fell, I reach not,
Unless caught by some spring of his own setting
(For, on my pain, he never dream'd of dying):
The plot was all his own, and he had cunning
Enough to save himself; but tis the property
Of guilty deeds to draw your wisemen downward.
Therefore the wonder ceases.—Oh this torment!

DUKE: Our guard below there!

(*Enter a* LORD *with a* GUARD.)

LORD: My Lord.
HIPPOLITO: Run and meet death then,
And cut off time and pain. [*Runs on a sword and dies.*]
LORD: Behold, my Lord,
H'as run his breast upon a weapon's point.
DUKE: Upon the first night of our nuptial honours,
Destruction play her triumph, and great mischiefs
Mask in expected pleasures, 'tis prodigious!
They're things most fearfully ominous: I like 'em not.
Remove these ruin'd bodies from our eyes. [GUARD *removes*
       the dead bodies.]
   BIANCA [*Aside*]: Not yet, no change? when falls he to the
       earth?
   LORD: Please but your Excellence to peruse that paper,
       [*Gives paper.*]
Which is a brief confession from the heart
Of him that fell first, ere his soul departed;
And there the darkness of these deeds speaks plainly.
'Tis the full scope, the manner, and intent;
His ward, that ignorantly let him down,
Fear put to present flight at the voice of him.
   BIANCA [*Aside*]: Nor yet?
   DUKE: Read, read; for I am lost in sight and strength.
   CARDINAL: My noble Brother!
   BIANCA: Oh the curse of wretchedness!
My deadly hand is fall'n upon my lord:
Destruction take me to thee, give me way;
The pains and plagues of a lost soul upon him,
That hinders me a moment.
   DUKE: My heart swells bigger yet; help here, break't ope,
My breast flies open next. [*Dies.*]
   BIANCA: Oh with the poison,
That was prepar'd for thee, thee, Cardinal!
'Twas meant for thee.
   CARDINAL: Poor prince!
   BIANCA: Accursed error!
Give me thy last breath, thou infected bosom,
And wrap two spirits in one poison'd vapour. [*Kisses* DUKE.]
Thus, thus, reward thy murderer, and turn death
Into a parting kiss: my soul stands ready at my lips,
Ev'n vext to stay one minute after thee.
   CARDINAL: The greatest sorrow and astonishment
That ever struck the general peace of Florence
Dwells in this hour.

BIANCA: So my desires are satisfied,
I feel death's power within me.
Thou has prevail'd in something (cursed poison)
Though thy chief force was spent in my lord's bosom;—
But my deformity in spirit's more foul;
A blemish'd face best fits a leprous soul.
What make I here? these are all strangers to me,
Not known but by their malice, now th'art gone;
Nor do I seek their pities. [*Drinks from the poisoned cup.*]
CARDINAL: O restrain
Her ignorant wilful hand!
BIANCA: Now do; 'tis done.
Leantio: now I feel the breach of marriage
At my heart-breaking. Oh the deadly snares
That women set for women, without pity
Either to soul or honour! Learn by me
To know your foes: in this belief I die,
Like our own sex we have no enemy!
LORD: See, my Lord,
What shift sh'as made to be her own destruction.
BIANCA: Pride, greatness, honours, beauty, youth, ambition,
You must all down together, there's no help for't:
Yet this my gladness is, that I remove,
Tasting the same death in a cup of love. [*Dies.*]
CARDINAL: Sin, what thou art, these ruins show too piteously.
Two kings on one throne cannot sit together,
But one must needs down, for his title's wrong;
So where lust reigns, that prince cannot reign long. (*Exeunt.*)

FINIS.

THE LADY
FROM THE SEA

Henrik Ibsen

Characters

DR. WANGEL, *district physician*
ELLIDA WANGEL, *his second wife*
BOLETTE } *daughters by his*
HILDA } *first marriage*
ARNHOLM, *headmaster of a school*
LYNGSTRAND
BALLESTED
A STRANGER
YOUNG PEOPLE OF THE TOWN
TOURISTS AND SUMMER VISITORS

The action takes place during the summer in a small town on a fjord in northern Norway.

ACT 1

DR. WANGEL'S *house. A spacious veranda to the left, with a garden to the front and side of the house. Below the veranda, a flagpole. In the garden to the right, an arbor, containing a table and chairs. A hedge with a small gate in the background. Beyond the hedge, a path along the shore, lined by trees. Through the trees the fjord can be seen, with high peaks and mountain ranges in the distance. It is a warm, brilliantly clear summer morning.*

BALLESTED, *middle-aged, wearing an old velvet jacket and a broad-brimmed artist's hat, stands under the flagpole, adjusting the ropes. The flag lies on the ground. Not far from him is an easel with canvas in place. Beside it on a campstool are brushes, a palette, and a paint-box.*

BOLETTE WANGEL *comes out through the open door to the veranda. She is carrying a large vase of flowers, which she sets down on the table.*

BOLETTE: Well, Ballested—can you get it to work?

BALLESTED: Why, certainly, miss. It's nothing, really. If you'll pardon the question—are you expecting visitors today?

BOLETTE: Yes, we expect Mr. Arnholm here this morning. He arrived in town last night.

BALLESTED: Arnholm? But wait—wasn't his name Arnholm, the man who was tutor here some years ago?

BOLETTE: Yes, that's the man.

BALLESTED: I see. So he's back in these parts again.

BOLETTE: That's why we want the flag up.

BALLESTED: Well, that makes sense, I guess.

(BOLETTE *goes back into the house. Afer a moment* LYNG-
STRAND *comes down the road from the right and stops, interested, as he catches sight of the easel and painting materials.
He is a slender young man, poorly but neatly dressed, and
has a rather frail appearance.*)

LYNGSTRAND (*from the other side of the hedge*): Good
morning.
BALLESTED (*turning*): What—! Good morning. (*Runs up
the flag.*) There—she's off. (*Fastens the rope and begins busy-
ing himself at the easel.*) Good morning, sir. I really don't
believe I've had the pleasure—
LYNGSTRAND: You must be a painter.
BALLESTED: Naturally. And why shouldn't I be a painter?
LYNGSTRAND: Yes, I can see you are. Would it be all right
if I just stopped in a moment?
BALLESTED: Maybe you'd like to look at it?
LYNGSTRAND: Yes, I really would, very much.
BALLESTED: Oh, there's nothing remarkable to see yet. But
please, if you want to, come in.
LYNGSTRAND: Thank you. (*He enters through the gate.*)
BALLESTED (*painting*): It's the fjord there between those
islands that I'm trying to get.
LYNGSTRAND: Yes, I see.
BALLESTED: But the figure's still lacking. In this town
there's not a model to be found.
LYNGSTRAND: Is there going to be a figure as well?
BALLESTED: Yes. In here by this rock in the foreground,
there'll be a mermaid lying, half dead.
LYNGSTRAND: Why half dead?
BALLESTED: She's wandered in from the sea and can't find
her way out again. And so, you see, she lies here, expiring in
the tide pools.
LYNGSTRAND: Yes, of course.
BALLESTED: It was the lady of this house who gave me the
idea.
LYNGSTRAND: What will you call the painting when it's fin-
ished?
BALLESTED: I've thought of calling it "The Dying Mer-
maid."
LYNGSTRAND: Very effective. You certainly can make
something fine out of this.
BALLESTED (*looking at him*): A fellow craftsman, per-
haps?
LYNGSTRAND: A painter, you mean?

BALLESTED: Yes.

LYNGSTRAND: No, I'm not that. But I'm going to be a sculptor. My name is Hans Lyngstrand.

BALLESTED: So you're going to be a sculptor? Yes, yes, sculpture's one of the better arts, too—quite elegant. I think I've seen you a couple of times on the street. Have you been in town very long?

LYNGSTRAND: No, I've been here only two weeks. But if I can manage it, I'd like to stay the whole summer.

BALLESTED: And savor the ocean bathing, hm?

LYNGSTRAND: Yes, I need to build up my strength a little.

BALLESTED: Not in delicate health, I hope.

LYNGSTRAND: Yes, my health's been a bit uncertain. But it's nothing really serious. It's my chest—just some trouble getting my breath.

BALLESTED: Pah—that's nothing! All the same, you still ought to see a good doctor.

LYNGSTRAND: I was thinking of Dr. Wangel, if I have the chance.

BALLESTED: Yes, do that. (*Looks off to the left.*) There's another steamer, jammed full of people. It's incredible how many more tourists have been coming here these last few years.

LYNGSTRAND: Yes, it seems like pretty heavy traffic to me.

BALLESTED: And with all the summer visitors, too. I'm often afraid our town's going to lose its character with all these strangers around.

LYNGSTRAND: Were you born here?

BALLESTED: No, I wasn't. But I've accli—acclimatized myself. I've grown attached to the place—time and habit, I guess.

LYNGSTRAND: Then you've lived here quite a while?

BALLESTED: Oh, some seventeen, eighteen years. I came with Skive's Theater Company. But then we ran into financial problems, and the company broke up and scattered to the winds.

LYNGSTRAND: But you stayed on.

BALLESTED: I stayed. And I did rather well for myself. Actually, in those days I was mainly a scene painter, if you want to know.

(BOLETTE *comes out with a rocking chair, which she sets down on the veranda.*)

BOLETTE (*speaking toward the room within*): Hilda—see if you can find the embroidered footstool for Father.

LYNGSTRAND (*going over to the veranda to greet her*): Good morning, Miss Wangel!

BOLETTE (*by the railing*): Oh my, is it you, Mr. Lyngstrand? Good morning. Excuse me a moment—I just have to— (*Goes within.*)

BALLESTED: Do you know the family?

LYNGSTRAND: Not really. I've only met the girls here and there in company. And then I talked a while with Mrs. Wangel at the last concert in the park. She said I was welcome to come and call on them.

BALLESTED: Ah, you know what—you ought to cultivate that connection.

LYNGSTRAND: Yes, I was thinking of making a visit. Sort of a courtesy call, you might say. Now if I could only find some excuse—

BALLESTED: Some—what? Excuse! (*Glances off to the left.*) Damnation! (*Gathering his things together.*) The steamer's already docked. I'm due at the hotel. It might be some of the new arrivals will need me. Actually, if you want to know, I'm working as a barber and a hairdresser, too.

LYNGSTRAND: You're really very versatile.

BALLESTED: In small towns you have to know how to ac— acclimatize yourself in various fields. If you ever need anything in the way of hair preparations—a little pomade or something, then ask for Ballested, the dance instructor.

LYNGSTRAND Dance instructor—?

BALLESTED: Director of the Wind Ensemble, if you like. We're giving a concert in the park this evening. Good-bye— good-bye!

(*He carries his painting materials through the garden gate and goes off to the left.* HILDA *comes out with the footstool.* BOLETTE *brings more flowers.* LYNGSTRAND *nods to* HILDA *from below in the garden.*)

HILDA (*by the railing, without returning his greeting*): Bolette said that you'd ventured inside today.

LYNGSTRAND: Yes, I took the liberty of coming inside just a little.

HILDA: Have you had your morning walk already?

LYNGSTRAND: Oh, no—I didn't get very far today.

HILDA: Did you have a swim then?

LYNGSTRAND: Yes, I was in for a short while. I saw your mother down there. She went into her bathhouse.

HILDA: Who did?

LYNGSTRAND: Your mother.

HILDA: You don't say. (*She places the footstool in front of the rocking chair.*)

BOLETTE (*breaking in*): Did you see anything of Father's boat out on the fjord?

LYNGSTRAND: Yes, I thought I saw a sailboat heading inshore.

BOLETTE: That must be Father. He's been on a sick call out in the islands. (*She straightens up the table.*)

LYNGSTRAND (*Taking one step up the stairs to the veranda*): How marvelous, with all these flowers——!

BOLETTE: Yes, doesn't it look nice?

LYNGSTRAND: Oh, it looks lovely. It looks as if there were a holiday in the house.

HILDA: That's just what it is.

LYNGSTRAND: I thought as much. It has to be your father's birthday today.

BOLETTE (*warningly to* HILDA): Uh-uh!

HILDA (*paying no attention*): No, Mother's.

LYNGSTRAND: Oh, it's your mother's?

BOLETTE (*in a low, angry voice*): Really, Hilda——!

HILDA (*likewise*): Leave me alone! (*To* LYNGSTRAND.) I suppose you'll be going home for lunch now?

LYNGSTRAND (*stepping down off the stairs*): Yes, I guess I better get something to eat.

HILDA: You must find it a pretty good life at the hotel.

LYNGSTRAND: I'm not living at the hotel any longer. It was too expensive.

HILDA: Where are you living now?

LYNGSTRAND: I'm boarding up at Mrs. Jensen's.

HILDA: Which Mrs. Jensen?

LYNGSTRAND: The midwife.

HILDA: Pardon me, Mr. Lyngstrand—but I'm really much too busy to——

LYNGSTRAND: Oh, I know I shouldn't have said that.

HILDA: Said what?

LYNGSTRAND: What I said.

HILDA (*measuring him with a cool look*): I absolutely don't understand you.

LYNGSTRAND: No, no, Well then I'll be saying good-bye to you both for now.

BOLETTE (*coming forward to the stairs*): Good-bye, good-bye, Mr. Lyngstrand. You really must excuse us today. But some other time—when you really can stay a while—and if you'd like to—then you must stop by again and see Father and—and the rest of us.

LYNGSTRAND: Oh, thank you. I'd like that very much.

(*He bows and goes out by the gate. As he passes along the road to the left, he nods and smiles again up to the veranda.*)

HILDA (*in an undertone*): *Adieu, monsieur!* Do give my best to Mother Jensen.

BOLETTE (*softly, shaking her by the arm*): Hilda—! You naughty child! Are you crazy! He could have heard you!

HILDA: Ffft! Who cares!

BOLETTE (*looking off to the right*): There's Father.

(DR. WANGEL, *dressed for travel and carrying a small bag, comes up the footpath from the left.*)

WANGEL: So, my little girls, you have me back! (*He comes in through the gate.*)

BOLETTE (*going toward him across the garden*): Oh, how lovely that you're here.

HILDA (*also going down to him*): Are you taking the rest of the day off, Father?

WANGEL: Oh, no, I'll still have to go down to the office for a spell. Say, do you know if Arnholm's come?

BOLETTE: Yes, he arrived last night. We had word from the hotel.

WANGEL: Then you haven't seen him yet?

BOLETTE: No. But he's sure to be out here this morning.

WANGEL: Yes, he undoubtedly will.

HILDA (*tugging at him*): Father, now you must look around.

WANGEL (*glancing over at the veranda*): Yes, child, I can see. It's really quite festive.

BOLETTE: Yes, don't you think we've made it attractive?

WANGEL: Well, I should say so! Are—are we alone here, just the three of us?

HILDA: Yes, she went in—

BOLETTE (*hurriedly*): Mother's in swimming.

WANGEL (*looks fondly at* BOLETTE *and pats her head, then says somewhat hesitantly*): But listen, you girls—do you want to leave all these things here, like this, all day long? And the flag up, too, all day?

HILDA: Oh, but Father, of course! What else do you think!

WANGEL: Hm—all right, but you see—

BOLETTE (*nodding and winking at him*): Can't you imagine how we went and did all this for Mr. Arnholm's sake. When such a good old friend comes back to visit you the very first time—

HILDA (*smiling and shaking him*): Just think—he used to be Bolette's tutor, Father!

WANGEL (*with a half smile*): What a pair of sly ones you are! Well, after all—it's only natural that we go on remembering her, although she's no longer with us. But even so—Hilda, see here. (*Handing over his bag.*) This goes down to the office. No, children—I don't like this. It just isn't right, you understand. Every year we shouldn't have to— Well, what can one say! I don't know that it'll ever be different.

HILDA (*starts through the garden, left, with the bag, then stops and turns, pointing*): See that man there, walking this way? That must be your tutor.

BOLETTE (*following her gaze*): Him? (*laughs.*) Oh, you are the limit! You think that decrepit specimen is Arnholm!

WANGEL: Not so fast, there. So help me if it isn't him! Yes, it most certainly is!

BOLETTE (*staring, hushed in astonishment*): My Lord, yes, I think you're right—!

(ARNHOLM, *in elegant morning dress, with gold-rimmed glasses and a thin cane, appears on the path from the right. He looks rather tired, as if overworked. Approaching the garden he waves a friendly greeting and enters through the gate.*)

WANGEL (*going toward him*): Welcome, my dear old friend! Welcome back to the old grounds!

ARNHOLM: Thank you, Dr. Wangel! Many, many thanks. (*They shake hands and walk up through the garden together.*) And these are the children! (*Taking their hands and looking at them.*) Why, I can hardly recognize them.

WANGEL: No, I'm not surprised.

ARNHOLM: Oh, well—perhaps Bolette. Yes, Bolette I would have known.

WANGEL: Just barely, I imagine. It's been nine, ten years now since you saw her last. Ah, yes, a great deal has changed here since then.

ARNHOLM (*looking around*): As a matter of fact, I was thinking just the opposite. Except that the trees have grown considerably—and an arbor has been built over there—

WANGEL: Oh, no, if you mean outwardly—

ARNHOLM (*with a smile*): And then not to mention that now you have two grown-up, marriageable daughters in the house.

WANGEL: Oh, there's only one who's marriageable yet.

HILDA (*in an undertone*): Father, honestly!

WANGEL: But now I think we'll set ourselves up on the veranda. It's cooler than here. If you will.

ARNHOLM: Thank you, Doctor.

(*They mount the stairs,* WANGEL *motioning* ARNHOLM *into the rocking chair.*)

WANGEL: There now. You just sit perfectly quiet and relax. Because, really, you look quite done in from the trip.

ARNHOLM: Oh, that's nothing. In these surroundings here—

BOLETTE (*to* WANGEL): Shouldn't we bring you some soda water and lemonade? And perhaps you'd like it inside? It's going to be very hot out.

WANGEL: Yes, do that, girls. Some soda water and lemonade. And then maybe a little cognac.

BOLETTE: Cognac, too?

WANGEL: Just a little. In case somebody wants it.

BOLETTE: All right, then. Hilda, you go down to the office with the bag.

(BOLETTE *goes into the house, closing the door after her.* HILDA *takes the bag and goes through the garden around the house to the left.*)

ARNHOLM (*who has followed* BOLETTE *with his eyes*): What an attractive— How attractively your two daughters have turned out!

WANGEL (*sitting*): Yes, don't you think?

ARNHOLM: Why, Bolette is simply astonishing. And Hilda too. But—about yourself, now, Doctor. Have you decided to stay here permanently?

WANGEL: Yes, so it seems. After all, I was born and raised in these parts, as they say. And then I had those years of marvelous happiness here with her—who was taken from us so soon. And who you remember from you time here, Arnholm.

ARNHOLM: Yes—yes.

WANGEL: And now I've been made happy again by my second wife. I must say, in the sum of things, fate's been kind to me.

ARNHOLM: But no children in your second marriage?

WANGEL: We had a little boy about two, two and a half years ago. But we didn't keep him long. He died when he was some four, five months old.

ARNHOLM: Is your wife not home today?

WANGEL: Oh, yes, she'll be along any time. She went down

for a swim. It's her regular practice now, every day—and in all sorts of weather.

ARNHOLM: Not for reasons of health, I hope.

WANGEL: No, not exactly. Although she's definitely shown signs of nervousness in the past two years. Off and on, I mean. I really can't make out just what the trouble is. But this bathing in the sea—it's become almost the one ruling passion of her life.

ARNHOLM: I remember something of the kind from before.

WANGEL (*with an almost imperceptible smile*): That's right, you know Ellida from the time you were teaching out at Skjoldvik.

ARNHOLM: Of course. She often visited the rectory where I boarded. And then I nearly always saw her whenever I was out at the lighthouse visiting her father.

WANGEL: I can tell you, the life out there has left its mark on her. The people in town here can't understand her. They call her "the lady from the sea."

ARNHOLM: They do?

WANGEL: Yes. So, if you would—talk to her now about the old days, Arnholm. It would do her a world of good.

ARNHOLM (*looking skeptically at him*): Have you really any reason to think so?

WANGEL: I'm sure of it.

ELLIDA'S VOICE (*from the garden, off to the right*): Are you there, Wangel?

WANGEL (*rising*): Yes, dear.

(ELLIDA WANGEL, *wearing a large, light robe, her hair wet and falling loose over her shoulders, comes through the trees near the arbor.* ARNHOLM *gets up.*)

WANGEL (*smiling and reaching his hands out toward her*): Well, there's our mermaid!

ELLIDA (*moving quickly to the veranda and taking his hands*): Thank goodness you're here! When did you come?

WANGEL: Just now. Only a moment ago. (*Gesturing toward* ARNHOLM.) But aren't you going to greet an old acquaintance—?

ELLIDA (*holding her hand out to* ARNHOLM): So, we finally got you here. Welcome! And forgive me that I wasn't home—

ARNHOLM: Don't mention it. No standing on ceremony—

WANGEL: Was the water nice and fresh today?

ELLIDA: Fresh! Good Lord, this water's never fresh. So stale and tepid. Ugh! The water's sick here in the fjord.

ARNHOLM: Sick?

ELLIDA: Yes, it's sick. And I think it makes people sick, too.

WANGEL (*smiling*): Well, you're a fine testimonial for a summer resort.

ARNHOLM: It seems more likely to me, Mrs. Wangel, that you have a peculiar tie to the sea and everything connected with it.

ELLIDA: Oh, yes, it's possible. At times I almost think so— But just look, how festive the girls have made things in your honor!

WANGEL (*embarrassed*): Hm— (*looks at his watch.*) Now I will have to run—

ARNHOLM: Is this really in my honor—?

ELLIDA: Obviously. We don't have displays like this every day. Phew! It's stifling under this roof! (*Going down into the garden.*) Come on over here. At least there's the semblance of a breeze. (*She settles herself in the arbor.*)

ARNHOLM (*following after*): The air here seems quite refreshing to me.

ELLIDA: Yes, you're used to that foul city air. I've heard it's just dreadful there in the summer.

WANGEL (*who also has gone down into the garden*): Ellida dear—now it's up to you to entertain our friend for a while.

ELLIDA: You have work to do?

WANGEL: Yes, I have to go down to my office. And then I want to change my clothes. But I won't be long—

ARNHOLM (*sitting down in the arbor*): Don't rush yourself, Doctor. I'm sure your wife and I will find much to talk about.

WANGEL (*nods*): I'm counting on that. Well—till later, then. (*He goes out through the garden to the left.*)

ELLIDA (*after a short pause*): Isn't it lovely to sit here?

ARNHOLM: I think it's lovely now.

ELLIDA: We call this place the summerhouse. *My* summerhouse, because I had it built. Or rather Wangel did—for my sake.

ARNHOLM: Do you often sit here?

ELLIDA: Yes, most of the day.

ARNHOLM: I suppose, with the children?

ELLIDA: No, the children—they keep to the veranda.

ARNHOLM: And Wangel?

ELLIDA: Oh, Wangel goes back and forth. First he's here with me, and then he's over with them.

ARNHOLM: Is it you who want it like that?

ELLIDA: I think all parties concerned prefer it that way.

We can talk across to each other—whenever we have something to say.

ARNHOLM (*after a moment's thought*): The last time we
saw each other—out at Skjoldvik, I mean—hm—it seems so
long ago now—

ELLIDA: It's all of ten years since you came out to see us.

ARNHOLM: Yes, about that. But when I remember you out
there at the lighthouse—! "The pagan"—as the old priest used
to call you, because your father gave you the name of a ship
instead of a proper Christian name—

ELLIDA: Well—?

ARNHOLM: The last thing I'd ever have believed was that I
would see you again down here, as Mrs. Wangel.

ELLIDA: No, at that time Wangel wasn't yet— The girls'
mother was still alive then. Their real mother, I mean.

ARNHOLM: Yes, I understand. But even if that hadn't
been— Even if he'd been quite unattached—I never would
have imagined that this could happen.

ELLIDA: Nor I, either. Not for anything—then.

ARNHOLM: Wangel is such a good man. So honest. So genuinely kind toward everyone—

ELLIDA (*with warm affection*): Yes, he is!

ARNHOLM: But to me, the two of you seem different as
night and day.

ELLIDA: You're right. We are.

ARNHOLM: Well, but how did this happen then? How did it
happen!

ELLIDA: Oh, Arnholm, don't ask me that. I'd never be able
to explain it. And even if I could, you'd never understand one
particle of it.

ARNHOLM: Hm. (*His voice dropping slightly.*) Have you
ever told your husband anything about me? I mean, about
that futile gesture I once let myself be charmed into?

ELLIDA: Certainly not! I've said nothing at all to him
about—what you mean.

ARNHOLM: I'm glad. Because I've been feeling a bit oppressed by the idea that—

ELLIDA: You needn't be. I've only told him what's perfectly
true, that I was very fond of you, and that you were the best
and truest friend I had up there.

ARNHOLM: Thank you. But tell me then—why did you
never write me after I left?

ELLIDA: I thought it might be painful for you to hear from
someone who—who couldn't respond as you wanted. It
seemed to me rather like reopening a wound.

ARNHOLM: Hm—yes, yes, you may be right.

ELLIDA: But why did you never write yourself?

ARNHOLM (*regarding her with a half-reproachful smile*): I make the overtures? Maybe arouse suspicion of trying to start things up again? After the kind of rejection I got?

ELLIDA: Yes, I can understand. But has there never been any other involvement since?

ARNHOLM: Never. I've stayed faithful to my memories.

ELLIDA (*half joking*): Oh, nonsense! Let the old memories go. You should be thinking instead of becoming a happily married man.

ARNHOLM: That'll have to be soon then. You realize I've already passed thirty-seven?

ELLIDA: Well, all the more reason to hurry up. (*She is silent a moment, then speaks in a low, serious voice.*) But listen, Arnholm—I want to tell you something now that I couldn't have mentioned then to save my life.

ARNHOLM: What's that?

ELLIDA: When you made what you just called your futile gesture—there was no other answer I *could* have given you.

ARNHOLM: I know you only had friendship to offer. I know that.

ELLIDA: But you didn't know that my whole being and all my thoughts were directed elsewhere at the time.

ARNHOLM: At the time!

ELLIDA: Yes.

ARNHOLM: But that's impossible! You're mistaken about the time! You hardly knew Wangel then.

ELLIDA: I don't mean Wangel.

ARNHOLM: You don't—? But up in Skjoldvik—I can't recall one single, solitary person you could possible have been interested in.

ELLIDA: No, I can imagine. Because it was all so utterly insane.

ARNHOLM: But then you must tell me more about this!

ELLIDA: Oh, it's enough for you to know I wasn't free then. And you know that now.

ARNHOLM: But if you *had* been free—?

ELLIDA: Yes?

ARNHOLM: Would you have answered my letter differently?

ELLIDA: How do I know? When Wangel came, I answered differently.

ARNHOLM: Then what's the good of telling me you weren't free?

ELLIDA (*rising with a troubled, anxious air*): Because I've got to confide in someone. No, no, don't get up.

ARNHOLM: Your husband knows nothing of this?

ELLIDA: I let him know from the first that I'd once set my heart on somebody else. He never asked to know more, and we've never discussed it since. After all, it was nothing but madness. And it was over before it started. That is—more or less.

ARNHOLM (*rises*): More or less? Not definitely!

ELLIDA: Yes, yes, definitely! Good Lord, Arnholm, it's not what you're thinking at all. It's something so incomprehensible, I don't know how to begin telling you. You'd only believe I was ill—or out of my mind.

ARNHOLM: My dear Ellida—there's no other way: you've got to tell me everything.

ELLIDA: All right! At least I can try. How would you, as a reasonable man, presume to account for—(*Looks away and breaks off.*) Wait a while. Someone's coming.

(LYNGSTRAND *appears on the road to the left and enters the garden. He is wearing a flower in his lapel and carries a large, colorful bouquet wrapped in paper and silk ribbons. He stops, with a hesitant, uncertain look, by the veranda.*)

ELLIDA (*coming forward in the arbor*): Are you looking for the girls, Mr. Lyngstrand?

LYNGSTRAND (*turning*): Oh, are you there, Mrs. Wangel? (*Bows and approaches.*) No, actually not. Not for the girls. For you, Mrs. Wangel. You suggested that I might come and call on you—

ELLIDA: I certainly did. You're always welcome here.

LYNGSTRAND: Thank you. And since it just so happens that you're having a celebration here today—

ELLIDA: Ah, you know about that?

LYNGSTRAND: Oh, yes. That's why I'd like to take the liberty of presenting you, Mrs. Wangel, with this— (*He bows and offers the bouquet.*)

ELLIDA (*smiling*): But my dear Mr. Lyngstrand, wouldn't it be better if you gave those beautiful flowers to Mr. Arnholm directly? Because, you see, it's really for his sake that—

LYNGSTRAND (*looking indecisively at them both*): Pardon me—but I don't know this gentleman. This is—I brought it for a birthday present.

ELLIDA: Birthday? Then you're mistaken, Mr. Lynstrand. It's no one's birthday here today.

LYNGSTRAND (*smiling broadly*): Oh, I know it is. But I never thought it was such a secret.

ELLIDA: Just what do you know?

LYNGSTRAND: That it's your birthday, Mrs. Wangel.

ELLIDA: Mine?

ARNHOLM (*looks inquiringly at her*): Today? No, it can't be.

ELLIDA (*to* LYNGSTRAND): Whatever gave you that idea?

LYNGSTRAND: It was Hilda who let it slip. I stopped by here a moment earlier today, and I happened to ask the girls why all the decorations, the flowers, the flag—

ELLIDA: Yes, and—?

LYNGSTRAND: And so Hilda answered: "Because today it's Mother's birthday."

ELLIDA: Mother's—! I see.

ARNHOLM: Aha! (*Exchanges an understanding look with* ELLIDA.) Well, Mrs. Wangel, since the young man already knows—

ELLIDA: Yes, now that you know, of course—

LYNGSTRAND (*presenting the bouquet again*): If you'll permit me to offer my best wishes—

ELLIDA (*taking the flowers*): Thank you very much. Please, come and sit for moment, Mr. Lyngstrand.

(ELLIDA, ARNHOLM, *and* LYNGSTRAND *sit down in the arbor.*)

ELLIDA: This business—about my birthday—it was supposed to have been a secret, Mr. Arnholm.

ARNHOLM: Yes, I'm sure of that. It wasn't for us outsiders.

ELLIDA (*laying the bouquet aside*): Yes, quite so. Not for outsiders.

LYNGSTRAND: I promise I won't tell a living soul.

ELLIDA: Oh, it's really not that important. But how are things going for you? I think you're looking better now than you did.

LYNGSTRAND: Yes, I believe I'm doing quite well. And then next year, if maybe I can get to the south of Europe—

ELLIDA: And you will, the girls tell me.

LYNGSTRAND: Yes, because I have a patron in Bergen who'll back me. And he's agreed to help me next year.

ELLIDA: How did you get to know him?

LYNGSTRAND: An, that was a rare piece of luck. I went to sea once on one of his ships.

ELLIDA: Really? So you had the sea in your blood?

LYNGSTRAND: No, not at all. But when my mother died, my father didn't want me lolling around the house any longer, so he packed me off to sea. Then on the home trip we went down in the English Channel. Yes, and that was lucky for me.

ARNHOLM: How so?

LYNGSTRAND: Well, because it was through the shipwreck that I got the condition here in my chest. I stayed so long in the icy waters before they pulled me out that I had to quit the sea. Yes, it was really my good fortune.

ARNHOLM: You believe that?

LYNGSTRAND: Yes. Because this condition is hardly dangerous. And now I can be a sculptor, which I want more than anything else. Imagine—a chance to work in that beautiful clay, to feel it so supple under your fingers, and to model it into form.

ELLIDA: What kind of form? Mermen and mermaids? Or the old Vikings—?

LYNGSTRAND: No, nothing like that. As soon as I'm able, I want to try for a large work—a group, as they call it.

ELLIDA: Oh, yes. But what will this group portray?

LYNGSTRAND: It'll be based on something out of my own experience.

ARNHOLM: Good—stay close to that.

ELLIDA: But what will it be?

LYNGSTRAND: Well, my idea was to have the figure of a young woman, a sailor's wife, stretched out, lying in a strangely troubled sleep. And she would be dreaming, too. I really believe I can develop it so you can actually see that she's dreaming.

ARNHOLM: But isn't there more to the idea?

LYNGSTRAND: Oh, yes, there'll be one other figure. A kind of specter, you might say. It would be her husband, that she'd been unfaithful to while he was away. And he's been drowned at sea.

ARNHOLM: What—?

ELLIDA: He's been drowned?

LYNGSTRAND: Yes. He was drowned on a voyage. But then the strange thing is that he comes home all the same. It's night, and now he stands there over her bed, looking down at her. He'll stand there, dripping wet, like a man dragged out of the sea.

ELLIDA (*leaning back in her chair*): What an astonishing conception! (*Shuts her eyes.*) Yes, I can see it as clear as crystal.

ARNHOLM: But how on earth, Mr.—Mr.—! You said it was something you'd experienced yourself.

LYNGSTRAND: That's right. I did experience all this—at least up to a point.

ARNHOLM: You witnessed a dead man that—

LYNGSTRAND: Well now, I didn't mean experience, strictly speaking. Not actuality. But something very much like it—

ELLIDA (*with lively anticipation*): Tell me more—all you can—about this! I want to know everything.

ARNHOLM (*smiling*): Yes, this is just the thing for you. It has the spell of the sea.

ELLIDA: What was it, Mr. Lyngstrand?

LYNGSTRAND: We were to sail for home from a town called Halifax when, as it happened, the boatswain took sick, and we had to leave him behind in the hospital there. So we signed on an American as a replacement. This new boatswain—

ELLIDA: The American?

LYNGSTRAND: Yes. One day he borrowed a stack of old newspapers from the captain, and he used to read them by the hour. He said he wanted to learn Norwegian.

ELLIDA: Yes? And then!

LYNGSTRAND: Then one evening we were running in a tremendous gale. All the crew were on deck—except the boatswain and me. He'd turned his ankle so he couldn't walk on it, and I was on the sick list, laid up in my bunk. Well, so he was sitting there in the forecastle, reading in one of those old papers again—

ELLIDA: Yes! Go on!

LYNGSTRAND: Then all of a sudden I heard him give out almost a kind of howl. And when I looked at him, I could see that his face had gone chalk-white. Then he twisted and tore the paper in his hands and ripped it to a thousand little pieces. But he did it all so quietly, so quietly.

ELLIDA: Did he say anything? Did he speak?

LYNGSTRAND: Not at first. But after a time he said, as if to himself: "Married. To another man. While I was away."

ELLIDA (*closing her eyes, in a near whisper*): He said that?

LYNGSTRAND: Yes. And, you know—he said it in perfect Norwegian. He must have a rare gift for learning languages, that man.

ELLIDA: And then what? What happened after?

LYNGSTRAND: Well, then came this incredible thing that I'll never forget as long as I live. For he went on, again very quietly, and said: "But she's mine, and mine she'll always be. And if I go home and fetch her, she'll have to go off with me, even if I came as a drowned man up out of the dark sea."

ELLIDA (*pouring herself a glass of water, her hand trembling*): Phew—how humid it is today—!

LYNGSTRAND: And he said that with such a power of will I thought he'd be the man to do it, too.

ELLIDA: Do you have any idea—what became of this man?

LYNGSTRAND: Oh, I'm sure he's no longer alive.

ELLIDA (*quickly*): Why do you think so?

LYNGSTRAND: Well, because we went down in the Channel right after. I got away in the longboat with the captain and five others. The mate went with the dinghy, along with the American and another man.

ELLIDA: And nothing's been heard of them since?

LYNGSTRAND: No, not a word. My patron mentioned it again just recently in a letter. But that's exactly why I feel such an urge to turn all this into a work of art. I can see the unfaithful wife so vividly in my mind. And then the avenger, drowned, and yet coming back from the sea. I can picture them both so clearly.

ELLIDA: And I, too. (*Rising.*) Come, let's go in. Or better, down to Wangel. I think it's stifling here. (*She goes out of the arbor.*)

LYNGSTRAND (*who likewise has risen*): For my part, I'll have to be saying good-bye. This was only meant for a short visit on account of your birthday.

ELLIDA: As you wish. (*Giving him her hand.*) Good-bye, and thank you for the flowers.

(LYNGSTRAND *bows and leaves through the gate and off to the left.*)

ARNHOLM (*rises and goes over to* ELLIDA): It's plain to see this has struck you to the heart, Ellida.

ELLIDA: Yes, that's a good way of putting it—although—

ARNHOLM: But, after all, is it really any more than you should have expected?

ELLIDA (*staring at him*): Expected!

ARNHOLM: Yes, I'd say so.

ELLIDA: Expect someone to return again—! Return like that!

ARNHOLM: What in the world—! Is it that crazy sculptor's story—?

ELLIDA: Perhaps he's not so crazy, Arnholm.

ARNHOLM: Is it this nonsense about a dead man that's shaken you so? And I was thinking—

ELLIDA: What?

ARNHOLM: I was thinking, of course, that you were simply putting on an act. That actually you were sitting here suffering because you'd discovered that a family ritual was being kept secret from you. That your husband and his children had a private life that you weren't part of.

ELLIDA: Oh, no. That's as it has to be. I have no right to demand that my husband be mine and mine alone.

ARNHOLM: I'd say you have that right.

ELLIDA: Yes. But, even so, I don't. That's the point. I also have a life—that the others aren't part of.

ARNHOLM: You! (*Lowering his voice.*) Does that mean—? Do you— not really love your husband?

ELLIDA: Yes, yes! With all my heart, I've learned to love him! And that's just what makes it so terrible—so baffling— so utterly inconceivable—!

ARNHOLM: Now you *must* tell me your troubles, freely and openly, Ellida! Will you do that?

ELLIDA: Oh, my dear friend, I can't. Not now, in any case. Perhaps later.

(BOLETTE *comes out on the veranda and down into the garden.*)

BOLETTE: Father's back from the office. Couldn't we all sit inside?

ELLIDA: Yes, let's do that.

(WANGEL, *in fresh clothes, comes with* HILDA *around the house from the left.*)

WANGEL: There! Now I'm totally at your service! How about a nice glass of something cool to drink?

ELLIDA: Just a moment. (*She goes into the arbor and gets the bouquet.*)

HILDA: Oh, look! What lovely flowers! Where did you get them?

ELLIDA: From Mr. Lyngstrand, dear.

HILDA (*startled*): From Lyngstrand?

BOLETTE (*Uneasily*): Was Lyngstrand here—again?

ELLIDA (*with a half smile*): Yes. He stopped by with these. For a birthday present, you know.

BOLETTE (*glancing at* HILDA): Oh—!

HILDA (*under her breath*): The beast!

WANGEL (*painfully embarrassed, to* ELLIDA): Uh—yes, you see—I should explain, Ellida, my dear—dearest—

ELLIDA (*interrupting*): Come along, girls! We can put my flowers in water with the others. (*She goes up onto the veranda.*)

BOLETTE (*softly to* HILDA): She really *is* kind at heart.

HILDA (*in an angry whisper*): Flimflam! She's just bewitching Father.

WANGEL (*on the veranda, presses* ELLIDA'S *hand*): Thank you! Thank you for that, Ellida!

ELLIDA (*arranging the flowers*): Nonsense. Shouldn't I play my part too in celebrating—Mother's birthday?

ARNHOLM: Hm!

(*He goes up and joins* WANGEL *and* ELLIDA. BOLETTE *and* HILDA *remain below in the garden.*)

ACT 2

In a local park, high on a wooded hill behind the town. A cairn of stones and a weather vane stand in the near background. Large stones, serving as seats, are grouped about the cairn and in the foreground. Far below, the outer fjord can be seen in the distance, with islands and jutting headlands. The open sea is not visible. It is one of the light summer nights of the north. There is a red-gold tinge to the twilight sky and over the mountain peaks far off on the horizon. The sound of four-part singing drifts faintly up the hill from the right. Young men and women from the town come in couples up from the right and, conversing casually, pass the cairn and go out, left. A moment latter BALLESTED *appears, guiding a party of foreign tourists with their ladies. He is loaded down with shawls and traveling bags.*

BALLESTED (*pointing upward with his stick*): Sehen Sie, meine Herrschaften—dort over there liegt eine andere hill. Das willen wir also besteigen, und so herunter— (*He continues in French and leads the group out to the left.*)

(HILDA *comes briskly up the slope on the right, stops and looks back. After a moment* BOLETTE *comes up after her.*)

BOLETTE: But, Hilda, why should we run away from Lyngstrand?

HILDA: Because I can't stand climbing hills like that. So slow! Look! Look at him, creeping along!

BOLETTE: Oh, you know how sickly he is.

HILDA: Do you think it's very serious?

BOLETTE: Yes, I think so, definitely.

HILDA: He was in to see Father this afternoon. I'd give any-thing to know what Father thinks.

BOLETTE: He told me it was a hardening of the lungs—or something like that. And Father said he hasn't too long to live.

HILDA: No! He said that? Imagine—I guessed the same, exactly.

BOLETTE: But, for heaven's sake now, don't show anything.

HILDA: Oh, what an idea! (*Lowering her voice.*) There, now Hans has finally made it. Hans—doesn't he just look like his name should be Hans?

BOLETTE (*whispers*): Will you behave yourself! You're going to get it!

(LYNGSTRAND *comes in from the right, carrying a parasol.*)

LYNGSTRAND: You girls will have to forgive me that I can't go as fast as you can.

HILDA: Did you get yourself a parasol too, now?

LYNGSTRAND: It's your mother's. She said I should use it for a stick. I forgot to bring one.

BOLETTE: Are they down there still? Father and the oth-ers?

LYNGSTRAND: Yes. Your father stopped in at the restau-rant a moment, and the others are sitting outside, listening to the music. But your mother said they'll be up later.

HILDA (*stands staring at him*): You really look tired now.

LYNGSTRAND: Yes, I almost think I'm a bit tired out. I re-ally do believe I'll have to sit down a while. (*He sits on a stone in the foreground, right.*)

HILDA (*standing in front of him*): Did you know there's going to be a dance later, down by the bandstand?

LYNGSTRAND: Yes, I heard some talk about that.

HILDA: Don't you think it's fun, going dancing?

BOLETTE (*who has begun picking wild flowers in the heather*): Now, Hilda—let Mr. Lyngstrand get his breath.

LYNGSTRAND (*to* HILDA): Yes, I'm sure I'd love dancing— if I only could.

HILDA: You've never learned?

LYNGSTRAND: No, I haven't, actually—but that's not what I meant. I meant, I can't because of my chest.

HILDA: Because of what you call your "condition"?

LYNGSTRAND: Yes, that's it.

HILDA: Does having your "condition" make you very un-happy?

LYNGSTRAND: Oh, no, I can't really say that. (*Smiles.*) Because I think it's why people are always being so kind and considerate—and so charitable to me.

HILDA: Yes, and then it's not at all serious, either.

LYNGSTRAND: No, not in the least. Your father was quite reassuring on that.

HILDA: Then as soon as you're able to travel, it'll pass off.

LYNGSTRAND: Oh, yes. It'll pass off.

BOLETTE (*with flowers*): Here you are, Mr. Lyngstrand—these go in your buttonhole.

LYNGSTRAND: Ah, thank you so much! This is really too kind of you.

HILDA (*looking downward to the right*): They're coming up the path.

BOLETTE (*also looking down*): If they only know where to turn off. No, they're missing it.

LYNGSTRAND (*gets up*): I'll run down to the bend and call them.

HILDA: You'll really have to shout.

BOLETTE: No, it's not worth it. You'll only tire yourself out again.

LYNGSTRAND: Oh, it's easy going downhill. (*He hurries off to the right.*)

HILDA: Yes—downhill. (*Looking after him.*) He's even jumping! And it never occurs to him that he's got to climb back up again.

BOLETTE: Poor thing—

HILDA: If Lyngstrand proposed to you, would you accept him?

BOLETTE: Are you out of your mind?

HILDA: I mean, naturally, if he didn't have this condition in his chest. And if weren't going to die so soon. Would you have him then?

BOLETTE: I think you better have him.

HILDA: Not on your life! He doesn't have a pin to his name. He hasn't even got enough to live on himself.

BOLETTE: Then why are you so taken up with him?

HILDA: Oh, I'm interested in his disease, that's all.

BOLETTE: I've never noticed you pitying him for that.

HILDA: I don't, either. But I think it's fascinating.

BOLETTE: What?

HILDA: To watch him and to get him to say it isn't serious and that he's going to travel abroad and be an artist. He really believes every bit of it, and it fills him with such a joy. And yet it's all going to come to nothing, absolutely nothing.

Because he won't live long enough. When I think of it, it seems so thrilling.

BOLETTE: Thrilling!

HILDA: Yes, I do think it's thrilling. That's my privilege.

BOLETTE: Hilda, you really are a nasty brat!

HILDA: That's what I want to be. Just for spite! (*Looking down.*) Well, at last! Arnholm doesn't like all this climbing. (*Turns.*) That's for sure. You know what I saw about Arnholm at lunch?

BOLETTE: What?

HILDA: He's beginning to lose his hair—right up here, in the middle of his head.

BOLETTE: What nonsense! It's not true.

HILDA: Oh, yes. And then he has wrinkles here around his eyes. Oh, Bolette, how could you have had such a crush on him when he was your tutor!

BOLETTE (*smiling*): Yes, would you believe it? I remember crying my heart out once because he said he thought Bolette was an ugly name.

HILDA: Imagine! (*Looking down again.*) Well, will you look at that! There goes our "lady from the sea," babbling away to Arnholm. Father's all by himself. Hm—I wonder if those two don't have eyes for each other.

BOLETTE: You should be ashamed of yourself, really! How can you stand there and talk about her like that? Just when we were getting along so well—

HILDA: That's right—dream on, my little goose! Oh, no, we'll never get along with her, never. She's not our kind. And we're not hers, either. God knows why Father ever dragged her into the house—! I wouldn't be surprised if, one fine day she was to go quite mad.

BOLETTE: Mad! How'd you get that idea?

HILDA: Oh, it's not so inconceivable. After all, her mother went crazy. She died insane, I know that.

BOLETTE: Good grief, what you don't have your nose in! But just don't go around talking about it. Try to be good now—for Father's sake. Do you hear me, Hilda?

(WANGEL, ELLIDA, ARNHOLM, *and* LYNGSTRAND *come up from the right.*)

ELLIDA (*pointing off into the distance*): It lies out there.

ARNHOLM: That's right. It must be in that direction.

ELLIDA: Out there, the sea.

BOLETTE (*to* ARNHOLM): Don't you think it's pretty up here?

ARNHOLM: I think it's magnificent. The view's superb.

WANGEL: Yes, I expect you've never been up here before.

ARNHOLM: No, never. I think in my time it was nearly inaccessible. Not even a footpath then.

WANGEL: And no park, either. This has all come about in the last few years.

BOLETTE: The view is even more marvelous over there from Lodskoll.

WANGEL: Perhaps we should go there, Ellida?

ELLIDA (*sitting down on a stone to the right*): Thanks, but not for me. You others can go. I don't mind sitting here for a while.

WANGEL: Well, then I'll stay with you. The girls can show Arnholm around.

BOLETTE: Would you like to go with us, Mr. Arnholm?

ARNHOLM: Yes, very much. Is there a path over there too?

BOLETTE: Oh, yes. A fine, wide path.

HILDA: The path's so wide, two people can easily go arm in arm.

ARNHOLM (*lightly*): Can I believe that, my little Hilda? (*To* BOLETTE.) Shall the two of us see if she's right?

BOLETTE (*suppressing a smile*): All right. Let's. (*They go out, left, arm in arm.*)

HILDA (*to* LYNGSTRAND): Shall we go too—?

LYNGSTRAND: Arm in arm—?

HILDA: Well, why not? Suits me.

LYNGSTRAND (*takes her arm and laughs delightedly*): This really is droll!

HILDA: Droll—?

LYNGSTRAND: I mean, it looks exactly as if we were engaged.

HILDA: You've never gone strolling before with a girl on your arm, Mr. Lyngstrand? (*They go out to the left.*)

WANGEL (*standing by the cairn*): So, Ellida dear, now we have time to ourselves—

ELLIDA: Yes, come and sit here by me.

WANGEL (*sitting*): How free and calm it is. Now we can little.

ELLIDA: What about?

WANGEL: About you. And about our life together. I see all too well that it can't go on like this.

ELLIDA: What would you have instead?

WANGEL: Full confidence between us. A closeness of man and wife—like the old days.

ELLIDA: Oh, I wish it could be! But it's impossible.

WANGEL: I think I understand. From certain remarks you've dropped now and then, I think I know.

ELLIDA (*passionately*): But you don't! Don't say you understand—!

WANGEL: And yet, I do. Ellida, you're such an honest person. So loyal.

ELLIDA: Yes—loyal.

WANGEL: Any relationship in which you could feel secure and happy would have to be complete and unreserved.

ELLIDA (*looking tensely at him*): And so?

WANGEL: You were never made to be a man's second wife.

ELLIDA: Why do you say that—now?

WANGEL: I've often had my misgivings. Today made it clear. The children celebrating the birthday anniversary—you saw me as a kind of accomplice. And—well, a man's memories can't be erased. Not mine, anyway. I'm not like that.

ELLIDA: I know that. Oh, I know it so well.

WANGEL: But you're mistaken, all the same. For you it's almost as if the children's mother were still alive. As if she were there, invisible, among us. You think my feelings are divided equally between you and her. It's that thought that unsettles you. You find something almost immoral in our relationship. And that's why you no longer can—or no longer want to live with me as a wife.

ELLIDA (*rising*): Is this how you see it, Wangel? Like this?

WANGEL: Yes, today I finally saw the whole thing, down to the bottom.

ELLIDA: Down to the bottom, you say. Oh, don't be too sure.

WANGEL (*rising*): I know quite well there's still more to it.

ELLIDA (*anxiously*): More?

WANGEL: Yes. The fact is, you can't bear these surroundings. The mountains oppress and weigh down your spirit. There's not enough light for you here. Not enough space. Not enough strength and sweep to the wind.

ELLIDA: You're right. Night and day, winter and summer I feel it— this overpowering homesickness for the sea.

WANGEL: Ellida dear, I know that. (*Putting his hand on her head.*) It's why the poor sick child will be going back home again.

ELLIDA: What do you mean?

WANGEL: Just what I said. We're moving away.

ELLIDA: Away!

WANGEL: Yes. Away somewhere by the open sea. Someplace where you can find a true home after your own heart.

ELLIDA: Oh, don't even think of it! It's impossible. You'd never be happy anywhere on earth but here.

WANGEL: Let that take care of itself. Besides—do you think I could live here happily—without you?

ELLIDA: But I'm here. And I'll stay here. I'm yours.

WANGEL: Are you mine, Ellida?

ELLIDA: Oh, don't talk about this other. Here's where you have everything you live for. Your whole lifework is right here.

WANGEL: I said, let that take care of itself. We're moving. Going somewhere out there. It's all settled now, Ellida.

ELLIDA: But what do you think we'll gain by that?

WANGEL: You'll regain your health and your peace of mind.

ELLIDA: By some remote chance. But what of you? Think of yourself. What would you gain?

WANGEL: You, back again.

ELLIDA: But you can't! No, no, you can't do that, Wangel! That's just what's so terrible—and so desolating to think about.

WANGEL: It's worth the risk. If you're going around thinking like this, then there's really no other solution for you than—a move. And the sooner, the better. It's all settled, you hear.

ELLIDA: No! In heaven's name then, I'd better tell you everything straight out—just as it is.

WANGEL: Yes, if you only would!

ELLIDA: I don't want you unhappy for my sake. Especially when it won't get us anywhere.

WANGEL: You gave me your word now that you'll tell me everything— just as it is.

ELLIDA: I will, as best I can. And as much as I understand it. Come here and sit by me.

(*They sit on the stones.*)

WANGEL: Well, Ellida? So—?

ELLIDA: That day when you came out to the lighthouse and asked if I'd be yours—you spoke to me so openly and so honestly about your first marriage. It had been so very happy, you said.

WANGEL: And it was.

ELLIDA: Yes, dear, I believe you. That's not why I bring it up now. I only want to remind you that, on my side also, I was straightforward with you. I told you quite frankly that once in my life I had loved someone else. That it had developed into—into a kind of engagement between us.

WANGEL: A kind of—?

ELLIDA: Yes, something of the sort. Well, it lasted no time at all, hardly. He went away. And so I took it as over and done with. I told you all that.

WANGEL: But, Ellida dear, why drag this up? Really, it has nothing to do with me. And I've never so much as asked you once who he was.

ELLIDA: No, you haven't. You're always so considerate of me.

WANGEL (*smiling*): Oh, in any case—I think I could more or less guess the name.

ELLIDA: The name!

WANGEL: Up there around Skjoldvik there weren't so many to choose from. As a matter of fact, there was actually only one choice—

ELLIDA: You're thinking it was—Arnholm.

WANGEL: Well, wasn't it?

ELLIDA: No.

WANGEL: It wasn't? Well, then I'm really at a loss.

ELLIDA: Do you remember once in late autumn a large American ship that put in to Skjoldvik for repairs?

WANGEL: Yes, I remember very well. They found the captain in his cabin one morning, murdered. I went out myself and did the postmortem.

ELLIDA: That's right, you did.

WANGEL: It was the mate, supposedly, who killed him.

ELLIDA: Who can tell! It was never proved.

WANGEL: There's not much doubt about it, all the same. Why else should he go off and drown himself?

ELLIDA: He didn't drown himself. He shipped out, to the north.

WANGEL (*surprised*): How do you know?

ELLIDA (*with an effort*): You see—it was the mate that I was—engaged to.

WANGEL (*springing up*): What are you saying! Impossible!

ELLIDA: Yes—but true. He was the one.

WANGEL: But, Ellida, how on earth—! How could you do such a thing! Get engaged to someone like him! A total stranger—! What was his name?

ELLIDA: At that time he called himself Freeman. Later, in his letters, he signed himself Alfred Johnston.

WANGEL: And where was he from?

ELLIDA: From Finmark, he said. But actually he was born

in Finland and came to Norway as a child—with his father, I think.

WANGEL: A Quain, then.

ELLIDA: Yes, I guess that's what they're called.

WANGEL: What else do you know about him?

ELLIDA: Only that he went to sea quite young. And that he'd made some long voyages.

WANGEL: Nothing else?

ELLIDA: No. We never talked of his past.

WANGEL: What did you talk of?

ELLIDA: Mainly about the sea.

WANGEL: Ah—! About the sea.

ELLIDA: About the storms and the calms. The dark nights at sea. And the sea in the sparkling sunlight, that too. But mostly we talked of whales and dolphins, and of the seals that would lie out on the skerries in the warm noon sun. And then we spoke of the gulls and the eagles and every kind of seabird you can imagine. You know—it's strange, but when we talked in such a way, then it seemed to me that all these creatures belonged to him.

WANGEL: And you yourself—?

ELLIDA: Yes, I almost felt that I belonged among them, too.

WANGEL: I see. So that's how you got engaged.

ELLIDA: Yes. He said I must.

WANGEL: Must? Had you no will of your own?

ELLIDA: Not when he was near. Oh—afterward I thought it was utterly incomprehensible.

WANGEL: Were you often together with him?

ELLIDA: No, not very often. One day he came out for a look around the lighthouse. That's how we met. And later we saw each other occasionally. But then came this thing with the captain, and he had to leave.

WANGEL: Yes, tell me a bit more about that.

ELLIDA: It was early one morning, just getting light—when I had a message from him. In it he said that I should meet him out at Bratthammer—you know, that headland between the lighthouse and Skjoldvik.

WANGEL: Of course—I remember it well.

ELLIDA: I was to go there right away, he wrote, because he had to speak to me.

WANGEL: And you went?

ELLIDA: Yes, I had to. Well, he told me then that he'd stabbed the captain that night.

WANGEL: He said it himself! Confessed!

ELLIDA: Yes. But he'd only done what was necessary and right, he said.

WANGEL: Necessary and right? Then why did he kill him?

ELLIDA: He wouldn't discuss it. Only that it was nothing for me to hear.

WANGEL: And you believed him, on his word alone?

ELLIDA: I never thought to doubt him. Well, anyway he had to get away. But just before he was to say good-bye— you'll never guess what he did.

WANGEL: Well, tell me.

ELLIDA: He took a key-ring out of his pocket, and then pulled a ring that he'd always worn from his finger. I also had a little ring, and he took that too. He slipped both of them together onto the key-ring—and then he said that we two would marry ourselves to the sea.

WANGEL: Marry—?

ELLIDA: Yes, that's what he said. And then he threw the rings together, with all his strength, as far as he could out in the ocean.

WANGEL: And you, Ellida? You accepted all this?

ELLIDA: Yes, can you imagine—I felt then as if it were fated to be. But then, thank God—he went away!

WANGEL: And when he'd gone—?

ELLIDA: Oh, I came to my senses soon enough—and saw how mad and meaningless it had all been.

WANGEL: But you mentioned some letters before. So you *have* heard from him since.

ELLIDA: Yes, I've heard from him. First I got a few short lines from Archangel. He wrote only that he was going on to America. And he enclosed an address where I could write him.

WANGEL: And did you?

ELLIDA: At once. I wrote, of course, that everything had to be ended between us. That he was no longer to think of me, just as I would never again think of him.

WANGEL: And he wrote back, even so?

ELLIDA: Yes, he wrote back.

WANGEL: And what did he say to your terms?

ELLIDA: Not a word. It was as if I'd never broken with him at all. His answer was cool and calm, that I should wait for him. When he could provide for me, he would let me know, and then I should come to him at once.

WANGEL: So he wouldn't let you go?

ELLIDA: No. I wrote him again. Almost word for word the same as before—but in even stronger terms.

WANGEL: Did he give up then?

ELLIDA: Oh, no, nothing like that. He wrote as calmly as ever. Not a word that I'd broken it off. Then I realized it was useless, so I never wrote him again.

WANGEL: Or heard from him, either?

ELLIDA: Yes, I had three more letters from him. He wrote me once from California, and another time from China. The last letter I had was from Australia. He said then that he was going to the gold mines. I haven't heard from him since.

WANGEL: That man has had an unearthly power over you, Ellida.

ELLIDA: Yes. Yes, he's horrible!

WANGEL: But you mustn't think of him anymore. Never! My dearest Ellida, promise me that! Now we have to try a better cure for you. Fresher air than here in the fjords. The sting of the salt sea breeze. What do you say?

ELLIDA: Oh, don't talk about it! Or think of it even! There's no help for me here. I can feel it in my bones—I won't get rid of this out there either.

WANGEL: Oh what? Just what do you mean?

ELLIDA: I mean the horror. The fantastic hold on my mind—

WANGEL: But you *have* gotten rid of it. Long ago. When you broke with him. It's over and done with now.

ELLIDA (*springing to her feet*): No, that's just the thing, it isn't.

WANGEL: Not over!

ELLIDA: No, Wangel—it's not over. And I'm afraid it never will be.

WANGEL (*in a strangled voice*): Are you saying, then, that in your heart of hearts, you'll never be able to forget this man?

ELLIDA: I *had* forgotten him. But suddenly one day it was as if he returned.

WANGEL: When was that?

ELLIDA: About three years ago now—or a little more. It was while I was carrying the child.

WANGEL: Ah—then! Yes, now I begin to understand.

ELLIDA: No, dear, you're wrong! This thing that's happened to me—oh, I don't think it can ever be understood.

WANGEL (*looking sorrowfully at her*): To think—that here you've gone for three whole years loving another man. Another man. Not me—but somebody else!

ELLIDA: Oh, you're so absolutely wrong. I love no one else but you.

WANGEL (*quietly*): Why, then, in all this time, have you not wanted to live with me as my wife?

ELLIDA: Because of the terror I feel of him, of the stranger.

WANGEL: Terror—?

ELLIDA: Yes, terror. A terror so huge that only the sea could hold it. All right, I'll tell you, Wangel—

(*The young people of the town come back from the left, nod as they pass and go out to the right. Along with them come* ARNHOLM, BOLETTE, HILDA, *and* LYNGSTRAND.)

BOLETTE (*as they go by*): Well, are you still enjoying the view?

ELLIDA: Yes, it's so cool and nice up here.

ARNHOLM: We've decided to go dancing.

WANGEL: Very good. We'll be down right away.

HILDA: See you soon then.

ELLIDA: Mr. Lyngstrand—oh, just a moment.

(LYNGSTRAND *stops.* ARNHOLM, BOLETTE, *and* HILDA *go out to the right.*)

ELLIDA (*to* LYNGSTRAND): Are you going dancing, too?

LYNGSTRAND: No, Mrs. Wangel, I don't think I should.

ELLIDA: Yes, you'd better be careful. That chest trouble—you're not fully over it, you know.

LYNGSTRAND: Not entirely, no.

ELLIDA (*somewhat hesitantly*): How long can it be now since you made that trip—?

LYNGSTRAND: When I got this condition?

ELLIDA: Yes, the voyage you told about this morning.

LYNGSTRAND: Oh, I guess that was around—let me see—yes, it's a good three years ago now.

ELLIDA: Three years.

LYNGSTRAND: Or a shade more. We left America in February, and we went down in March. It was the equinoctial gales that finished us off.

ELLIDA (*looking at* WANGEL): So it was at that time—

WANGEL: But, Ellida dear—?

ELLIDA: Well, don't let us keep you, Mr. Lyngstrand. Go on now. But don't dance.

LYNGSTRAND: No, I'll just look on. (*He goes out, right.*)

WANGEL: Ellida, why did you question him about the voyage?

ELLIDA: Johnston was with him on board, I'm positive of that.

WANGEL: Why do think so?

ELLIDA (*without answering*): It was then that he learned

I'd married someone else while he was away. And then—at that same moment, this thing came over me.

WANGEL: This terror?

ELLIDA: Yes. Sometimes, suddenly, I can see him standing large as life in front of me. Or actually—a little to one side. He never looks at me. He's simply there.

WANGEL: How does he seem to look?

ELLIDA: Exactly as I saw him last.

WANGEL: Ten years ago?

ELLIDA: Yes, out at Bratthammer. And clearest of all I can see the stickpin he wore, with a great blue-white pearl in it. That pearl is like the eye of a dead fish. And it seems to be staring at me.

WANGEL: In God's name—! Ellida, you're ill—much more than I thought. Or than you can possible know.

ELLIDA: Yes! Yes, help me! I feel it's tightening—tightening around me. More and more.

WANGEL: And you've been going about in this state for three whole years, bearing your suffering in secret, without confiding in me.

ELLIDA: But I couldn't tell you! Not till now, not till I had to—for your sake. If I'd confessed all this to you, I'd also have had to tell you—what's unspeakable.

WANGEL: Unspeakable—?

ELLIDA (*averting her face*): No, no, no! Don't talk! Just one other thing, then I'm through. Wangel—how can we ever fathom this—this—mystery about the child's eyes—?

WANGEL: My dearest Ellida, I promise you, that was nothing but your own imagination. The child had exactly the same eyes as all other normal children.

ELLIDA: He did not! And you can't see it! His eyes changed color with the sea. When the fjord lay still in the sunlight, his eyes were like that. And in the storms, too—oh, I saw it well enough, even if you didn't.

WANGEL (*indulgently*): Well—so be it. But even so—what then?

ELLIDA (*quietly, coming closer*): I've seen eyes like that before.

WANGEL: When? And where?

ELLIDA: Out on Bratthammer—ten years ago.

WANGEL (*stepping back*): What do you—?

ELLIDA (*whispers, with a shudder*): The child had the stranger's eyes.

WANGEL (*with an involuntary cry*): Ellida—!

ELLIDA (*clasping her hands in misery about her head*): Now you can understand why I never again *want*—why I never again *dare* to live with you as your wife! (*She turns quickly and runs off down the hill to the right.*)

WANGEL (*hurrying after her and calling*): Ellida—Ellida! My poor, miserable Ellida!

ACT 3

A remote corner of DR. WANGEL'S *garden. It is a damp, marshy place, overshadowed by large old trees. To the right the edge of a stagnant pond is visible. A low picket fence separates the garden from the footpath and the fjord in the background. Beyond the fjord on the horizon, high peaks and mountain ranges. It is late afternoon, near evening.* BOLETTE *sits, sewing, on a stone bench to the left. On the bench lie a couple of books and a sewing basket.* HILDA *and* LYNGSTRAND, *both with fishing rods, walk along the edge of the pond.*

HILDA (*making a sign to* LYNGSTRAND): Don't move! There, I can see a big one.

LYNGSTRAND (*looking*): Where?

HILDA (*pointing*): Can't you see—down there. And there! Holy God, look at that one! (*Peering off through the trees.*) Ahh! Here he comes to scare them away.

BOLETTE (*glancing up*): Who's coming?

HILDA: Your tutor, ma'am.

BOLETTE: My—?

HILDA: Well, I'll bet you he's never been *mine*.

(ARNHOLM *comes through the trees from the right.*)

ARNHOLM: Are there fish in the pond now?

HILDA: Yes, some enormously old carp.

ARNHOLM: Really? So the old carp are still alive?

HILDA: Yes, they're tough, all right. But we're going to pull in a few of them.

ARNHOLM: You'd probably do better out by the fjord.

LYNGSTRAND: No, the pond is—I think it's more mysterious.

HILDA: Yes, it's more thrilling here. Have you been in the water?

ARNHOLM: Moments ago. I'm just now coming from the bathhouse.

HILDA: You stick close to the shore, I guess.

ARNHOLM: Yes, I'm not very much of a swimmer.

HILDA: Can you swim on your back?

ARNHOLM: No.

HILDA: I can. (*To* LYNGSTRAND.) Let's try over there on the other side.

(*They go around the pond off to the right.*)

ARNHOLM (*going closer to* BOLETTE): Sitting all by yourself, Bolette?

BOLETTE: Oh, yes, I do that quite often.

ARNHOLM: Isn't your mother here in the garden?

BOLETTE: No, she's gone for a walk with Father.

ARNHOLM: How is she this afternoon?

BOLETTE: I'm not quite sure. I forgot to ask.

ARNHOLM: What are the books you have there?

BOLETTE: Oh, one of them's something on plant life. And the other's a geography book.

ARNHOLM: Do you like reading that sort of thing?

BOLETTE: Yes, when I can find time for it. But I have to put the housework first.

ARNHOLM: But doesn't your mother—your stepmother—help you with that?

BOLETTE: No, that's up to me. I had to look after it the two years that Father was alone. And it's gone on that way since.

ARNHOLM: But you're as fond of reading as ever.

BOLETTE: Yes, I read every book I can get hold of and that I think I can learn from. One wants so much to know something about the world. Because here we live so completely cut off from everything that's going on. Well, almost completely.

ARNHOLM: Now, Bolette, you mustn't say that.

BOLETTE: It's true. I don't think we live very differently from the carp down there in the pond. They have the fjord so close to them, and there the shoals of great, wild fish go streaking in and out. But these poor, tame pet fish know nothing of that, and they'll never be part of that life.

ARNHOLM: I hardly think they'd do very well out there.

BOLETTE: As well as here, I expect.

ARNHOLM: Besides, you really can't say you're so very removed from life here. Not in the summer, at least. Nowadays it seems like this place is a rendezvous for the whole live world. Almost *the* social capital for tourists.

BOLETTE (*smiling*): Oh, yes, since you're here only as one of the tourists, it's easy enough for you to make fun of us.

ARNHOLM: I make fun—? What gives you that idea?

BOLETTE: Oh, because all that rendezvous and tourist capital talk is something you've heard in town. They always say things like that.

ARNHOLM: Well, as a matter of fact—so I'd noticed.

BOLETTE: But actually there's not a word of truth in it. Not for us year-round people. What good is it to us if the great, strange world goes by on its way up to see the midnight sun? We never go along. We never see the midnight sun. Oh, no; we live our snug little lives out here, in our fish pond.

ARNHOLM (*sitting down beside her*): Tell me, Bolette—I'm wondering, as you go about your life here, isn't there something—I mean some definite thing—that you long for?

BOLETTE: Yes—perhaps.

ARNHOLM: And what's that? Tell me.

BOLETTE: Mostly to get away.

ARNHOLM: That most of all?

BOLETTE: Yes. And afterward, a chance to learn. To get to know something about—just everything.

ARNHOLM: In those days when I was tutoring you, your father often said you'd be going on to the university.

BOLETTE: Oh, poor Father—he says so many things. But when it comes right down to it—there's no real willpower in him.

ARNHOLM: Yes. I'm afraid you're right; there isn't. But have you ever spoken to him about it? I mean, quite seriously and unequivocally?

BOLETTE: No, I haven't exactly.

ARNHOLM: But you know, you absolutely should. Before it's too late, Bolette. Why haven't you?

BOLETTE: Oh, I suppose it's because there's no real willpower in me, either. That's one trait I've picked up from him.

ARNHOLM: Hm—don't you think you're being unfair to yourself?

BOLETTE: I wish I were, but—no. Besides, Father has so little time to think of me and my future. And not much interest, either. That kind of thing he'd rather avoid, if he possibly can. Because he's so involved with Ellida—

ARNHOLM: Involved—? How—?

BOLETTE: I mean, he and my stepmother—(*Breaking off.*) Father and Mother have their own world, you can see that.

ARNHOLM: Well, so much the better, then, if you get away from here.

BOLETTE: Yes, but I don't think I have any right to go—to leave Father.

ARNHOLM: But, Bolette dear, you're going to have to someday, anyway, So I'd say, the sooner the better.

BOLETTE: Oh, I guess it's the only thing. I ought to think of myself, too. Try to get some kind of work. When Father goes, I'll have no one to turn to. But poor Father—I dread leaving him.

ARNHOLM: Dread——?

BOLETTE: Yes, for his sake.

ARNHOLM: But, good Lord, your stepmother! She'll be with him.

BOLETTE: That's true. But she simply hasn't any grasp of all those things that Mother took on so well. There's so much this one just doesn't see. Or maybe doesn't want to see—or bother with. I don't know which it is.

ARNHOLM: Hm. I think I know what you mean.

BOLETTE: Poor Father—he's weak in certain respects. Perhaps you've noticed it yourself. Then too, he hasn't enough work to fill up his time. And she's so incapable of giving him any support. But that's partly his own fault.

ARNHOLM: How so?

BOLETTE: Oh, Father only wants to see happy faces around him. There has to be sunshine and joy in the house, he says. So I'm afraid that many times he's given her medicine that in the long run does her no good.

ARNHOLM: Do you really think so?

BOLETTE: I can't think anything else. She acts so strange at times. (*Heatedly.*) But it does seem so unfair that I should have to stay on here at home! It's really no earthly use to Father. And I have obligations to myself, too.

ARNHOLM: You know, Bolette—we have to talk all this over more fully.

BOLETTE: Oh, that's not going to help any. I'm just fated to stay in my fish pond, that's all.

ARNHOLM: Nonsense! It depends completely on you.

BOLETTE (*suddenly buoyant*): You really think so?

ARNHOLM: Yes, I know so. The whole thing is there, right in your own hands.

BOLETTE: Oh, if that could be true—! Would you maybe put in a good word for me with Father?

ARNHOLM: Of course. But first of all I want to speak frankly and freely, with you, Bolette. (*Glancing off to the left.*) Shh! Don't give it away. We'll come back to this later.

(ELLIDA *appears from the left, hatless, with a large scarf thrown over her head and shoulders.*)

ELLIDA (*nervously animated*): It's lovely here! Simply beautiful!

ARNHOLM (*getting up*): Have you been out walking?

ELLIDA: Yes, a long, long glorious walk through the hills with Wangel. And now we're going out for a sail.

BOLETTE: Won't you sit down?

ELLIDA: No, thanks. I won't sit.

BOLETTE (*moving along the bench*): There's plenty of room.

ELLIDA: No, no, no—I won't sit. Won't sit.

ARNHOLM: That walk certainly did you good. You look so elated.

ELLIDA: Oh, I feel so marvelously well! So indescribably happy! And safe! So safe— (*Looking off to the left.*) What's that big steamer coming in there?

BOLETTE (*rises and looks out*): It must be the large English one.

ARNHOLM: It's putting in by the buoy. Does it usually stop here?

BOLETTE: Just half an hour. It goes farther on up the fjord.

ELLIDA: And then tomorrow—out again. Out on the great open sea. Straight over the sea. Imagine—just to be on board! If one could! If only one could!

ARNHOLM: Have you never taken a long sea voyage, Mrs. Wangel?

ELLIDA: Never at all. Only these short trips here in the fjord.

BOLETTE (*with a sigh*): Ah, yes, we have to make do with dry land.

ARNHOLM: Well, after all, it's our natural home.

ELLIDA: I don't believe that in the slightest.

ARNHOLM: But—we belong to the land, no?

ELLIDA: No. I don't believe it. I believe that, if only mankind had adapted itself from the start to a life on the sea—or perhaps *in* the sea—then we would have become something much different and more advanced than we are now. Both better—and happier.

ARNHOLM: You really believe that?

ELLIDA: I don't see why not. I've often discussed it with Wangel.

ARNHOLM: Yes, and he—?

ELLIDA: He thinks it's entirely possible.

ARNHOLM (*playfully*): Well—maybe. But what's done is done. So once and for all we took the wrong turn and became land animals, instead of sea creatures. Considering the circumstances, it's a little late now to amend the error.

ELLIDA: Yes, there's the unhappy truth. And I think people have some sense of it, too. They bear it about inside them like a secret sorrow. And I can tell you—there, in that feeling, is the deepest source of all the melancholy in man. Yes—I'm sure of it.

ARNHOLM: But, my dear Mrs. Wangel—I never got the impression humanity was so very melancholy. Quite the contrary, I think the majority take life for the best, as it comes—and with a great, quiet, instinctive joy.

ELLIDA: Oh no, that isn't true. The joy—it's much like our joy in these long, light summer days and nights. It has the hint in it of dark times to come. And that hint is what throws a shadow over our human joy—like the drifting clouds with their shadows over the fjord. Everything lies there so bright and blue—and then all of a sudden—

ARNHOLM: You shouldn't give way to these sad thoughts now. A moment ago you were so gay, so elated—

ELLIDA: Yes. Yes, so I was. Oh, this—I'm so stupid. (*Looking around uneasily.*) If Wangel would only come. He promised me he would, definitely. But he still hasn't come. He must have forgotten. Oh, my dear Arnholm, please, try to find him for me, won't you?

ARNHOLM: Yes, gladly.

ELLIDA: Tell him he has to come right away. Because now I can't see him—

ARNHOLM: Can't see him—?

ELLIDA: Oh, you wouldn't understand. When he's not near me, then often I can't remember how he looks. And then it's as if I'd lost him for good. It's a horrible feeling. Please, go! (*She walks aimlessly about by the pond.*)

BOLETTE (*to* ARNHOLM): I'll go with you. You won't know where—

ARNHOLM: Don't bother. I'll manage—

BOLETTE (*in an undertone*): No, no, I'm worried. I'm afraid he's gone on the ship.

ARNHOLM: Afraid?

BOLETTE: Yes, he likes to see if there are people he knows. And then there's the bar on board—

ARNHOLM: Oh, yes. Well, come on then.

(*He and* BOLETTE *go off, left.* ELLIDA *stands a moment, staring down into the pond. Intermittently she speaks in bro-*

*ken whispers to herself. Outside, on the path behind the
fence, a STRANGER, dressed for traveling, comes from the
left. He has bushy, reddish hair and a beard. He has a Scotch
tam on his head and a musette bag on a strap over his shoulder. The* STRANGER *walks slowly along the fence, scanning
the garden. When his eyes fall on* ELLIDA, *he stops and stares
at her with an intense, probing gaze.)*

STRANGER (*in a low voice*): Good evening, Ellida!

ELLIDA (*turning with a cry*): Oh, my love—you've come
at last!

STRANGER: Yes, at last.

ELLIDA (*looks with astonishment and terror at him*): Who
are you? What do you want here?

STRANGER: You know well enough.

ELLIDA (*starting*): What's that! Why are you speaking to
me? Who are you looking for?

STRANGER: I've been looking for you.

ELLIDA (*with a shudder*): Ah—! (*stares at him, falters
back and breaks out in a half-stifled cry.*) The eyes! The
eyes!

STRANGER: Well—you're finally beginning to know me
again? I knew you at once, Ellida.

ELLIDA: The eyes! Don't look at me like that! I'll cry for
help!

STRANGER: Shh, shh! Don't be afraid. I won't hurt you.

ELLIDA (*her hands over her eyes*): I said, don't look at me
that way!

STRANGER (*leaning his arms on the fence*): I came on the
English ship.

ELLIDA (*glancing fearfully at him*): What do you want of
me?

STRANGER: I promised you I'd return as soon as I could—

ELLIDA: Go! Go away! Don't ever come back—ever! I
wrote you that everything was over between us! Completely!
You know that!

STRANGER (*unperturbed, not answering her*): I wanted to
come before this. But I couldn't. Now, at last, I'm able. And
so you have me, Ellida.

ELLIDA: What is it you want of me? What are you thinking
of? What have you come here for?

STRANGER: You must know that I've come to take you.

ELLIDA (*wincing in fright*): To take me! Is that your idea!

STRANGER: Why, of course.

ELLIDA: But—you must know that I'm married.

STRANGER: Yes, I know.

ELLIDA: And yet—even so, you've come here to—to take me!

STRANGER: That's what I'm doing.

ELLIDA (*pressing her fists to her head*): Oh, it's monstrous! It's horrible—horrible!

STRANGER: Do you think you won't come?

ELLIDA (*in confusion*): Don't look at me that way!

STRANGER: I'm asking if you don't want to come.

ELLIDA: No, no, no! I don't! Never! I don't want to, I tell you! I neither can nor will! (*More quietly.*) Nor dare to.

STRANGER (*climbing over the fence and entering the garden*): All right, Ellida—then let me just say one thing to you before I move on.

ELLIDA (*tries to run, but cannot, and stands as if paralyzed by fright, supporting herself against a tree by the pond*): Don't touch me! Stay away from me! Not—nearer! Don't touch me, you hear!

STRANGER (*cautiously coming a few steps closer*): You needn't be afraid of me, Ellida.

ELLIDA (*covering her eyes with her hands*): Don't look at me like that!

STRANGER: Don't be afraid. Don't be afraid.

(DR. WANGEL *comes through the garden from the left.*)

WANGEL (*still half hidden by the trees*): Well, you've been waiting a mighty long while for me.

ELLIDA (*rushes to him and clings tightly to his arm, crying out*): Oh, Wangel—save me. Save me—if you can!

WANGEL: Ellida—what in God's name—!

ELLIDA: Save me, Wangel! Can't you see him? He's standing right over there!

WANGEL: That man? (*Approaching him.*) If I may—who are you? And why are you here in the garden?

STRANGER (*indicating* ELLIDA *with a nod*): I want to talk to her.

WANGEL: I see. So it was you— (*To* ELLIDA.) I heard some stranger had been up at the house, asking for you.

STRANGER: Yes, it was me.

WANGEL: And what do you want with my wife? (*Turning.*) Do you know him, Ellida?

ELLIDA (*quietly, wringing her hands*): Do I know him? Yes, yes!

WANGEL (*brusquely*): Well?

ELLIDA: It's him, Wangel! He's the man! The one I told you about—!

WANGEL: What? What did you say? (*Turning.*) Are you the Johnston who once—

STRANGER: You can call me Johnston—it's all right with me. But that's not my name.

WANGEL: It's not?

STRANGER: Not any longer, no.

WANGEL: And what is it you want with my wife? Because you know, of course, that the lighthouse keeper's daughter has been married for some time now. And I guess you must also know who she's married to.

STRANGER: I've known for more than three years.

ELLIDA (*in suspense*): How did you find out?

STRANGER: I was on my way home to you, when I came on an old newspaper—one from these parts—and it told there about the wedding.

ELLIDA (*staring into space*): The wedding—so that was it—

STRANGER: I found it so strange. Because those rings in the sea—they were a wedding, too, Ellida.

ELLIDA (*hiding her face in her hands*): Ah—!

WANGEL: How dare you?

STRANGER: Had you forgotten?

ELLIDA (*feeling his eyes on her*): Stop looking at me like that!

WANGEL (*moving up to him*): Better deal with me, not her. All right, short and sweet—since you know the situation, what business do you have around here? Why have you sought out my wife?

STRANGER: I promised Ellida I'd come to her as soon as I could.

WANGEL: Ellida—again!

STRANGER: And Ellida promised faithfully to wait till I came.

WANGEL: I hear you calling my wife by her first name. That kind of familiarity isn't appreciated around here.

STRANGER: I understand. But, after all, she belongs to me first—

WANGEL: To you! The nerve—!

ELLIDA (*retreating behind* WANGEL): Oh—! He'll never let go!

WANGEL: To you! You say she belongs to you!

STRANGER: Did she tell you anything about the two rings? Mine and Ellida's?

WANGEL: She did. But what of it? She put an end to that long ago. You've had her letters. You should know.

STRANGER: Ellida and I both agreed that joining our rings would have all the binding force of an actual marriage.

ELLIDA: But I don't want it, you hear me! I never want to see you again! Keep your eyes off me! I don't want this!

WANGEL: You must be crazy if you think you can come here and base your rights on such adolescent games.

STRANGER: It's true, I have no rights—in your sense.

WANGEL: Then what do you intend to do? You certainly can't imagine you could take her away from me forcibly—against her will?

STRANGER: No. What good would that be? If Ellida goes off with me, she'll have to come of her own free will.

ELLIDA (*with a start, crying out*): My own free will—!

WANGEL: How can you think—!

ELLIDA (*to herself*): My own free will—!

WANGEL: You must be out of your head! Get on your way. We've nothing more to do with you.

STRANGER (*looking at his watch*): It's almost time for me to be on board again. (*Approaching a step.*) Well, Ellida— I've kept my promise. (*Closer still.*) I've kept the word I gave you.

ELLIDA (*shrinking aside*): Oh, don't—don't touch me!

STRANGER: And now you've got till tomorrow night to think it over.

WANGEL: There's nothing here to think over. Let's see you clear out!

STRANGER (*still to* ELLIDA): I'll be going up the fjord now with the ship. Tomorrow night I'll come by here again—and I'll look for you. You must wait for me here in the garden. Because I'd rather settle this matter with you alone, you understand?

ELLIDA (*in a low, tremulous voice*): Oh, you hear that, Wangel?

WANGEL: Don't worry. I think we can forestall that visit.

STRANGER: Good-bye until then, Ellida. Till tomorrow night.

ELLIDA (*imploringly*): No, no—not tomorrow night! Not ever again!

STRANGER: And if, by that time, you've made up your mind to follow me over the sea—

ELLIDA: Don't look at me that way!

STRANGER: Then be ready to leave right away.

WANGEL: Go up to the house, Ellida!

ELLIDA: I can't. Oh, help me! Save me, Wangel!

STRANGER: Because you have to remember one thing: if you don't go with me tomorrow, it's all over.

ELLIDA (*trembling as she looks at him*): All over? Forever?

STRANGER (*nods*): It can never be altered then, Ellida. I'll never be back in these parts again. You won't see me anymore. Or hear from me, either. Never. Then I'll be dead and gone from you forever.

ELLIDA (*her breathing labored*): Oh—!

STRANGER: So think over carefully what you'll do. Goodbye. (*Goes to the fence, climbs over, stops and says.*) Yes, Ellida—be ready to travel tomorrow night. I'm coming to take you away. (*He goes slowly and calmly off down the path to the right.*)

ELLIDA (*looking after him a moment*): He said, of my own free will! Imagine—he said I should go with him of my own free will.

WANGEL: Don't get upset. He's gone now—and you won't see him anymore.

ELLIDA: How can you say that? He's coming back tomorrow night.

WANGEL: Let him come. He's not seeing you, at any rate.

ELLIDA (*shaking her head*): Ah, Wangel, don't think you can stop him.

WANGEL: Oh, yes, dear, I can—just leave it to me.

ELLIDA (*deep in thought, not hearing him*): After he's been here tomorrow night—and after he's sailed off to sea with the ship—

WANGEL: Yes?

ELLIDA: I wonder if he'll never—never come back?

WANGEL: Ellida dear, that you can be quite sure of. What would he be doing here afterward? Now that he's heard from your own lips that you've no more interest in him at all. That closes the case.

ELLIDA (*to herself*): Tomorrow, then. Or never.

WANGEL: And even if he did come back—

ELLIDA: Then what?

WANGEL: Then it's within our power to render him harmless.

ELLIDA: Don't you believe it.

WANGEL: I'm telling you, we have that power! If you can't have peace from him any other way, he's going to pay for the murder of the captain.

ELLIDA (*passionately*): No! No, not that! We know nothing about the captain's murder! Nothing at all!

WANGEL: We don't know? He confessed to you himself!

ELLIDA: No, nothing of that! If you say anything, I'll deny it. Don't cage him in! He belongs to the open sea. He belongs out there.

WANGEL (*gazes at her and says slowly*): Ah, Ellida—Ellida!

ELLIDA (*clinging to him passionately*): Oh, my dearest own— save me from that man!

WANGEL (*gently freeing himself*): Come! Come with me!

(LYNGSTRAND *and* HILDA, *both with fishing rods, appear from the right by the pond.*)

LYNGSTRAND (*goes quickly up to* ELLIDA): You know what, Mrs. Wangel—it's the most amazing thing!

WANGEL: What is?

LYNGSTRAND: Just think—we saw the American.

WANGEL: The American?

HILDA: Yes, I saw him, too.

LYNGSTRAND: He passed up behind the garden and then onto that big English steamer.

WANGEL: How do you know this man?

LYNGSTRAND: I once went to sea with him. I was positive he'd been drowned—and there he was, live as could be.

WANGEL: You know anything more about him?

LYNGSTRAND: No. But he must have come back to have revenge on his faithless wife.

WANGEL: What did you say?

HILDA: Lyngstrand's going to make him into a piece of sculpture.

WANGEL: I don't understand one word—

ELLIDA: You can hear it all later.

(ARNHOLM *and* BOLETTE *come along the path from the left outside the fence.*)

BOLETTE (*to those in the garden*): Come and see! It's the English steamer sailing up the fjord.

(*A large steamer glides slowly by in the distance.*)

LYNGSTRAND (*to* HILDA, *near the fence*): Tonight he'll be standing over her.

HILDA (*nods*): Over the faithless wife—yes.

LYNGSTRAND: Imagine—as midnight strikes.

HILDA: I think it's just thrilling.

ELLIDA (*watching the ship*): Tomorrow, then—

WANGEL: And then, never again.

ELLIDA (*in a low, uncertain voice*): Oh, Wangel—save me from myself.

WANGEL (*looking anxiously at her*): Ellida—I feel something behind this.

ELLIDA: Yes. You can feel the undertow.

WANGEL: The undertow—?

ELLIDA: That man is like the sea.

(*She goes slowly and pensively out through the garden to the left.* WANGEL *walks uneasily beside her, observing her searchingly.*)

ACT 4

DR. WANGEL'*s conservatory. Doors right and left. In the rear wall, between the two windows, a glass door, open, leading out to the veranda. Beyond, some of the garden can be seen. A sofa and table in the left foreground. To the right a piano, and farther back a large flower stand. In the center of the room, a round table with chairs grouped about it. On the table a blossoming rose tree, and various potted plants elsewhere around the room. It is morning.*

By the table to the left, BOLETTE *sits on the sofa, occupied with some embroidery.* LYNGSTRAND *is seated on a chair at the upper end of the table. Below in the garden* BALLESTED *sits painting.* HILDA *stands next to him, looking on.*

LYNGSTRAND (*sits for a time in silence, his arms resting on the table, studying the way* BOLETTE *works*): It must really be very hard to sew a border like that, Miss Wangel.

BOLETTE: Oh, no, it's not so difficult—if you just keep your counting straight—

LYNGSTRAND: Counting? You mean you're counting as well?

BOLETTE: Yes, the stitches. See here.

LYNGSTRAND: Why, of course! That's amazing! You know, it's almost a kind of art. Can you also sketch?

BOLETTE: Oh, yes—if I can copy something.

LYNGSTRAND: Otherwise, no?

BOLETTE: Otherwise no.

LYNGSTRAND: Then it's not a real art, after all.

BOLETTE: No, I guess it's mostly a kind of—handiwork.

LYNGSTRAND: But I do think that you could maybe learn an art.

BOLETTE: When I haven't any talent?

LYNGSTRAND: In spite of that—if you were to spend your time in the company of a real, authentic artist—

BOLETTE: You think I could learn from him?

LYNGSTRAND: I don't mean learn in the conventional sense. But I think it would dawn on you little by little—almost like a kind of miracle, Miss Wangel.

BOLETTE: That would be something.

LYNGSTRAND (*after a moment*): Have you ever thought imminently—I mean—have you ever thought deeply and seriously about marriage, Miss Wangel?

BOLETTE (*giving him a quick glance*): About—? No.

LYNGSTRAND: I have.

BOLETTE: Oh? Have you really?

LYNGSTRAND: Oh, yes. I think very often about things like that. Most of all, about marriage. And then, of course, I've read about it, too, in quite a few books. I think that marriage has to be accounted almost a kind of miracle. The way a woman little by little makes herself over until she becomes like her husband.

BOLETTE: Takes on his interests, you mean?

LYNGSTRAND: Yes, exactly!

BOLETTE: Well, but his powers too? His skills, and his talents?

LYNGSTRAND: Hm—yes, I wonder if all that couldn't as well—

BOLETTE: Then perhaps you also believe that whatever a man has studied, or though out for himself—that this, too, can become part of his wife?

LYNGSTRAND: That too, yes. Little by little, almost miraculously. But I'm quite sure it can only happen in a marriage that's faithful and loving and truly happy.

BOLETTE: Has it ever occurred to you that perhaps a man could also be absorbed that way, over into his wife? Become like her, I mean?

LYNGSTRAND: A man? No, I never thought of that.

BOLETTE: But why couldn't it work as well one way as the other?

LYNGSTRAND: No, because a man has his vocation to live for. And that's the thing that makes a man strong and stable, Miss Wangel. He has a calling in life, you see.

BOLETTE: All men? Every last one?

LYNGSTRAND: Oh, no. I was thinking particularly of artists.

BOLETTE: Do you think it's right for an artist to go and get married?

LYNGSTRAND: Yes, of course I think so. If he can find someone that he cares for deeply—

BOLETTE: All the same, I think he'd do best simply to live for his art alone.

LYNGSTRAND: Well, naturally he will. But he can do that just as well if he's also married.

BOLETTE: Yes, but what about her?

LYNGSTRAND: Her? Who?

BOLETTE: The one that he marries. What's she going to live for?

LYNGSTRAND: She'll live for his art, also. I think that a woman must feel a profound happiness in that.

BOLETTE: Hm—I wonder really—

LYNGSTRAND: Oh, yes, that you can believe. Not only from all the honor and esteem that she'll win through him—because I think that ought to be reckoned about the least of it. But that she can help him to create—that she can ease his work for him by being there and making him comfortable and taking care of him and seeing that his life is really enjoyable. I think that must be thoroughly satisfying for a woman.

BOLETTE: Why, you have no idea how self-centered you are!

LYNGSTRAND: I—self-centered! My Lord in heaven, if you only knew me a little better—! (*Leaning closer to her.*) Miss Wangel, once I'm gone—and I will be soon enough—

BOLETTE (*looking compassionately at him*): Please, don't start thinking sad thoughts.

LYNGSTRAND: There's nothing so sad about that.

BOLETTE: What do you mean then?

LYNGSTRAND: I'll be leaving now in about a month's time. First from here, and then, soon after, I'll be traveling south.

BOLETTE: Oh, I see. Of course.

LYNGSTRAND: Miss Wangel, will you think of me then, every so often?

BOLETTE: Yes, of course I will.

LYNGSTRAND (*happily*): Promise me that!

BOLETTE: Yes, I promise.

LYNGSTRAND: By all that's holy—Bolette?

BOLETTE: By all that's holy. (*In a changed tone.*) But what can it come to, really? It won't lead to anything at all.

LYNGSTRAND: How can you say that! For me it will be so beautiful to know that you're here at home, thinking of me.

BOLETTE: Yes, but what else?

LYNGSTRAND: Well, beyond that I really don't know exactly—

BOLETTE: Nor I either. It has so much working against it. Everything works against it, I think.

LYNGSTRAND: But miracles can happen, you know. A marvelous spell of good fortune—something like that. Because I really believe that luck is with me.

BOLETTE (*vivaciously*): Yes, that's right! You believe it, don't you!

LYNGSTRAND: I believe it unshakably, beyond all doubt. And then—in a few years—when I come home again as a famous sculptor, comfortably fixed, in the fullness of health—

BOLETTE: Yes. Yes, that's what we're hoping for you.

LYNGSTRAND: You can count on it. If only you'll think warm, faithful thoughts of me while I'm away in the south. And now I have your word for that.

BOLETTE: You have my word. (*Shaking her head.*) But it can never lead anywhere, all the same.

LYNGSTRAND: Oh, yes, at the least it's sure to do one thing—make my work as an artist go easier and faster.

BOLETTE: You really think so?

LYNGSTRAND: Yes, I can feel it intuitively. And then I should think it would be quite exhilarating for you, too—out here so remote from everything—to know secretly that you were helping me to create.

BOLETTE (*looks at him*): And you, for your part—?

LYNGSTRAND: I—?

BOLETTE (*glancing out toward the garden*): Shh! Talk about something else. Mr. Arnholm's coming.

(ARNHOLM *comes into view below in the garden from the left. He stops and speaks with* BALLESTED *and* HILDA.)

LYNGSTRAND: Are you fond of your old teacher, Bolette?

BOLETTE: Fond of him?

LYNGSTRAND: Yes, I mean, do you think a lot of him?

BOLETTE: Why, of course. He's been wonderful to have as an adviser and a friend. He never fails to be helpful whenever he can be.

LYNGSTRAND: But isn't it surprising that he's never married?

BOLETTE: You think it's so very surprising?

LYNGSTRAND: Yes. Because they tell me he's quite well off.

BOLETTE: I suppose he is. But then it hasn't been so easy for him to find someone who'll have him.

LYNGSTRAND: Why?

BOLETTE: Well, almost all the young girls he knows have been his students. He says that himself.

LYNGSTRAND: So—what's the difference?

BOLETTE: But, my Lord, you don't go marrying someone who's been your teacher!

LYNGSTRAND: Don't you think that a young girl can fall in love with her teacher?

BOLETTE: Not after she's really grown up.

LYNGSTRAND: What an amazing idea!

BOLETTE(*warning him*): Shh, shh, shh!

(BALLESTED *has, in the meantime, been gathering his things together; he carries them off to the right in the garden,* HILDA *helping him.* ARNHOLM *comes up onto the veranda and enters the room.*)

ARNHOLM: Good morning, my dear Bolette. Good morning, Mr.—Mr.—hm!

(*He looks irritated and nods coolly to* LYNGSTRAND, *who gets up and bows.*)

BOLETTE (*rising and going to* ARNHOLM): Good morning, Mr. Arnholm.

ARNHOLM: How's everything here today?

BOLETTE: Just fine, thank you.

ARNHOLM: I suppose your stepmother's down swimming again today?

BOLETTE: No, she's up in her room.

ARNHOLM: Not feeling well?

BOLETTE: I don't know. She's locked herself in.

ARNHOLM: Hm—has she?

LYNGSTRAND: Mrs. Wangel had a horrible shock from that American yesterday.

ARNHOLM: What do you know about that?

LYNGSTRAND: I told Mrs. Wangel that I'd seen him go walking large as life past the garden.

ARNHOLM: Oh, I see.

BOLETTE (*to* ARNHOLM): You and Father were certainly up late last night.

ARNHOLM: Yes, rather late. We got into a serious discussion.

BOLETTE: Did you get to talk a little about me and my plans?

ARNHOLM: No, Bolette dear. I hadn't a chance—he was completely caught up in something else.

BOLETTE (*sighs*): Ah, yes—he always is.

ARNHOLM (*gives her a meaningful look*): But later today

the two of us will have to talk some more about all this. Where's your father now? Gone out, perhaps?

BOLETTE: Oh, no, he must be down at the office. Let me go fetch him.

ARNHOLM: Please don't. I'd just as soon go down there.

BOLETTE (*hearing sounds to the left*): Wait a bit, Mr. Arnholm. I think that's Father on the stairs. Yes. I guess he's been up to see her.

(DR. WANGEL *comes in through the door, left.*)

WANGEL (*shaking hands with* ARNHOLM): Well, my friend—you're here already? It was good of you to come so early. I want to talk some more with you.

BOLETTE (*to* LYNGSTRAND): Maybe we should go out in the garden a while with Hilda?

LYNGSTRAND: Oh, I'd like to, very much.

(*He and* BOLETTE *go down into the garden and out through the trees in the background.*)

ARNHOLM (*having followed them with his eyes, turns to* WANGEL): Do you know that young man fairly well?

WANGEL: No, not at all.

ARNHOLM: But then what do you think of him hanging around the girls so much?

WANGEL: Does he? I really hadn't noticed.

ARNHOLM: Seems to me, you ought to keep an eye on him.

WANGEL: Yes, you're entirely right. But, my Lord, what can a poor man do? The girls are so used to looking after themselves. They can't be told anything, by me or Ellida.

ARNHOLM: Not by her, either?

WANGEL: No. Besides, I can hardly expect her to get mixed up in these matters. They're beyond her competence. (*Breaking off.*) But we're not here to talk about that. Tell me—have you thought anymore about this business—about everything I told you?

ARNHOLM: I've thought of nothing else since I left you last night.

WANGEL: And what do you think ought to be done?

ARNHOLM: I think that you, as a doctor, must know far better than I.

WANGEL: Oh, if you only knew how hard it is for a doctor to prescribe for someone he loves! And then this is no ordinary illness. No ordinary doctor can help here—and no ordinary medicines.

ARNHOLM: How is she today?

WANGEL: I was up to see her just now, and she seemed quite calm. But behind all her moods there's something mysterious that I just can't fathom. And then she's so erratic—so elusive—so thoroughly unpredictable.

ARNHOLM: That goes with the morbid state of her mind.

WANGEL: Only in part. If you come right down to it, she was born that way. Ellida's one of the sea people. There's the crux of it.

ARNHOLM: What do you really mean by that?

WANGEL: Haven't you ever noticed that the people who live out close by the sea are almost like a race to themselves? It's as though they lived the sea's own life. There's the surge of the waves—the ebb and the flow—in their thoughts and their feelings both. And they never can be transplanted. Oh, I should have remembered that. It was a plain sin against Ellida to take her away from there and bring her inland.

ARNHOLM: You've come to that conclusion?

WANGEL: Yes, more and more I have. But I should have seen it from the start. Oh, basically I knew it, all right. But I didn't want to look at it. Because I loved her so much, you see. So first and foremost I thought of myself. I was just inexcusably selfish then!

ARNHOLM: Hm—any man would be a bit selfish under those circumstances. As a matter of fact, that's a flaw I don't think I've noticed in you, Doctor.

WANGEL (*pacing about restlessly*): Oh, yes! And I've gone on being selfish, too. I'm so very much older than she is. I should have been something of a father to her—and a guide. I should have done my best toward helping her mind develop and grow. But unhappily nothing came of it. I hadn't the willpower for it. I wanted her just as she was. But then she grew worse and worse. And here I was, not knowing what I should do. (*Quieter.*) That was why, in my perplexity, I wrote you and asked you here for a visit.

ARNHOLM (*staring astounded at him*): What! Is that why you wrote?

WANGEL: Yes. But don't give it away.

ARNHOLM: But of all things—what earthly good did you expect of me? I don't understand.

WANGEL: That's not surprising. You see, I was off on the wrong track. I thought that Ellida had once set her heart on you—and that secretly she still cared for you a little. I thought maybe it would do her good to see you again and talk of home and the old days.

ARNHOLM: It was your wife, then, that you meant when

you wrote that there was someone here thinking of me and—and perhaps longing to see me.

WANGEL: Yes, who else?

ARNHOLM (*quickly*): No, no, that's all right. I just hadn't understood.

WANGEL: It's not at all surprising, as I said. I was completely on the wrong track.

ARNHOLM: And you say that you're selfish!

WANGEL: Oh, I have a lot to atone for. I felt I shouldn't neglect anything that could possibly ease her mind a little.

ARNHOLM: How can you explain the power this stranger has over her?

WANGEL: Well—there may be aspects of the problem that just don't admit explanation.

ARNHOLM: You mean something that *can't* be explained, inherently—and permanently.

WANGEL: Something that can't, anyway—by what we know now.

ARNHOLM: Then you believe in such things.

WANGEL: I neither believe nor disbelieve. I simply don't know. So I leave it open.

ARNHOLM: Yes, but tell me one thing: this peculiar, grim insistence of hers about the child's eyes—

WANGEL (*fiercely*): I don't believe one word of it! I won't believe anything like that! It's pure imagination on her part—and nothing else.

ARNHOLM: Did you notice the man's eyes when you saw him yesterday?

WANGEL: Of course I did.

ARNHOLM: And you found no such resemblance?

WANGEL (*evasively*): Well, my Lord—what can I say? There wasn't much light when I saw him. And then I've always heard so much about that resemblance from Ellida—I really don't know if I was able to see him objectively.

ARNHOLM: Well, that's quite possible. But the other thing then. That all this anxiety and unrest came over her at exactly the time the stranger seems to have been on his voyage home?

WANGEL: Yes, you know—that's also something she must have dreamed up overnight. It never came on her as suddenly—all at once—as she's claiming now. Ever since she heard from this young Lyngstrand that Johnston—or Freeman—or whatever he's called—that he was on his way three years ago in March, she's honestly believed that all her mental turmoil dates from that very month.

ARNHOLM: You mean it doesn't?

WANGEL: Not by any means. There were ample warning signs long before that time. It *is* true that—as it happens— just in March three years ago, she had a rather violent siege of it—

ARNHOLM: Well, then—!

WANGEL: Yes, but that could easily be a sign of what she was going through, of her condition then. She was expecting at that time.

ARNHOLM: So—signs against signs.

WANGEL (*knitting his hands*): And then not to be able to help her! Not to know what to say! Not to see the way out!

ARNHOLM: If only you could bring yourself to move away and live elsewhere. Someplace where she'd be able to feel more at home.

WANGEL: Oh, don't you think I've suggested that, too? I proposed that we move back to Skjoldvik. But she won't.

ARNHOLM: Not even there?

WANGEL: No. She doesn't see any use to that. And maybe she's right.

ARNHOLM: Hm—you think so?

WANGEL: Yes. What's more—on second thought—I really don't know how I could carry through with it. For the girls' sakes, I scarcely think I could justify a move into such isolation. After all, they have to live where there are at least some prospects for a decent marriage.

ARNHOLM: Marriage? Are you already so concerned about that?

WANGEL: Well, my Lord—I do have to think about it! But then, on the other hand again, there's my poor, sick Ellida—! Ah, my dear Arnholm—in many ways, I really feel caught between fire and water.

ARNHOLM: You hardly need to worry about Bolette— (*Breaking off.*) I wonder where she's—where they've gone? (*He goes to the open door and looks out.*)

WANGEL (*over by the piano*): I'd gladly make any sacrifice for all three of them—if I only knew what.

(ELLIDA *comes through the door on the left.*)

ELLIDA (*hurriedly to* WANGEL): You mustn't go out this morning.

WANGEL: No, of course not. I'll stay home with you. (*Gesturing toward* ARNHOLM, *who approaches them.*) But aren't you going to greet our friend?

ELLIDA (*turning*): Oh, you're here, Mr. Arnholm. (*Gives him her hand.*) Good morning.

ARNHOLM: Good morning, Mrs. Wangel. Not taking your swim today?

ELLIDA: No, no! Don't even mention it. But won't you sit down just a moment?

ARNHOLM: No, thank you—not now. (*Looks at* WANGEL.) I promised the girls I'd meet them in the garden.

ELLIDA: Well, goodness knows if you'll find them. I never know where they've gone.

WANGEL: Oh, now, they're sure to be down by the pond.

ARNHOLM: Well, I guess I can follow their trail. (*He nods and crosses the veranda into the garden and off, right.*)

ELLIDA: What time is it, Wangel?

WANGEL((*looking at his watch*): A little after eleven.

ELLIDA: A little after. And at eleven—or half-past eleven tonight, the steamer will come. Oh, to be done with it!

WANGEL (*going closer to her*): Ellida dear—there's one thing I want to ask you about.

ELLIDA: What is it?

WANGEL: The night before last—up there in the park— you said, in these last three years, you'd seen him so often before you, large as life.

ELLIDA: Yes, that's true. I have.

WANGEL: But how did you see him?

ELLIDA: How did I see him—?

WANGEL: I mean—how did he look when you saw him?

ELLIDA: But you know yourself, Wangel, how he looks.

WANGEL: Did he look just like that in these visions of yours?

ELLIDA: Yes, exactly.

WANGEL: But how did it happen, then, that you didn't recognize him at once?

ELLIDA (*with a start*): I didn't?

WANGEL: No. You said yourself, later, that you didn't have any idea at first who this stranger was.

ELLIDA (*struck with wonder*): Yes, actually—you're right! But isn't that odd, Wangel? Imagine—that I didn't know him at once.

WANGEL: It was only by the eyes, you said—

ELLIDA: Yes—the eyes! The eyes!

WANGEL: But at the park you said he always appeared to you the way he looked when you parted—out there, ten years ago.

ELLIDA: I said that?

WANGEL: Yes.

ELLIDA: Then he must have looked about the same in those days as he does now.

WANGEL: No. Walking back, the night before last, you gave me quite a different picture of him. You said he had no beard ten years ago. He was dressed quite differently, too. And then the stickpin with the pearl—the man yesterday had nothing like that.

ELLIDA: No, that's right.

WANGEL (*looks searchingly at her*): Try to think back now, Ellida. Or—maybe you can't remember any longer how he looked when he stood with you on Bratthammer?

ELLIDA (*concentrating with her eyes closed*): Not very clearly. No—today I can't at all. Isn't that strange?

WANGEL: Not so strange, actually. There's a new image in you now, shaped out of reality—and it's eclipsing the old one so you can't see it anymore.

ELLIDA: Do you think so, Wangel?

WANGEL: Yes. And it's shutting out the sick fantasies, too. It's a good thing the reality came.

ELLIDA: Good? You call it good?

WANGEL: Yes. The fact that it came—may well be the cure you've needed.

ELLIDA (*sitting down on the sofa*): Wangel—come and sit here by me. I have to tell you all that's on my mind.

WANGEL: Yes, my dear, please do. (*He sits on a chair on the other side of the table.*)

ELLIDA: It was really a stroke of misfortune—for both of us—that we two, of all people, had to come together.

WANGEL (*startled*): What are you saying!

ELLIDA: Oh, yes—it was. And that was only natural. It could only end in misfortune—considering the way that we came together.

WANGEL: What was so wrong about the way we—!

ELLIDA: Now listen, Wangel—there's no need for us going around any longer, lying to ourselves—and to each other.

WANGEL: We're doing what! Lying?

ELLIDA: Yes. Or anyway, concealing the truth. Because the truth—the plain, simple truth is that you came out there and—and bought me.

WANGEL: Bought—! You say—bought!

ELLIDA: Oh, I wasn't one particle better than you. I met your offer—and sold myself to you.

WANGEL (*gives her a pained look*): Ellida—how can you be so heartless?

ELLIDA: But what else can I call it? You couldn't bear the emptiness in your house any longer. You were out after a new wife—

WANGEL: And a new mother for the children, Ellida.

ELLIDA: Perhaps that too—on the side. Although you had no idea if I'd fit that role. You'd no more than seen me, and talked a bit with me a couple of times. Then you wanted me, and so—

WANGEL: Yes, you can put it that way, if you choose.

ELLIDA: And I, on my side—I was helpless then, not knowing which way to turn—and so utterly alone. It was such good sense to accept your offer—since you proposed maintaining me for life.

WANGEL: It never struck me in terms of maintainance. I asked you, in all honesty, if you'd be willing to share with me and the children the little I had.

ELLIDA: Yes, so you did. But the point is, I never should have accepted. Never, for any price! I never should have sold myself! The meanest work—the poorest conditions would have been better—if I'd chosen them myself, by my own free will!

WANGEL (*rising*): Then these five, six years we've lived together—have they been such a total waste?

ELLIDA: Oh, you mustn't think that, Wangel! I've lived as well here with you as anyone could hope for. But I didn't come into your house by my own free will. That's the thing.

WANGEL (*studying her*): Not by your own free will!

ELLIDA: No. I didn't go with you freely.

WANGEL (*quietly*): Ah—I remember those words—from yesterday.

ELLIDA: Everything came together in those words—like a beam of light—and I can see things now, as they are.

WANGEL: What do you see?

ELLIDA: I see that this life we're living with each other—is really no marriage at all.

WANGEL (*bitterly*): What you say is true enough. The life we have *now* is no marriage.

ELLIDA: Nor earlier, either. Never. Not from the very start. (*Gazing into space.*) The first—*that* one might have been full and complete.

WANGEL: The first? What first do you mean?

ELLIDA: Mine—with him.

WANGEL (*stares bewildered at her*): I absolutely don't understand you.

ELLIDA: Oh, Wangel—let's not lie to each other. Or to ourselves, either.

WANGEL: All right! Go on.

ELLIDA: You see—we can never get away from one thing: that a promise freely given is just as binding as a marriage license.

WANGEL: But what in God's name—!

ELLIDA (*rising impetuously*): I want to be free to leave you, Wangel.

WANGEL: Ellida—! Ellida—!

ELLIDA: Yes, yes—give me my freedom! You have to believe me—things aren't going to change. Not after the way we met and married.

WANGEL (*mastering his feelings*): Have we really come to this point?

ELLIDA: We had to. There was no other way.

WANGEL (*looking sorrowfully at her*): Then all we've shared hasn't won you to me. You've never belonged to me—never.

ELLIDA: Oh, Wangel—if only I could love you as much as I want to! As completely as you deserve! But now I can tell—it's not going to be.

WANGEL: Divorce, then? That's what you want? An absolute divorce?

ELLIDA: You understand me so little. I'm not concerned about the formalities. This isn't a matter of outward things. What I want is simply that the two of us agree, of our own free will, to release each other.

WANGEL (*bitterly, nodding slowly*): Dissolve the contract—hm?

ELLIDA: Exactly. Dissolve the contract.

WANGEL: And then what, Ellida? Afterward? Have you thought over what lies ahead of us then? How life might turn out both for you and for me?

ELLIDA: That doesn't matter. Life will take care of itself. What I'm begging and pleading for, Wangel, is all that's important. Let me go free! Give me my full freedom back!

WANGEL: Ellida, this is a fearful thing you're asking. At least give me some time to collect my thoughts and come to a decision. Let's talk it over some more. And give yourself time to consider what you're doing.

ELLIDA: There isn't the time for that. I must have my freedom today.

WANGEL: Why so soon?

ELLIDA: Because he'll be here tonight.

WANGEL (*with a start*): He! Coming! What's this stranger got to do with it?

ELLIDA: I want to be free, completely, when I go to him.

WANGEL: And what—what good will that do you?

ELLIDA: I won't hide behind the fact of being another man's wife. I won't claim that I have no choice—because then there'd be no decision made.

WANGEL: You talk of choice! Choice, Ellida! Choice in this thing!

ELLIDA: Yes, I must have freedom of choice. Choice either way. To send him away alone—or, as well, to go with him.

WANGEL: Do you know what you're saying? To go with him! To put your whole fate in his hands!

ELLIDA: But I put my whole fate in your hands—without any question.

WANGEL: That's true. But he! He's a total stranger! You hardly know him.

ELLIDA: But I think I knew you even less—and still I went off with you.

WANGEL: At least at that time you knew something of what kind of life you'd be taking on. But here, with him? Just consider! What do you know about him? Nothing! Not even who he is—or what he is.

ELLIDA (*staring into space*): It's true. But that's exactly the horror of it.

WANGEL: Yes—well, it *is* horrible.

ELLIDA: And it's also why, it seems to me, I've got to face it.

WANGEL (*looking at her*): Because you find it horrible?

ELLIDA: Yes. Precisely.

WANGEL (*comes closer*): Tell me, Ellida—what do you really mean when you speak of the horror?

ELLIDA (*after a moment's thought*): It's something that—that terrifies and attracts.

WANGEL: Attracts, too?

ELLIDA: Attracts most of all—I think.

WANGEL (*deliberately*): Ellida—you belong to the sea.

ELLIDA: That's part of the horror.

WANGEL: And part of the horror in you. You both terrify—and attract.

ELLIDA: You think so, Wangel?

WANGEL: I've really never known you—at least, to any depth. I'm beginning to see that now.

ELLIDA: Then you have to set me free! Completely free from whatever's yours! I'm not the person you took me for. Now you can see it yourself. We can separate now as friends—by our own free choice.

WANGEL (*heavily*): It might be best for us both—if we parted—but even so, I just can't! You have for me this same horrifying spell, Ellida, this attraction—that's so powerful in you.

ELLIDA: You can say that?

WANGEL: Let's try to get through this day resolutely—with

calm in our spirits. I don't dare let you go or free you today. I can't take that liberty. Not for your sake, Ellida. I have my right and my duty to defend you.

ELLIDA: Defend me? Against what? There's no threat here from the outside. The horror goes deeper, Wangel. The horror—is the force of attraction in my own mind. And what can you do about that?

WANGEL: I can steady and strengthen you to fight against it.

ELLIDA: Yes—if I want to fight it.

WANGEL: You don't want to?

ELLIDA: That's it—I don't know!

WANGEL: It will all be settled tonight, Ellida—

ELLIDA (*in an outburst*): Yes, to think—! The decision is so near! And for the rest of my life!

WANGEL: And tomorrow—

ELLIDA: Yes, tomorrow! By then the future I was meant for may have been ruined!

WANGEL: You were meant for—?

ELLIDA: A whole, full life of freedom ruined, wasted—for me—and maybe for him.

WANGEL (*in a lower tone, gripping her by the wrist*): Ellida—do you love this stranger?

ELLIDA: Do I—? Oh, how do I know! I only know that for me he has a terrifying attraction, and that—

WANGEL: And that—?

ELLIDA (*tearing herself away*): That I think I belong with him.

WANGEL (*bowing his head*): I begin to understand nearly everything.

ELLIDA: And how can you help against this? What do you prescribe for me?

WANGEL (*looks sadly at her*): Tomorrow—he'll be gone. This misfortune will have blown over. And then I'll be willing to let you go free. We'll dissolve the contract then, Ellida.

ELLIDA: Oh, Wangel—! Tomorrow—then it's too late!

WANGEL (*looking out toward the garden*): The children! We ought to spare them at least—while we can.

(ARNHOLM, BOLETTE, HILDA, *and* LYNGSTRAND *appear in the garden.* LYNGSTRAND *excuses himself and goes out left. The others come into the room.*)

ARNHOLM: We've been making some marvelous plans—
HILDA: We'll be going out on the fjord tonight, and—
BOLETTE: No, don't say anything!

WANGEL: We've been making some plans here, too.

ARNHOLM: Oh—really?

WANGEL: Tomorrow Ellida's going away to Skjoldvik—for a while.

BOLETTE: Going away—?

ARNHOLM: Why, that's a fine idea, Mrs. Wangel.

WANGEL: She wants to go home again. Home to the sea.

HILDA (*darting several steps toward* ELLIDA): You're going? You're leaving us!

ELLIDA (*alarmed*): But, Hilda! What's got into you?

HILDA (*controlling herself*): Oh, it's nothing. (*Under her breath, turning away.*) Go! Go on then!

BOLETTE (*anxiously*): Father—I can see it in your face. You're going away, too—to Skjoldvik.

WANGEL: No, certainly not! I may be out there at times—

BOLETTE: But you'll come back to us—?

WANGEL: I'll be here, too.

BOLETTE: Yes, at times!

WANGEL: My dear child, it has to be. (*He crosses the room.*)

ARNHOLM (*in a whisper to* BOLETTE): We'll talk this over later. (*He follows* WANGEL. *They talk quietly together by the door.*)

ELLIDA (*to* BOLETTE, *her voice lowered*): What was that with Hilda? She looked so upset.

BOLETTE: Haven't you ever noticed what it is that Hilda longs for day and night?

ELLIDA: Longs for?

BOLETTE: Ever since you came to this house.

ELLIDA: No. No, what's that?

BOLETTE: One small expression of love from you.

ELLIDA: Ah—! Then—I do have some purpose here?

(*She clasps her hands tight over her head and stares intently off into space, as if riddled by conflicting thoughts and feelings.* WANGEL *and* ARNHOLM *come forward in hushed conversation.* BOLETTE *goes over and glances into the room to the right, then opens the door wide.*)

BOLETTE: Father dear—the food's on the table—if you'd like to—

WANGEL (*with forced composure*): Is it, dear? That's good. Arnholm, please! Now we'll go drink a parting cup to the health of—of our "lady from the sea."

(*They move toward the door on the right.*)

ACT 5

The far corner of DR. WANGEL's *garden by the carp pond. The deepening twilight of a summer night.* ARNHOLM, BO- LETTE, LYNGSTRAND, *and* HILDA, *in a boat, are punting along the bank from the left.*

HILDA: See, we can easily jump ashore from here!
ARNHOLM: No, no, don't!
LYNGSTRAND: I can't jump, Hilda.
HILDA: And you, Arnholm, can't you jump either?
ARNHOLM: I'd rather pass it up.
BOLETTE: Then let's put in by the bathhouse steps.

(*They pole off to the right. At the same time* BALLESTED *appears on the footpath from the right, carrying music scores and a French horn. He waves to those in the boat, turns and talks to them. Their answers are heard farther and farther off in the distance.*)

BALLESTED: What did you say—? Yes, that's right—for the English steamer. It's her last trip of the year. But if you want to relish the music, you better not wait too long. (*Shouts.*) What? (*Shaking his head.*) Can't hear you!

(ELLIDA, *with a shawl over her head, comes in from the left, followed by* DR. WANGEL.)

WANGEL: But, Ellida, dear—I tell you, there's still plenty of time.
ELLIDA: No, no—there isn't! He can come any moment.
BALLESTED (*outside the garden fence*): Well, good eve- ning, Doctor! Good evening, Mrs. Wangel!
WANGEL (*becoming aware of him*): Oh, is that you? Are we having music tonight?
BALLESTED: Yes. The Wind Ensemble's going to make it- self heard. There's no shortage of festivities these days. Tonight we're saluting the English ship.
ELLIDA: The English ship! Has she been sighted?
BALLESTED: Not yet. But she slips her way in, you know— between the islands. There's no sign of her—and then, sud- denly, there she is.

ELLIDA: Yes—that's just the way it is.

WANGEL (*half to* ELLIDA): Tonight's the last voyage. And then—no more.

BALLESTED: A doleful thought, Doctor. But all the more reasons, as I say, for making a celebration. Ah, me! These delightful summer days will soon be over. The sea-lanes will soon be locked in ice—as the old tragedy has it.

ELLIDA: The sea-lanes locked—yes.

BALLESTED: How sad to think. We've been summer's happy children now for weeks and months. It's hard to reconcile oneself with the dark days coming. Yes, I mean, it is at first. Because, you know, people learn to accli—acclimatize themselves, Mrs. Wangel. Yes, they really do.

(*He bows and goes out left.*)

ELLIDA (*looking out across the fjord*): Oh, this agonizing suspense! This feverish last half hour before the decision.

WANGEL: Then you definitely do want to talk to him yourself?

ELLIDA: I have to talk to him myself. It's the only way I can make a free choice.

WANGEL: You have no choice, Ellida. You haven't the right. I won't permit it.

ELLIDA: You can't keep me from choosing. Neither you nor anyone else. You can forbid me to go with him—if I choose that. You can hold me here by force—against my will. That you can do. But that I choose—choose from the depths of my being—choose him, and not you—if I have to—*that* you can never prevent.

WANGEL: No, you're right. I can't prevent you.

ELLIDA: So I have nothing at all to stop me. Not one earthly tie here at home. I've been so completely without roots in this house, Wangel. I have no place with the children—in their hearts, I mean. I never have. When I go—if I go—either with him tonight, or to Skjoldvik tomorrow—I won't even have a key to give up, or a set of instructions to leave behind about anything at all. That's how rootless—how totally outside of things I've been from the moment I came.

WANGEL: You wanted it that way round.

ELLIDA: No, I didn't. I had no wants this way or that. I've simply left everything just as it was on the day I arrived. It was you, and nobody else, who wanted it like that.

WANGEL: I tried to do what was best for you.

ELLIDA: Yes, Wangel—I know you did! But these things retaliate on us; they take revenge. Now I have nothing to hold me here—no foundation—no support—no impulse toward everything that should have been our dearest common bonds.

WANGEL: Yes, that's clear enough. So you'll have your freedom from tomorrow on. You can live your own life then.

ELLIDA: My own life, you call it! Oh, no, the real thread of my life snapped when I came here to live with you. (*Clenching her fists in a tremor of fear.*) And now, tonight—in half an hour, he'll be here, the man I broke faith with, the man whose word I should have kept sacred, as he kept mine. He's coming to ask me—this one last time—to start my life over—to live a life out of my own truth—the life that terrifies and attracts—and that I *can't* give up, not of my own free will!

WANGEL: Exactly why you need me, as your husband—and your doctor—to assume that power, and act in your own behalf.

ELLIDA: Yes, Wangel, I understand very well. Oh, don't think there aren't times when I'm sure there'd be peace and security for me in taking refuge completely in you—and trying to defy all the tempting, treacherous powers. But I can't. No, no—I can't do it!

WANGEL: Come, Ellida—let's walk up and down by the shore for a while.

ELLIDA: I'd like to. But I don't dare. He said I should wait for him here.

WANGEL: Come along. You have plenty of time.

ELLIDA: You think so?

WANGEL: More than enough, yes.

ELLIDA: Let's walk a bit then.

(*They go off in the foreground to the right. As they depart,* ARNHOLM *and* BOLETTE *appear by the upper bank of the pond.*)

BOLETTE (*noticing the others leaving*): Look—!

ARNHOLM (*softly*): Shh—let them go.

BOLETTE: Have you any idea what's been happening between them the last few days?

ARNHOLM: Have you noticed anything?

BOLETTE: I'll say!

ARNHOLM: Something special?

BOLETTE: Oh, this and that. Haven't you?

ARNHOLM: Oh, I really don't know—

BOLETTE: Yes, you know all right. But you won't come out with it.

ARNHOLM: I think it'll be good for your stepmother to take that little trip.

BOLETTE: You think so?

ARNHOLM: Yes, I'm wondering if it wouldn't be a good thing for all parties if she could get away now and then?

BOLETTE: If she goes home to Skjoldvik tomorrow, she'll never come back here again to us.

ARNHOLM: But, Bolette dear, where did you ever get that notion?

BOLETTE: I'm absolutely convinced. You just wait! You'll see—she won't come back again. At least, not while Hilda and I are around the house.

ARNHOLM: Hilda, too?

BOLETTE: Well, with Hilda it might work out. She's still not much more than a child. And then I think, underneath, she really worships Ellida. But with me, it's another story. A stepmother who's hardly much older than oneself—

ARNHOLM: Bolette—for you it might not be so long before you could get away.

BOLETTE (*fervently*): You mean it! Then you've talked it over with Father?

ARNHOLM: Yes, I've done that.

BOLETTE: well—and what did he say?

ARNHOLM: Hm—of course, right now your father's so absorbed in other things—

BOLETTE: Yes, that's what I told you before.

ARNHOLM: But I did get this much out of him: that you mustn't be counting on any help from him.

BOLETTE: None—!

ARNHOLM: He made his situation quite clear to me. Something of that order, he felt, would be totally out of the realm of possibility for him.

BOLETTE (*reproachfully*): And you can simply stand there and tease me.

ARNHOLM: I'm not teasing at all, Bolette. It's completely up to you whether or not you can break away.

BOLETTE: You say it's up to me?

ARNHOLM: That is, if you really want to enter the world—and learn about everything that interests you most—share in whatever you've longed for here at home—and live a more ample life. What do you say, Bolette?

BOLETTE (*clasping her hands*): My God in heaven—! But—it's all so impossible. If Father won't or can't, then—Because there's no one else I can turn to.

ARNHOLM: Couldn't you accept a helping hand from your old—I mean, your former teacher?

BOLETTE: From you, Mr. Arnholm! You'd be willing to—?

ARNHOLM: To stand by you? Yes, with all my heart. In both word and deed. You can rely on that. So—do you agree? Well? Is it a bargain?

BOLETTE: A bargain! To leave—to see the world—to learn what life really is! It's like some beautiful, unattainable dream.

ARNHOLM: But it all can come true for you now—if you'll try for it.

BOLETTE: So much happiness—it's breathtaking! And you'll help me to it. But—tell me, is it right to take such a gift from a stranger?

ARNHOLM: From me, Bolette, you certainly can. Whatever you need.

BOLETTE (seizing his hands): Yes, I almost believe I can! I don't know why it is, but— (In an outburst of feeling)—oh, I could both laugh and cry for joy! I feel so happy. Oh—so I am going to live, after all. I was beginning to feel so afraid that life would pass me by.

ARNHOLM: That's nothing you have to fear. But now you must tell me very frankly—if there's anything—anything to bind you here.

BOLETTE: Bind me? No, there isn't.

ARNHOLM: No one in particular?

BOLETTE: No one at all. Well, I mean—Father, of course, in a way. And Hilda, too. But—

ARNHOLM: Well—you'd be leaving your father sooner or later. And Hilda will be going her own way, too, before long. It's only a question of time, that's all. But otherwise you've no other ties? No other kind of relationship?

BOLETTE: No, nothing. So I can just as well leave as I wish.

ARNHOLM: Well, if that's the case—then you must leave with me.

BOLETTE (clapping her hands): Oh, God—I can't believe it!

ARNHOLM: Because I hope you have full confidence in me?

BOLETTE: Why, of course.

ARNHOLM: And you feel quite safe in trusting yourself and your future in my hands? You do, don't you?

BOLETTE: Naturally! Why shouldn't I? How can you ask? You're my old teacher—I mean, my teacher from the old days.

ARNHOLM: Not only that. That aspect of it I'd just as soon forget. But—well—anyway you're free, Bolette. There are no ties binding you. So I'm asking you then—if you'd—you'd be willing to join yourself to me—for life.

BOLETTE (*recoiling, startled*): Oh—what are you saying?

ARNHOLM: For the rest of your life, Bolette. If you'll be my wife.

BOLETTE (*half to herself*): No, no, no! This is impossible. Quite impossible.

ARNHOLM: Does it really seem so utterly impossible to you that—?

BOLETTE: But you don't mean—you can't mean what you're saying, Mr. Arnholm! (*Looking at him*) Or—anyway— Is that what you meant when you offered to do so much for me?

ARNHOLM: Now listen to me a minute. I've surprised you considerably, I guess.

BOLETTE: How could something like this—from you—how could it not surprise me?

ARNHOLM: Perhaps you're right. Of course you didn't—and couldn't—know that it was for your sake I made the trip here.

BOLETTE: You came here—for my sake!

ARNHOLM: Yes. Last spring I got a letter from your father. There were some lines in it that gave me the idea—hm—that your memories of me were a little more than—just friendly.

BOLETTE: How could Father write like that?

ARNHOLM: He didn't mean it at all that way. But I persuaded myself into imagining that a young girl was going around the house here, yearning for me to return— No, Bolette, now don't interrupt! And you have to understand—when someone like me, who's past the pride of his youth, has that kind of belief—of illusion—it makes a powerful impression. From then on, there grew in me a warm—and grateful affection for you. I felt I had to come to you—see you again—and tell you that I shared those feelings which I'd dreamed myself into believing you felt for me.

BOLETTE: But now you know it wasn't true! That it was a mistake!

ARNHOLM: It's no help, Bolette. Your image—as I carry it within me—will always be colored now by those mistaken emotions. Maybe you can't understand all this. But it's the way it is.

BOLETTE: Anything like this I never would have believed possible.

ARNHOLM: But now that you know it is—what do you say, Bolette? Won't you promise yourself in—in marriage to me?

BOLETTE: But, Mr. Armholm, to me it's simply unthinkable. You were my teacher. I can't imagine ever being in any other kind of relationship to you.

ARNHOLM: Well, all right—if you really don't think you can— But, in any case, the old relationship is still unchanged.

BOLETTE: What do you mean?

ARNHOLM: Naturally, I stand by my offer, just the same. I'll make sure that you get out and see something of the world—study what interests you—and have a secure and independent life. And I'll see that your future's taken care of. I want you to know you'll always find me a staunch, reliable friend.

BOLETTE: But—Mr. Arnholm—that's all become quite impossible now.

ARNHOLM: Is that impossible, too?

BOLETTE: Yes, isn't that obvious! After what you've told me here—and the answer I gave you—oh, how could you think me capable of helping myself at your expense! There's absolutely nothing I can take from you—nothing after this!

ARNHOLM: You mean you'd rather stay here at home and watch life slipping away from you?

BOLETTE: Oh, that's too horribly depressing to think about!

ARNHOLM: You want to throw away your chance to see the outside world and be part of everything you've longed for? To know there's so infinitely much to life—and that, after all, you've never really experienced any of it? Think well on what you're doing, Bolette.

BOLETTE: Yes, yes—you're very right, Mr. Arnholm.

ARNHOLM: And then when your father's no longer here—maybe to stand alone and helpless in the world. Or else to have to give yourself to another man for whom you—quite possibly—might also feel no affection.

BOLETTE: Oh, yes—I can see quite well how true it is—everything you say. But still—! Or—perhaps—

ARNHOLM (quickly): Well?

BOLETTE (looking irresolutely at him): Perhaps it isn't so utterly impossible, after all—

ARNHOLM: What, Bolette?

BOLETTE: It might do, then—to try what—what you suggested.

ARNHOLM: You mean that perhaps you'd be willing to—? That at least you'd give me the satisfaction of being able to help you as a friend?

BOLETTE: No, no! That's absolutely impossible! No—Mr. Arnholm—if, instead, you'll take me—

ARNHOLM: Bolette! Then you will?

BOLETTE: Yes—I think—I want that.

ARNHOLM: Then you *will* be my wife?

BOLETTE: Yes. If you still think that—that you want me.

ARNHOLM: If I still—! (*Seizes her hand.*) Oh thank you—
thank you, Bolette! All this that you've said—these doubts
you've had—they don't frighten me. If I don't have you
wholeheartedly now, I'll find the ways to win you. Oh, Bolette,
how I'll treasure you!

BOLETTE: Now I can live in the world, in the midst of life.
You promised me that.

ARNHOLM: And I'll keep my word.

BOLETTE: And I can study anything I want.

ARNHOLM: I'll teach you, just as I used to. Remember that
last school year—?

BOLETTE (*musing quietly*): Imagine—to be free—and to
come out—into the unknown. And not to worry about the
future, or scrimping to get along—

ARNHOLM: No, you won't have to waste your thoughts like
that anymore. Which ought to be quite a relief in itself, don't
you think?

BOLETTE: Yes, definitely.

ARNHOLM (*putting his arms around her waist*): Ah, wait
till you see how easy and comfortable we'll be with each
other. And how competently we'll manage things together,
Bolette!

BOLETTE: Yes, I'm beginning to think—I really believe—
this is going to work. (*Looks off to the right and hurriedly
frees herself.*) Ah! Don't say anything yet!

ARNHOLM: Dear, what is it?

BOLETTE: Oh, it's that poor— (*Pointing.*) See, there.

ARNHOLM: Is it your father—?

BOLETTE: No, it's that young sculptor. He's over there
walking with Hilda.

ARNHOLM: Oh, Lyngstrand. What's the matter with him?

BOLETTE: Well, you know how frail and sickly he is.

ARNHOLM: Yes, if it isn't all in his mind.

BOLETTE: No, it's serious enough. He can't live much longer. But maybe it's the best thing for him.

ARNHOLM: How could *that* be the best thing?

BOLETTE: Well, because—because nothing could ever come
of his art, anyway. Let's go before they get here.

ARNHOLM: With the greatest pleasure, dearest. Let's.

(HILDA *and* LYNGSTRAND *appear by the pond.*)

HILDA: Hey—hey! Won't your majesties wait for us?

ARNHOLM: We'd rather stay in the lead.

(*He and* BOLETTE *go out to the left.*)

LYNGSTRAND (*laughs quietly*): It's really delightful here around this hour. Humanity comes in couples. Everyone's two by two.

HILDA (*looking after them*): I could almost swear that he's been courting her.

LYNGSTRAND: Really? Have you noticed something?

HILDA: Oh, yes. It's not too difficult—if you've got eyes in your head.

LYNGSTRAND: Bolette wouldn't have him. I'm positive of that.

HILDA: No. She thinks he's beginning to look horribly old. And also that he's going to be bald soon.

LYNGSTRAND: Those aren't the only reasons. She wouldn't have him, anyhow.

HILDA: How do you know that?

LYNGSTRAND: Because there's someone else she's promised to give her thoughts to.

HILDA: Just her thoughts?

LYNGSTRAND: While he's away, yes.

HILDA: Oh, in other words, it's *you* that she's going to go thinking about!

LYNGSTRAND: Well, it might just be.

HILDA: Did she promise you that?

LYNGSTRAND: Yes, just think—she promised me that! But you mustn't ever tell her you know.

HILDA: Oh, so help me God, I'll be quiet as the grave.

LYNGSTRAND: I think it's awfully kind of her.

HILDA: And when you come back here again—will you get engaged to her? And marry her?

LYNGSTRAND: No, that wouldn't be too good a match. I don't dare think about marrying for the first few years. And when I finally do arrive, then I expect she'll probably be too old for me.

HILDA: But all the same, you want to have her going around thinking about you?

LYNGSTRAND: Well, it's very necessary for me. You know, as an artist. And it's easy enough for her to do, when she hasn't any real vocation in life, anyhow. But it's kind of her, all the same.

HILDA: Do you believe you can work better on your art if you know Bolette's up here thinking about you?

LYNGSTRAND: Yes, I'm convinced of it. To know that someplace on this earth there's a young woman of rare breeding, living quietly in her dreams—of me—why, I think that must be so—so— Well, I really don't know what to call it.

HILDA: You mean—thrilling?

LYNGSTRAND: Thrilling? Yes, it's thrilling; you could call it that. Or something like it. (*Looks at her a moment.*) You're so perceptive, Hilda. Amazingly perceptive. When I come home again, you'll be about the same age your sister is now. Maybe then you'll look like her as well. And maybe you'll have gotten her temperament, too. Almost as if you and she had grown together—in one form, so to speak.

HILDA: Would that please you?

LYNGSTRAND: I really don't know. Yes, I guess it would. But now—for this summer—I'd prefer you to be just yourself alone. Exactly what you are.

HILDA: You like me best that way?

LYNGSTRAND: Yes, I like you very well that way.

HILDA: Hm—tell me—as an artist, do you think it's right for me always to wear these light summer dresses?

LYNGSTRAND: Yes, I think they're just the thing for you.

HILDA: Do you find the bright colors becoming on me?

LYNGSTRAND: Very becoming on you, at least to my taste.

HILDA: But tell me—as an artist—how do you think I'd look in black?

LYNGSTRAND: In black, Hilda?

HILDA: Yes, all in black. Do you think it would set me off well?

LYNGSTRAND: Black really isn't quite the thing for summer. Although you certainly would look striking in black. Expecially with your complexion.

HILDA (*gazing into the distance*): In black right up to the neck. Black ruffles. Black gloves. And a long black veil hanging down behind.

LYNGSTRAND: If you were to dress up like that, Hilda—I'd wish myself into a painter—and I'd paint you as a young, beautiful, grieving widow.

HILDA: Or a young, grieving bride.

LYNGSTRAND: Yes, that would be even better. But you can't really want to dress like that?

HILDA: It's hard to say. But I think it's thrilling.

LYNGSTRAND: Thrilling?

HILDA: Thrilling to think of, yes. (*Points suddenly out to the left.*) Oh, look there!

LYNGSTRAND (*following her stare*): The English steamer!
And she's already docked.

(WANGEL *and* ELLIDA *appear by the pond.*)

WANGEL: No, Ellida, I tell you—you're wrong! (*Notices
the others.*) Well, are you two here? What's the word, Mr.
Lyngstrand—she's not in sight yet, is she?

LYNGSTRAND: The English ship?

WANGEL: What else!

LYNGSTRAND (*pointing*): She's right there, Doctor.

ELLIDA: Ah—! I knew it.

WANGEL: Already come!

LYNGSTRAND: Like a thief in the night, you could say.
Gliding soundlessly in—

WANGEL: You better take Hilda down to the pier. Hurry
up! She'll want to hear the music.

LYNGSTRAND: Yes, we were just now leaving, Doctor.

WANGEL: We may come along later. In a little while.

HILDA (*whispering to* LYNGSTRAND): See, still another couple.

(*She and* LYNGSTRAND *go out through the garden to the
left. During what follows, the music of a brass band is heard
far off out on the fjord.*)

ELLIDA: He's come! He's here! Yes, yes—I can feel that.

WANGEL: You'd best go inside, Ellida. Let me talk to him
alone.

ELLIDA: Oh—it's impossible! Impossible, I tell you!
(*Crying out.*) Oh—there he is, Wangel!

(*The* STRANGER *appears from the left and stops on the
footpath outside the fence.*)

STRANGER (*bowing*): Good evening. So you see I'm back,
Ellida.

ELLIDA: Yes. The hour has come.

STRANGER: Are you ready to leave, or not?

WANGEL: You can see yourself that she's not.

STRANGER: I'm not talking about traveling clothes and that
sort of thing—or whether her trunks are packed. Everything
she needs on the trip I have with me on board. I've also reserved her a cabin. (*To* ELLIDA.) I'm asking, then, if you're
ready to come with me—of your own free will?

ELLIDA: Oh, don't ask me! You mustn't!

(*A ship's bell sounds in the distance.*)

STRANGER: They're ringing the first warning. Now you've got to say yes or no.

ELLIDA (*wringing her hands*): To decide! Decide for the rest of my life! And never the chance to go back!

STRANGER: Never! In half an hour it'll be too late.

ELLIDA (*with a shy, inquiring look*): Why are you so determined not to let me go?

STRANGER: Don't you feel, as I do, that we belong together?

ELLIDA: You mean, because of the promise?

STRANGER: Promises bind no one. Neither man nor woman. I don't let you go—because I can't.

ELLIDA (*in a low, tremulous voice*): Why didn't you come before?

WANGEL: Ellida!

ELLIDA (*in an outburst*): Oh—this power that charms and tempts and allures me—into the unknown! All the force of the sea is in this man!

(*The* STRANGER *climbs over the fence.*)

ELLIDA (*retreating behind* WANGEL): What is it? What do you want?

STRANGER: I can see it and I hear it in you, Ellida—it will be me that you choose in the end.

WANGEL (*steps toward him*): My wife has no choice in this. I'll both decide—and defend—where she's concerned. Yes, defend! If you don't clear out of here—out of this country—and never come back—then you better know what you're in for!

ELLIDA: No, no, Wangel! Don't!

STRANGER: What will you do to me?

WANGEL: I'll have you arrested—as a criminal! Right now, before you board ship! I know all about the murder up at Skjoldvik.

ELLIDA: Oh, Wangel—how can you—?

STRANGER: I was prepared for that. And so— (*Draws a revolver from his breast pocket.*)—so I provided myself with this.

ELLIDA (*flinging herself in front of* WANGEL): No—don't kill him! Kill me instead!

STRANGER: I'm not killing either of you, so don't get excited. This is for my own use. I want to live and die a free man.

ELLIDA (*in a rising tumult of feeling*): I have to say this—
and say it so he can hear! Yes, you can lock me in here!
You've got the power and the means! And that's what you
want to do! But my mind—my thoughts—all my longing
dreams and desire—those you can never constrain! They'll go
raging and hunting out—into the unknown that I was made
for—and that you've shut out for me!

WANGEL (*in quiet pain*): I see it so well, Ellida. Inch by
inch you're slipping away from me. This hunger for the
boundless, the infinite—the unattainable—will finally drive
your mind out completely into darkness.

ELLIDA: Oh, yes, yes—I feel it—like black, soundless wings
hanging over me!

WANGEL: It's not going to come to that. There's no other
way to save you. At least, not that I can see. And so—so I
agree that—our contract's dissolved. Right now, this moment.
Now you can choose your own path—in full freedom.

ELLIDA (*stares at him briefly as if struck dumb*): Is that
true—true—what you're saying? You mean it—with all your
heart?

WANGEL: Yes, I mean it—with all my miserable heart.

ELLIDA: Then you *can*—? You can let this *be*?

WANGEL: Yes, I can. Because I love you so much.

ELLIDA (*her voice soft and tremulous*): Have I grown so
close—and so dear to you?

WANGEL: With the years and the living together, yes.

ELLIDA (*striking her hands together*): And I—who've been
so blind!

WANGEL: Your thoughts have gone other ways. But now—
now you're entirely free from me—my life—my world. Now
you can pick up the thread of your own true existence again.
Because now you can choose in freedom—on your own responsibility.

ELLIDA (*hands to her head, staring blankly at* WANGEL):
In freedom—responsible to myself! Responsible? How this—
transforms everything!

(*The ship's bell rings again.*)

STRANGER: Ellida, listen! It's ringing for the last time now.
Come!

ELLIDA (*turns, looks fixedly at him, and speaks in a firm
voice*): I could never go with you after this.

STRANGER: Never!

ELLIDA (*holding tight to* WANGEL): No—I'll never leave
you now!

WANGEL: Ellida—Ellida!

STRANGER: Then it's over?

ELLIDA: Yes. Over forever.

STRANGER: I see. There's something stronger here than my will.

ELLIDA: Your will hasn't a shred of power over me now. To me you've become a dead man who came up out of the sea—and who's drifting back down again. There's no terror in you now. And no attraction.

STRANGER: Good-bye, then. (*He vaults over the fence.*) From now on, you're nothing more than—a shipwreck I barely remember. (*Goes out to the left.*)

WANGEL (*looks at her a moment*): Ellida, your mind is like the sea—it ebbs and flows. What brought the change?

ELLIDA: Oh, don't you understand that the change came— that it *had* to come—when I could choose in freedom?

WANGEL: And the unknown—it doesn't attract you anymore?

ELLIDA: It neither terrifies nor attracts. I've been able to see deep into it—and I could have plunged in, if I'd wanted to. I could have chosen it now. And that's why, also, I could reject it.

WANGEL: I begin to understand you—little by little. You think and feel in images—and in visions. Your longing and craving for the sea—your attraction toward him, toward this stranger—these were the signs of an awakened, growing rage for freedom in you. Nothing else.

ELLIDA: Oh, I don't know what to say. Except that you've been a good doctor for me. You found, and you dared to use the right treatment—the only one that could help me.

WANGEL: Yes—when it comes to extreme cases, we doctors have to risk desperate remedies. But now—will you be coming back to me, Ellida?

ELLIDA: Yes, my dear, faithful Wangel—I'm coming back to you now. I can now, because I come to you freely—and on my own.

WANGEL (*regarding her warmly*): Ellida! Ellida! Ah—to think that now we can live wholly for one another—

ELLIDA: And with the shared memories of our lives. Yours—and mine.

WANGEL: Yes, darling, we will.

ELLIDA: And with our two children, Wangel.

WANGEL: You call them *ours!*

ELLIDA: They're not mine—but I'll win them to me.

WANGEL: Ours—! (*Joyfully and quickly kissing her hands.*) Oh—how can I thank you for that one word!

(HILDA, BALLESTED, LYNGSTRAND, ARNHOLM, *and* BOLETTE *come from the left into the garden. At the same time a number of the young people of the town, along with summer visitors, come along the footpath outside.*)

HILDA (*in a whisper to* LYNGSTRAND): Why, she and Father—they look as if they're just engaged!

BALLESTED (*having overheard*): But it's summertime, little one.

ARNHOLM (*glancing at* WANGEL *and* ELLIDA): There, she's casting off now—for England.

BOLETTE (*going to the fence*): Here's the place to see her best.

LYNGSTRAND: The last sailing of the year.

BALLESTED: The sea-lanes will soon be locked in ice, as the poet says. It's sad, Mrs. Wangel. And now we'll lose you, too, for a while. Tomorrow, I hear, you're off for Skjoldvik.

WANGEL: No, not anymore. We changed our minds this evening.

ARNHOLM (*looking from one to the other*): No—really!

HILDA (*goes to* ELLIDA): You'll stay with us, after all?

ELLIDA: Yes, Hilda dear—if you'll have me.

HILDA (*struggling between joy and tears*): Oh—if I'll have—what an idea!

ARNHOLM (*to* ELLIDA): Well, this is quite a surprise—!

ELLIDA (*smiling gravely*): You see, Mr. Arnholm—you remember, we talked about it yesterday. Once you've really become a land animal, then there's no going back again—into the sea. Or the life that belongs to the sea, either.

BALLESTED: But that's just how it is with my mermaid.

ELLIDA: Yes, much the same.

BALLESTED: Except for the difference—that the mermaid dies of it. But people, human beings—they can acclam—acclimatize themselves. Yes, yes—that's the thing, Mrs. Wangel. They can ac-cli-matize themselves.

ELLIDA: Yes, they can, Mr. Ballested—once they're free.

WANGEL: And responsible, Ellida.

ELLIDA (*quickly takes his hand*): How very true!

(*The great steamer glides silently out over the fjord. The music can be heard closer in toward shore.*)

MISS JULIE

August Strindberg

Characters

MISS JULIE, *aged 25.*
JEAN, *a valet, aged 30.*
KRISTIN, *a cook, aged 35.*

The action takes place in the count's kitchen on Midsummer Eve

(*A large kitchen. The ceiling and side walls are concealed by hangings and draperies. The wall at the back runs obliquely up the stage from the left. On it, to the left, are two shelves with utensils of copper, brass, iron, and tin. The shelves are fringed with crinkled paper. A little to the right, three-fourths of the great arched doorway, with two glass doors, through which are seen a fountain with a Cupid, lilac shrubs in flower, and the tops of some Italian poplars.*

To the left of the stage is the corner of a large tiled range and a part of the chimney-hood.

On the right protrudes one end of the servants' dinner table of white pine, with some chairs beside it.

The stove is decorated with birch boughs: the floor strewn with twigs of juniper.

On the end of the table is a large Japanese spice-jar filled with lilac blossoms.

A refrigerator, a scullery table, and a washstand.

A large, old-fashioned bell above the door, and on the left of the door a speaking-tube.

KRISTIN *is standing by the stove, frying something in a frying pan. She is wearing a light cotton dress and a cook's apron.* JEAN *comes in, dressed in livery and carrying a pair of large riding boots, with spurs, which he puts down on a conspicuous part of the floor.*)

JEAN: Miss Julie's mad again to-night: absolutely mad!
KRISTIN: So you're back again, are you?
JEAN: I took the Count to the station, and as I passed the barn on my way home I went in and danced, and who should I see but the young lady leading the dance with the game-keeper. But the moment she catches sight of me she rushes straight up to me and asks me to dance the ladies' waltz. And

[241]

her sadism w/ men : her need to Dominate

then she danced like—well, I've never seen the like of it. She's mad!

KRISTIN: That she's always been, but never like this last fortnight since the engagement was broken off.

JEAN: I wonder what really was at the bottom of that affair! A fine fellow, wasn't he, though not well off. Oh, but they're so full of whims! (*Sits down at the end of the table.*) Anyhow, it's curious that a young lady—ahem!—should prefer to stay at home with the servants—eh?—rather than go with her father to see her relations?

KRISTIN: I expect she feels a bit shy after that set-to with her young man.

JEAN: Very likely! Anyhow, he could hold his own—that young fellow! Do you know how it happened, Kristin? I saw it myself, though I didn't want to let them see I did.

KRISTIN: You saw it, did you?

JEAN: I did. They were in the stable-yard one evening and our young lady was "training" him, as she called it. D'you know what that was? Why, she was making him jump over her riding-whip the way you teach a dog to jump. Twice he jumped, and got a cut with the whip each time; but the third time he snatched the whip from her and broke it into a thousand pieces. And then he went off.

KRISTIN: So that's how it was! Well, I never!

JEAN: Yes, that's how that was! But what have you got for me there, Kristin?

KRISTIN (*putting what she has cooked on a plate and placing it in front of* JEAN): Oh, just a little kidney that I cut from the veal!

JEAN (*smelling the food*): Splendid! My great *délice!* (*Feeling the plate*) But you might have warmed the plate!

KRISTIN: Well, if you aren't more fussy than the Count himself—when you give your mind to it! (*Pulls his hair gently.*)

JEAN (*annoyed*): Don't go pulling my hair! You know how sensitive I am.

KRISTIN: There, there now! It was only love, you know!

(JEAN *begins to eat.* KRISTIN *opens a bottle of beer.*)

JEAN: Beer? On Midsummer Eve? No, thank you! I've got something better than that! (*Opens a drawer in the table and takes out a bottle of red wine with yellow seal.*) Yellow seal, you observe! Now give me a glass. A wineglass, of course, when one drinks *neat!*

KRISTIN (*goes back to the stove and puts a small saucepan on it*): Lord help the woman who gets *you* for a husband! Such an old fusser!

JEAN: Oh nonsense! You'd be glad enough to get such a smart fellow as I am! I don't think it's done you much harm *my* being known as your sweetheart! (*Tastes the wine.*) Fine! Remarkably fine! Might be just a shade warmer! (*Warms the glass in his hands.*) We bought this at Dijon, four francs the litre—without the bottle; and then there was the duty!— What are you cooking there—making that infernal smell?

KRISTIN: Oh, some devil's stuff Miss Julie wants for Diana.

JEAN: You should be more refined in your language, Kristin! But why should you have to cook for that cur on the eve of a holiday? Is the dog ill then?

KRISTIN: Yes, she's ill! She's been sneaking about with the pug at the lodge—and now things have gone wrong—and that, you see, the young lady won't hear of.

JEAN: The young lady is too stuck up in some ways and not enough in others—just like the Countess was while she was alive. She was at home in the kitchen and the cowsheds, yet she would never go out driving with one horse only; she went about with dirty cuffs, but she would have the coronet on the buttons. Our young "lady—to come back to her— doesn't take any care about herself or her person. I might almost say that she's not refined. When she was dancing in the barn just now she snatched away the gamekeeper from Anna's side and actually asked him to dance with her. We shouldn't do that sort of thing ourselves; but that's what happens when the gentry try to behave like common people: they *become* common. But she's a fine woman! Magnificent! Ah, what shoulders! And—and so on!

KRISTIN: Now then, don't overdo it! Clara has dressed her, and I know what she says.

JEAN: Oh, Clara! You're always jealous of each other! But I've been out riding with her. . . . And look at her dancing!

KRISTIN: Now then, Jean! Won't you dance with me when I'm ready?

JEAN: Of course I will.

KRISTEN: Promise?

JEAN: Promise? If I say I will, of course I will! Well, thanks for the supper. It was very nice! (*Replaces the cork in the bottle*.)

JULIE (*in the doorway, speaking to someone outside*): Go on. I'll join you in a minute.

(JEAN *slips the bottle into the drawer and rises respectfully.* JULIE *comes in and goes up to* KRISTIN *by the looking-glass.*)

Well, have you finished it?

(KRISTIN *makes a sign that* JEAN *is present.*)

JEAN (*gallantly*): Have the ladies some secret between them? SHOCKING

JULIE (*striking him in the face with her handkerchief*): Don't be inquisitive!

JEAN: Oh, what a lovely smell of violets!

JULIE (*coquettishly*): What impudence! So you're an expert in scents too, are you? Dancing you're certainly good at. . . . There now, don't peep! Go away!

JEAN (*pertly, but politely*): Is it some witches' broth for Midsummer Eve you ladies are brewing? Something to tell one's fortune by in the star of fate, and so behold one's future love?

JULIE (*sharply*): You'd want good eyes to see *that!* (*To* KRISTIN) Put it into a pint bottle and cork it well. Now come and dance a schottische with me, Jean.

JEAN (*hesitating*): I don't want to be rude to anybody, but I'd promised Kristin this dance—

JULIE: Well, but she can have another instead—can't Kristin? Won't you lend me Jean?

KRISTIN: That's not for me to say. Since the young lady is so condescending it isn't for him to say no. Be off, now! And be thankful for the honour.

JEAN: Speaking frankly—no offence meant of course—I'm wondering if it's wise of Miss Julie to dance twice running with the same partner, especially as people here are only too ready to put their own construction on—

JULIE (*flaring up*): What do you mean? What sort of construction? What are you hinting at?

JEAN (*submissively*): As you won't understand I must speak more plainly. It doesn't look well to prefer one of your dependents to others who are expecting the same unusual honour—

JULIE: Prefer! What an idea! I'm surprised at you! I, the mistress of the house, honour the servants' ball with my presence, and now that I really do want to dance I intend to dance with someone who can guide and not make me look ridiculous.

JEAN: Just as you wish, Miss Julie! I am at your service.

JULIE (*gently*): Don't take it as a command! To-night we're happy people enjoying a holiday, and all questions of rank are set aside! Now give me your arm. Don't worry, Kristin! I shan't take your sweetheart away from you!

(JEAN *offers her his arm and leads her out.*)

PANTOMIME: *Played as though the actress were really alone. When desirable she turns her back on the audience. Does not look towards the spectators. Does not hurry, as though she were afraid the audience might become impatient.*

KRISTIN *alone. Soft violin music in the distance, in schottische time.* KRISTIN, *humming the tune, clears the table where* JEAN *has been sitting, washes the plate at the scullery board, dries it, and puts it into a cupboard.*

After that she removes her apron, takes out a small looking-glass from a table drawer, and leans it against the jar of lilac on the table. Lights a candle and heats a hairpin, with which she curls her front hair.

Then she goes to the door and listens. Comes back to the table. Discovers the handkerchief which MISS JULIE *has left behind; picks it up and smells it. Then she spreads it out abstractedly, pulls it straight, smooths it and folds it in four, and so on.*)

JEAN (*coming in alone*): Well, she really *is* mad! The way she danced! With everybody standing behind the doors grinning at her. What do you think about it, Kristin?

KRISTIN: Oh, she's not very well just now. And that always makes her a bit queer. But won't you come and dance with me now? STRIND.S REF TO PERIOD DISGUISED HERE

JEAN: You aren't angry with me for throwing you over—

KRISTIN: Of course not—not for a little thing like that. Besides, I know my place—

JEAN (*putting his arm round her waist*): You're a sensible girl, Kristin, and you ought to make a good wife—

JULIE (*comes in, unpleasantly surprised; with assumed jocularity*): Well, you *are* a nice cavalier, running away from your lady!

JEAN: On the contrary, Miss Julie; I have, as you see, hurried back to find the one I deserted!

JULIE (*changing her note*): Do you know there's not a

man that can dance like you!—But why are you in livery on a holiday evening? Take it off at once!

JEAN: Then I must ask you to go away for a moment; my black coat is hanging up here. (*Indicates the place and goes towards the right.*)

JULIE: Are you shy because of me? Just changing your coat? Go into your room then, and come back. Or you can stay here, and I'll turn my back.

JEAN: With your permission, Miss Julie! (*Goes towards the right. One of his arms is visible while he changes his coat.*)

JULIE (*to* KRISTIN): Tell me, Kristin: is Jean engaged to you that he's so intimate?

KRISTIN: Engaged? Yes, if you like! We call it that.

JULIE: Call?

KRISTIN: But you've been engaged yourself, my lady, and—

JULIE: Yes, we were properly engaged—

KRISTIN: But it didn't come to anything for all that—

(JEAN *comes in, in a black frock-coat and black bowler.*)

STARTS THE SCENE OF TEASING

JULIE: *Trés gentil, monsieur Jean! Trés gentil!*

JEAN: *Vous voulez plaisanter, madame!*

JULIE: *Et vous voulez parler français!* Where did you learn that?

JEAN: In Switzerland, while I was acting as *sommelier* at one of the largest hotels in Lucerne.

JULIE: But you look like a gentleman in that frock-coat! *Charmant!* (*Sits down at the table.*)

JEAN: Oh, you flatter me!

JULIE (*offended*): Flatter you?

JEAN: My natural modesty does not permit me to think that you are paying genuine compliments to one in my position. Consequently I take the liberty of assuming that you were exaggerating, or, in other words, flattering.

JULIE: Where did you learn to make speeches like that? I suppose you've been to the theatre a great deal?

JEAN: I have indeed! I've been about a lot, I have!

JULIE: But you were born in this neighbourhood?

JEAN: My father was a labourer on the district attorney's estate close by. I must have seen you as a child, though you never took any notice of me!

JULIE: Well, really!

JEAN: Yes, I remember one occasion especially. . . . No, I can't tell you about that!

Builds in intensity
→ to p 250 with her slapping
him
Miss Julie   [247]

JULIE: Oh, but do! Yes, just for once!

JEAN: No, I really cannot now! Another time, perhaps.

JULIE: Another time means no time. Is it so risky now?

JEAN: Not risky at all; but I'd rather not. Look at her there! (*Points to* KRISTIN, *who has fallen asleep on a chair by the stove.*)

JULIE: She'll make a nice sort of wife! Perhaps she snores too?

JEAN: No, but she talks in her sleep.

JULIE (*sarcastically*): How do you know she talks in her sleep?

JEAN (*impudently*): I've heard her!

(*A pause during which they look at each other.*) Sexual tension

JULIE: Why don't you sit down?

JEAN: I cannot take that liberty in your presence!

JULIE: But if I order you to?

JEAN: Then I obey.

JULIE: Sit down, then! No, wait! Can you give me something to drink first?

JEAN: I don't know what we've got here in the refrigerator. I fancy it's only beer.

JULIE: Don't say *only* beer! My tastes are simple and I prefer it to wine.

JEAN (*takes a bottle of beer from the refrigerator and opens it; fetches a glass and a plate from the cupboard and serves the beer*): Allow me!

JULIE: Thank you! Won't you have some yourself?

JEAN: I am not very fond of beer, but if your ladyship commands—

JULIE: Commands? I imagine that a polite cavalier would keep his lady company.

JEAN: Very true! (*Opens a bottle and fetches a glass.*)

JULIE: Drink my health now!

(JEAN *hesitates.*)

I really believe the fellow's shy!

JEAN (*kneeling, and raising his glass with mock solemnity*): To the health of my lady!

JULIE: Bravo! Now you must kiss my shoe too, and then everything will be quite perfect.

(JEAN *hesitates. Then he takes hold of her foot boldly and kisses it lightly.*) very sexual instead of very menial

Splendid! You ought to have been an actor.

JEAN (*getting up*): This can't go on any longer, my lady! Somebody may come in and see us.

JULIE: What would that matter?

JEAN: People would talk—that's all! If you only knew how their tongues went, up there just now, you—

JULIE: What sort of things did they say? Tell me! Sit down, please.

JEAN (*sitting down*): I don't want to hurt you, but they made use of expressions—which threw suspicions of a kind which ... well, you can imagine that for yourself. You are no longer a child, and when a lady is seen drinking alone with a man—not to say a servant—at night—well—

JULIE: Well, what? Besides, we're not alone. Kristin is here.

JEAN: Yes, asleep!

JULIE: Then I'll wake her up. (*Gets up.*) Kristin! Are you asleep?

KRISTIN (*in her sleep*): Bla-bla-bla-bla!

JULIE: Kristin!—What a sleeper!

KRISTIN (*in her sleep*): The Count's boots are clean—put the coffee on—in one moment—heigh-ho—pouff!

JULIE (*taking her by the nose*): Do wake up!

JEAN (*sternly*): One shouldn't disturb a sleeper!

JULIE (*sharply*): What?

JEAN: A woman who has stood by the stove all day long may well be tired at night. Besides, one ought to respect sleep. . . .

JULIE (*changing her tone*): A pretty thought: it does you credit! Thank you. (*Gives* JEAN *her hand.*) Now come out and pick a few lilacs for me.

(*During the following scene* KRISTIN *wakes up and walks sleepily to the right on her way to bed.*)

JEAN: With you, my lady?

JULIE: With me.

JEAN: That won't do! It simply won't!

JULIE: I can't understand your ideas. Is it possible that you're imagining something?

JEAN: Not I: the people.

JULIE: What? That I'm in love with my valet?

JEAN: I'm not a conceited man, but one has seen such cases—and to the people nothing is sacred!

JULIE: You're an aristocrat, I suppose!

JEAN: Yes. I am.

JULIE: I'm stepping down—

JEAN: Take my advice, my lady, and don't step down! No one will believe that you step down of your own accord. People will always say that you're falling down.

JULIE: I have a higher opinion of the people than you have. Come and put it to the test! Come! (*She holds him fast with her eye.*)

JEAN: You're very strange, you know!

JULIE: Perhaps, but so are you! Besides, everything is strange! Life, humanity, everything—slush that is whirled, whirled along the water, till it sinks, sinks! There's a dream of mine which comes back to me now and then; I remember it now. I have climbed to the top of a pillar, and am sitting there without seeing any possibility of getting down. When I look down I get dizzy, and yet get down I must, though I haven't the courage to throw myself down. I can't hold on, and I long to be able to fall; but I don't fall. And yet I have no peace till I am down, no rest till I am down, down, on the ground! And if I did reach the ground I should want to be down in the earth. . . . Have you ever felt like that?

JEAN: No. I usually dream that I'm lying under a tall tree in a dark wood. I want to be up, up at the top, to look out over the bright landscape where the sun is shining, and plunder the bird's nest where the golden eggs lie. So I climb and climb, but the stem of the tree is so thick and so smooth, and it's such a long way to the first branch. But I know that if I could only reach the first branch I should get to the top as easily as if I were on a ladder. I have never reached it yet; but reach it I shall, if only in my dreams!

JULIE: Here I am, chattering to you about dreams! Come now. Just into the park.

(*She offers him her arm and they go towards the door.*)

JEAN: We must sleep on nine midsummer flowers to-night: then our dreams will come true. Miss Julie!

(JULIE *and* JEAN *turn round at the door.* JEAN *puts his hand up to one eye.*)

JULIE: Let me see what you've got in your eye!

JEAN: Oh, it's nothing—just a speck of dust; it'll soon be gone.

JULIE: My sleeve must have brushed against it. Sit down and I'll help you. (*She takes him by the arm and makes him sit down; takes hold of his head and bends it backward; tries*

to remove the dust with the corner of her handkerchief.) Sit
still now, quite still! (*Slaps him on the hand.*) Do what I tell
you now! I do believe he's trembling, the great big fellow!
(*Feels his biceps.*) And such arms too!

JEAN (*warningly*): Miss Julie!   *The temptress*

JULIE: Yes, *Monsieur* Jean!

JEAN: *Attention! Je ne suis qu'un homme!*

JULIE: *Will* you sit still!— There! Now it's out! Kiss my
hand and say thank you!

JEAN (*getting up*): Miss Julie, listen to me. Kristin has
gone to bed now. Will you listen to me!

JULIE: Kiss my hand first!

JEAN: Listen to me!

JULIE: Kiss my hand first!

JEAN: Very well: but you'll have only yourself to blame!

JULIE: For what?

JEAN: For what? Are you a child at twenty-five? Don't
you know it's dangerous to play with fire?

JULIE: Not for me; I'm insured!   *The arrogance*

JEAN (*bluntly*): No, that you're not! And even if you are,
there are inflammable stores close by!

JULIE: Yourself, I suppose?

JEAN: Yes. Not because it is I, but because I'm a young
man—

JULIE: Of prepossessing appearance—what incredible conceit! A Don Juan perhaps? Or a Joseph? On my soul, I think
you must be a Joseph!

JEAN: Do you think so?

JULIE: I almost fear it!

(JEAN *goes boldly up to her and tries to clasp her round
the waist to kiss her.*)   *Her ambivalence*

(*Boxing his ears.*) Impudence!

JEAN: Is that serious or a joke?

JULIE: Serious!

JEAN: Then what happened just before was also serious!
Your play is much too serious, and that's the danger of it!
Now I'm tired of play and I beg leave to return to my work.
The Count's boots must be ready in time, and it's long past
midnight.

JULIE: Put those boots away!

JEAN: No. This is my work and I must do it. I never un-
dertook to be your playfellow, and I never can be that. I
consider myself too good for it!

JULIE: You are proud!

NOW HE'S READY! TO PLAY THE GAME

JEAN: In some ways, in other ways not.

JULIE: Have you ever been in love?

JEAN: We don't use that word, but I've been fond of several girls, and once I got ill because I couldn't have the one I wanted: ill, mark you, like the princes in the *Thousand and One Nights* who couldn't eat or drink from sheer love!

JULIE: Who was it?

(JEAN *is silent.*)

Who was it?

JEAN: You can't make me say that.

JULIE: If I ask you as an equal, as a—friend! Who was it?

JEAN: It was you!

JULIE (*sitting down*): How priceless! . . .

JEAN: Yes, if you like! It was ridiculous! That, you see, was the story which I wouldn't tell you just now, but now I will.

ABOVE = BELOW - CLEAN - DIRTY

Do you know how the world looks from below? You don't. Like hawks and falcons, whose backs one rarely sees because they usually hover above us! I used to live in the labourer's cottage with seven brothers and sisters and a pig, out in the grey fields where there wasn't a single tree! But from the windows I could see the Count's park wall with apple trees above it. It was the Garden of Eden; and a multitude of frowning angels with flaming swords stood there keeping watch over it. But none the less I and some other boys found the way to the Tree of Life.— You despise me now?

JULIE: Oh, all boys steal apples.

JEAN: You may say that now, but you despise me all the same. No matter! One day I went into the Paradise with my mother to weed the onion beds. Close to the garden stood a Turkish pavilion, shaded by jasmine and overgrown with honeysuckle. I had no idea what it might be used for, but I had never seen such a beautiful building. People went in and out of it, and one day the door was left open. I crept up and saw the walls covered with pictures of kings and emperors, and there were red curtains on the windows, with fringes on them—now you understand what I mean. I— (*Breaks off a lilac blossom and hoods it under* JULIE'S *nose*)—I had never been inside the castle, never seen anything but the church— but this was more beautiful; and whatever course my thoughts took they always went back—to that. Then gradually arose the desire to taste, just for once, the full pleasure of—*enfin*, I crept in, saw, and admired. Then I heard someone coming!

There was only one exit for members of the family, but for me there was another and I had to choose that.

(JULIE, *who has taken up the lilac blossom, lets it drop on the table.*)

So I took to my heels, plunged through a raspberry bed, darted across some strawberry beds, and came up on to the rose terrace. There I caught sight of a pink dress and a pair of white stockings—that was you. I lay down under a heap of weeds—right under it, I tell you—under prickly thistles and damp, evil-smelling earth. And I watched you going about among the roses, and I thought to myself: "If it's true that a thief may enter into heaven and dwell with the angels, it's curious that a labourer's child here on God's earth cannot come into the castle park and play with the Count's daughter!"

JULIE (*sentimentally*): Do you think all poor children think the the same as you did then?

JEAN (*doubtfully at first, then with conviction*): All poor—yes—of course! Of course!

JULIE: It must be terrible to be poor!

JEAN (*with deep distress, much exaggerated*): Oh, Miss Julie! Oh!—A dog may lie on the Countess's sofa, a horse be stroked on the nose by a young lady; but a servant—(*Changes his tone.*) Well, now and then you find a man with enough stuff in him to pull himself up into the world; but how often does that happen? However, do you know what I did next? I jumped into the millstream with my clothes on, was pulled out, and got a thrashing. But the following Sunday, when my father and all the others went off to my grandmother's, I contrived to stay at home. So I washed with soap and hot water, put on my best clothes, and went to church in order to see you! I saw you and went home, determined to die; but I wanted to die beautifully and comfortably, without pain. And then I remembered that it was dangerous to sleep under an elder bush. We had a large one, just then in bloom. I robbed it of all it had, and then made my bed in the oats-chest. Have you noticed how smooth oats are? Soft to the touch as the human skin! . . . Well, I shut the lid and closed my eyes; then fell asleep, and woke up feeling really ill. But I didn't die, as you see.

What I wanted—I really don't know! There was no hope of winning you—but you were a sign to me of the hopelessness of getting out of the circle in which I was born.

JULIE: You tell stories charmingly, you know! Did you ever go to school?

JEAN: Only for a short time. But I've read a good many novels, and gone to theatres. Besides that, I've listened to the conversation of refined people; and I've learnt most from them.

JULIE: So you stand about listening to what we say!

JEAN: Certainly! And I've heard a lot, I have, sitting on the coach-box or rowing the boat. Once I heard your ladyship and a girl friend . . .

JULIE: Oh? And what did you hear?

JEAN: Well, it's not very easy to tell you; but I must say I was rather surprised; I couldn't think where you'd learnt all those words. Perhaps, at bottom, there isn't so much difference as one thinks between one human being and another.

JULIE: For shame! We don't behave like you when we're engaged.

JEAN (*looking hard at her*): Is that a fact? Really, I shouldn't bother to make yourself out so innocent. . . .

JULIE: The man I gave my love to was a scoundrel.

JEAN: That's what you always say—afterwards.

JULIE: Always?

JEAN: Always, I believe—since I've heard the expression several times before on similar occasions.

JULIE: What sort of occasions?

JEAN: Like the one in question! The last time—

JULIE (*getting up*): I won't hear any more!

JEAN: *She* didn't want to either—strange to say. Now may I go to bed?

JULIE (*gently*): Go to bed on Midsummer Eve?

JEAN: Yes! Dancing with the riff-raff up there doesn't really amuse me.

JULIE: Get the key of the boat-house and take me out for a row on the lake; I want to see the sunrise!

JEAN: Is that prudent?

JULIE: That sounds as if you were anxious about your reputation!

JEAN: Why not? I don't want to be ridiculous. I don't want to be discharged without a character when I want to settle down. Moreover, I feel that I am more or less under an obligation to Kristin.

JULIE: Oh, so it's Kristin then. . . .

JEAN: Yes, but you too. Take my advice and go to bed!

JULIE: Am I to obey you?

JEAN: For once; for your own sake! I implore you! The night is far gone, sleepiness intoxicates, and one's head grows hot! Go to bed! Besides, if I'm not mistaken, I hear the people coming this way to look for me. If they find us here you're lost!

(*The Chorus approaches, singing*:)

> Two wives from the woods came walking,
>   Tridiridi-ralla tridiridi-ra.
> And one had a hole in her stocking,
>   Tridiridi-ralla-la.
>
> Their talk was of hundreds of dalers,
>   Tridiridi-ralla tridiridi-ra.
> Yet between them they'd hardly a daler,
>   Tridiridi-ralla-ra.
>
> No garland need I give you,
>   Tridiridi-ralla tridiridi-ra.
> For another, alas, I must leave you,
>   Tridiridi-ralla, ra!

condescending

JULIE: I know my people and I love them, as they love me. Let them come and you'll see!

JEAN: No, Miss Julie, they don't love you. They accept your food, but they spit at it! Believe me! Listen to them; just listen to what they're singing! No, don't listen to them!

JULIE: What are they singing?

JEAN: Some scurrilous verses! About you and me!

JULIE: Abominable! How disgraceful! And how sneaking!

JEAN: The rabble are always cowardly. In this sort of fight one can only run away!

JULIE: Run away? But where? We can't go out by the door! And we can't get into Kristin's room!

JEAN: Very well! Into mine then! Necessity knows no law. Besides, you can trust me, your true, sincere, and respectful friend!

JULIE: But think—think if they should look for you there!

JEAN: I shall bolt the door, and if they try to break in I shall shoot! Come! (*On his knees.*) Come!

JULIE (*meaningly*): Will you promise? ...

JEAN: I swear it!

(JULIE *goes out quickly to the right*, JEAN *follows her excitedly.*)

(BALLET. *The peasants enter, in holiday attire, with flowers in their hats. A fiddler leads the procession. A barrel of small*

*beer and a keg of spirits, decorated with greenery, are placed
on the table. Glasses are fetched and drinking begins. Then
they form a circle and sing and dance to the tune "Two
wives from the woods came walking."*

When this is finished they leave the room, singing.

JULIE *comes in alone; gazes on the havoc made of the
kitchen; claps her hands together. Then she takes her pow-
der-puff and powders her face.)* She's been seduced

JEAN (*comes in excitedly*): There, you see! And you heard
too! Do you think it possible to remain here?

JULIE: No, I do not. But what are we to do?

JEAN: Run away, travel, far away from here!

JULIE: Travel? Yes, but where?

JEAN: To Switzerland, to the Italian lakes; you've never
been there, have you?

JULIE: No. Is it nice there?

JEAN: Ah! It's eternal summer—orange trees, laurels! Glorious!

JULIE: But what are we to do when we get there?

JEAN: I'll start a hotel: first-class accommodation and
first-class customers. his plan in life anyway

JULIE: A hotel?

JEAN: Yes, there's life for you! New faces continually, and
new languages; not a minute's leisure for brooding or nerves;
no worrying about something to do—the work makes itself:
bells that ring night and day, whistling trains and 'buses coming and going; and gold pieces rolling along the counter.
There's life for you!

JULIE: Yes, that is life. And what about me?

JEAN: Mistress of the house, chief ornament of the firm.
With your looks ... and your style—oh—success is a certainty! Magnificent! You sit like a queen in the office and set
your slaves in motion by pressing an electric button; the
guests file past your throne and shyly place their treasures on
your table—you can't imagine how people tremble when they
get a bill in their hands—I'll salt the accounts and you shall
sugar them with your prettiest smiles—ah, let's get away
from here. (*Takes a time-table out of his pocket.*) At once,
by the next train! We're in Malmö at six-thirty; Hamburg
eight-forty in the morning; Frankfort-Basle in a day, and
Como, by the St. Gothard line, in—let me see—three days.
Three days!

JULIE: That's all very well! But, Jean—you must give me

courage—tell me that you love me! Come and put your arms around me!

JEAN (*hesitating*): I should like to—but I dare not! Not again in this house. I love you, Miss Julie! Without doubt—can you doubt it?

JULIE (*shyly, with true womanly feeling*): Miss Julie! Call me Julie! There are no longer any barriers between us two!—Call me Julie!

JEAN (*uneasily*): I cannot! There are barriers still between us, as long as we stay in this house. There is the past, there is the Count—I have never met any one for whom I felt such respect: I've only to see his gloves lying on a chair and I feel small: I've only to hear his bell upstairs and I start like a shying horse: and now when I see his boots standing there so stiff and proud, I feel my back beginning to bend! (*Kicks the boots.*) Superstition, prejudice, taught us from childhood—but as easily forgotten again. Only come to another country, a republic, and they'll bow to the earth before my porter's livery. Bow to the earth, I tell you! But *I* shall not! I am not born to bow to the earth; for there's stuff in me—there is character; and if only I can set my foot on the first branch you shall see me climb! To-day I'm a valet, but next year I shall be a man of property: in ten years I shall be living on my own dividends; and then I shall go to Roumania, get myself an order, and may—mark you. I say *may*—end my days as a Count!

JULIE: Splendid! Splendid!

JEAN: Oh, in Roumania one can buy the title, so you'll be a Countess after all! My Countess!

JULIE: What does all that matter to me? I'm putting it all behind me now! Say that you love me, or—if you don't—what am I?

JEAN: I'll say it, a thousand times—later on! But not here! And above all, no sentiment, if everything is not to be lost! We must take the matter coolly like sensible people. (*Takes a cigar, cuts it and lights it.*) Now you sit there, and I'll sit here; then we can talk as if nothing had happened.

JULIE (*in despair*): My God! Have you no feelings, then?

JEAN: I? No man is more full of feeling than I am; but I'm able to control myself.

JULIE: Just now you could kiss my shoe—and now?

JEAN (*hardly*): Yes, then! Now we've got something else to think of.

JULIE: Don't speak cruelly to me!

JEAN: No, but sensibly. One folly has been committed—don't commit more! The Count may be here any moment, and before he comes our fates must be settled. What do you think of my plans for the future? Do you approve of them?

JULIE: They seem to me quite reasonable; but just one question: so large an undertaking requires considerable capital; have you got that?

JEANS (*chewing his cigar*): Have I? Certainly I have! I have my professional skill, my unrivalled experience, my knowledge of languages! That's the sort of capital that counts, I should think!

JULIE: But you can't even buy a railway ticket with that.

JEAN: No doubt; that's why I'm looking for a partner—one who can advance the capital required!

JULIE: Where can you find one at a moment's notice?

JEAN: It's for you to find one, if you want to be my partner.

JULIE: I can't do that, and I've nothing of my own. (*A pause.*)

JEAN: Then the whole thing falls to the ground—

JULIE: And—

JEAN: All remains as before!

JULIE: Do you think I'm going to remain under this roof as your mistress? Do you think I'll have the people pointing their fingers at me? Do you think I can look my father in the face after this? No! Take me away from here—away from this humiliation and disgrace! O God, God, what have I done? (*Weeps.*)

JEAN: So that's the tune now—what have you done? What many have done before you! *TRUE? TO WHAT DEGREE?*

JULIE (*screaming hysterically*): And now you despise me! I'm falling, I'm falling! *WHY?*

JEAN: Fall down to my level, and I'll lift you up again!

JULIE: What dreadful power drew me towards you? The attraction of the weak to the strong? Of the falling to the rising? Or was it love? *This* love? Do you know what love is?

JEAN: Do I? You bet I do! Do you think I've never been with a girl before?

JULIE: What a way to speak! What thoughts to have!

JEAN: That's how I've been brought up and that's what I am! Now don't be hysterical, and don't give yourself airs, for we're both in the same boat now! There, little girl, let me give you a glass of something special!

(*Opens the table drawer and takes out the bottle of wine; fills the two glasses which had been used before.*)

all a phoney trick: cheapens it, vulgarizes it, lets you realize how manipulative Jean is / how ruthless he is in return to her teasing

JULIE: Where did you get that wine from?

JEAN: The wine-cellar!

JULIE: My father's burgundy!

JEAN: Isn't it good enough for his son-in-law?

JULIE: And I drink beer myself!

JEAN: That merely shows your tastes are worse than mine.

JULIE: Thief!

JEAN: Are you going to give me away?

JULIE: Oh, oh! The accomplice of a house-thief! Have I been drunk, have I been walking in dreams to-night? Midsummer Eve! The feast of innocent pleasures. . . .

JEAN: Innocent; h'm!

JULIE (*pacing backwards and forwards*): Is there a human being on earth so wretched as I am now?

JEAN: Why should you be? After such a conquest! Think of Kristin in there! Can't you imagine that she has her feelings too?

JULIE: I thought so just now, but I no longer think so! No, a menial is a menial—

JEAN: And a whore's a whore! *Bold language*

JULIE (*on her knees, with hands clasped together*): O God in heaven, put an end to my miserable life! Take me away from this filth in which I am sinking! Save me! Save me!

JEAN: I can't deny that I feel sorry for you! When I lay in the onion bed and saw you in the rose-garden, I . . . I can tell you now . . . I had the same ugly thoughts as other boys.

JULIE: You, who wanted to die because of me!

JEAN: In the oats-chest? That was all humbug.

JULIE: In other words, a lie!

JEAN (*beginning to feel sleepy*): Next door to it! Probably I read the story in some paper—about a chimney-sweep who shut himself up in a woodchest full of lilac blossoms because he was sued in some maintenance case. . . .

JULIE: So that's the sort of man you are. . . .

JEAN: I had to invent something; it's always the pretty speeches that capture women! *The movement from attraction to revulsion*

JULIE: Scoundrel!

JEAN: Filth!

JULIE: And now you've seen the hawk's back!

JEAN: Not exactly its *back!*

JULIE: And I was to be the first branch . . .

JEAN: But the branch was rotten . . .

JULIE: I was to be the signboard at the hotel . . .

JEAN: And I the hotel . . .

JULIE: Sit inside your office, lure your customers, falsify their accounts . . .

The power struggle based on BIRTH and on SEX —

JEAN: *I* was to do that.

JULIE: To think that a human soul could be so steeped in filth!

JEAN: Wash it then!

JULIE: You lackey, you menial, stand up when I'm speaking!

JEAN: You mistress of a menial, you lackey's wench, hold your jaw and get out! Are you the one to come and lecture me on my coarseness? No one in my class has ever behaved so coarsely as you have to-night. Do you think any servant girl attacks a man as you did? Have you ever seen a girl of my class throw herself at a man like that? I have only seen that sort of thing among beasts and fallen women!

JULIE (*crushed*): That's right; strike me; trample on me; I deserve it all. I'm a vile creature; but help me! Help me out of this, if there *is* any way out!

JEAN (*more gently*): I've no wish to lower myself by denying my own share in the honour of being the seducer. But do you imagine that any one in my position would have dared to look at you if you hadn't invited it yourself? Even now I am astounded . . .

JULIE: And proud . . .

JEAN: Why not? Though I must confess the conquest was too easy to carry me off my feet.

JULIE: Go on striking me!

JEAN (*getting up*): No! Rather forgive me for what I have said! I don't strike the defenceless—least of all a woman. I can't deny that in one way I an glad to have discovered that what dazzled us below was merely tinsel: to have discovered that the hawk's back, too, was only grey, that the delicate complexion was a mere powder, that the polished nails might have black edges, that the handkerchief was dirty, scented though it was! . . . On the other hand, it pains me to find that what I myself was striving to reach was not something higher, something more substantial; it pains me to see you sunk to a level far below that of your own cook; it pains me like the sight of autumn flowers lashed to pieces by the rain and turned into mud.

JULIE: You speak as if you already stood above me?

JEAN: And so I do. I could make you a Countess, you see, but you could never make me a Count.

JULIE: But I am a child of a Count; you can never be that!

JEAN: True, but I might be the father of Counts—if . . .

JULIE: But you are a thief. I am not that.

JEAN: There are worse things than being a thief! There are

lower levels than that! Besides, when I serve a house I regard myself to some extent as a member of the family, or one of the children; one doesn't count it theft when children filch a berry from loaded bushes! (*His passion wakens again.*) Miss Julie, you're a splendid woman, far too good for a man like me! You've been the prey of an intoxication, and you want to conceal the mistake by persuading yourself that you love me! That you do not do, unless possibly my outward appearance attracts you—in which case your love is no higher than mine—but I could never be content with being a mere animal for you, and your love I can never awaken.

JULIE: Are you sure of that?

JEAN: You mean that it might be possible!—My ability to love you, yes, without doubt! You are beautiful, you are re-fined—(*goes up to her and takes her hand*)—cultivated, amia-ble when you like, and the flame that is roused by you in a man will probably never be quenched. (*Puts his arm around her waist.*) You're like mulled wine with strong spices in it, and a kiss from you . . . (*He tries to lead her out; but she frees herself gently.*) *woman - what does she want*

JULIE: Leave me! You won't win me in that fashion!

JEAN: *How* then?—Not in that fashion! Not by caresses and pretty speeches; not by thought for the future, by saving you from disgrace! *How* then?

JULIE: How? How? I don't know. Not in any way! I loathe you as I loathe rats, but I can't escape you!

JEAN: Escape *with* me!

JULIE (*drawing herself up*): Escape? Yes, we must escape! But I'm so tired! Give me a glass of wine.

(JEAN *fills her glass.*)

(*Looking at her watch*) But we must talk first; we've still a little time left. (*Drinks the wine and holds out her glass for more.*)

JEAN: Don't drink so immoderately—it will go to your head!

JULIE: What if it does?

JEAN: What if it does? It's vulgar to get drunk! What was it you wanted to say?

JULIE: We must fly! But we must talk first; that is, I must talk; so far you have done all the talking. You've told me the story of your life; now I want to tell you mine; then we shall know each other thoroughly before we begin our travels to-gether.

JEAN: One moment! Pardon me! Consider whether you

won't regret it afterwards when you've laid bare the secrets of your life.

JULIE: Aren't you my friend?

JEAN: Yes, sometimes. But don't rely on me.

JULIE: You don't really mean that. Besides, my secrets are already common property. You see, my mother was of plebeian birth, the daughter of quite simple people. She was brought up according to the theories of her time as regards equality, woman's liberty, and all that sort of thing; and she had a decided objection to marriage. So when my father made love to her she said she could never marry him, but she did marry him all the same. I came into the world—against my mother's wishes, so far as I can make out. My mother wanted to bring me up as a child of nature: I was even to learn everything a boy learns, to become a proof that a woman is as good as a man. I had to go about dressed as a boy and learn how to handle a horse; but I wasn't allowed in the cowshed. I was made to groom and harness and go out hunting; I even had to try and learn farming! On our estate men were given women's work to do, and women men's—the result being that the property was on the verge of ruin and we became the laughing-stock of the neighbourhood. In the end my father must have wakened from the spell; he rebelled, and everything was altered to suit his wishes. My mother was taken ill—what it was I don't know—but she frequently had convulsive attacks, used to hide in the attic or in the garden, and sometimes stayed out all night. Then came the great fire which you have heard about. The house, the stables, and the farm-buildings were burnt down, and in circumstances which led one to suspect that the fire was no accident; for the disaster occurred the very day after the quarterly insurance premium had expired, and the new premium sent by my father was delayed by the messenger's carelessness, so that it arrived too late. (*She fills her glass and drinks.*)

JEAN: Don't drink any more!

JULIE: Oh, what does it matter? We had absolutely nowhere to go, and had to sleep in the carriages. My father didn't know where to get money for rebuilding the house. Then my mother advised him to try and borrow from a friend whom she had known in her youth, a brick-manufacturer near here. My father borrowed the money, without having to pay any interest, which surprised him. And so the estate was rebuilt. (*Drinks again.*) Do you know who burnt it down?

JEAN: The Countess, your mother!

JULIE: Do you know who the brick-manufacturer was?

the liberated emancipated women is a
cruel vindictive bitch who destroys
lives & property and who teaches
hate.

JEAN: Your mother's lover?

JULIE: Do you know who the money belonged to?

JEAN: Wait a little—no, I don't know!

JULIE: It was my mother's!

JEAN: The Count's, then—if there was no settlement?

JULIE: There was no settlement. My mother had a little money of her own, which she didn't want to be under my father's control, so she deposited it with—her friend!

JEAN: Who pinched it!

JULIE: Quite so! He kept it! All this comes to my father's knowledge; he can't bring an action; nor pay his wife's lover; nor prove that the money was hers! That was my mother's revenge on him for assuming control over the household. At that time he was on the point of shooting himself! Rumour said that he tried and failed. But he took a new lease of life, and my mother had to pay dearly for her conduct! You can imagine what those five years were for me! I sympathized with my father, but I took my mother's side nevertheless, because I didn't know the circumstances. From her I had learnt to mistrust and hate men—for she hated men, as you know—and I swore to her that I would never be the slave of a man.

JEAN: So you became engaged to the district attorney!

JULIE: Merely that he should be my slave.

JEAN: And that he wouldn't be?

JULIE: Oh, he wanted it all right, but he didn't get the chance. I got bored with him!

JEAN: I saw that—in the stable-yard!

JULIE: What did you see?

JEAN: What I did!— How he broke off the engagement.

JULIE: That is a lie! It was I who broke it off! Has he been saying that he did it—the scoundrel?

JEAN: Oh, I don't think he was a scoundrel! You hate men, Miss Julie?

JULIE: Yes, for the most part! But sometimes—when weakness comes—oh, the shame of it!

JEAN: You hate me too?

JULIE: Beyond words! I should like to have you killed like a wild beast.

JEAN: Just as one shoots a mad dog. Is that what you mean?

JULIE: Yes, just that!

JEAN: But now there's nothing here to shoot with—and no dog! What are we to do then?

JULIE: Travel!

JEAN: And plague each other to death?

JULIE: No—enjoy ourselves, for a day or two, for a week, for as long as one can enjoy oneself, and then—die—

JEAN: Die? How stupid! In that case I think it's better to start a hotel—

JULIE (*paying no attention*):—by Lake Como, where the sun is always shining, where the laurels are green at Christmas and the oranges glow.

JEAN: Lake Como is a rainy hole, and I never saw any oranges there except at the grocer's. But it's a good place for strangers, as there are lots of villas to be let to loving couples, a most paying industry—do you know why? Why, because the contract is for six months and they leave after three weeks!

JULIE: Why after three weeks?

JEAN: They quarrel, of course! But the rent has to be paid just the same! Then one lets again. So it goes on and on, for there's love enough—even if it doesn't last very long!

JULIE: You don't want to die with me?

JEAN: I don't want to die at all! Not only because I am fond of life, but because I regard self-murder as a crime against the Providence which has given us life.

JULIE: You believe in God—you?

JEAN: Certainly I do! And I go to church every other Sunday.— And now, to tell the truth, I'm tired of all this and I'm going to bed.

JULIE: Indeed! And you think I shall be content with that? Do you know what a man owes the woman he has brought to shame?

JEAN (*takes out his purse and throws a silver coin on the table.*): There you are! I don't want to have any debts!

JULIE (*pretending not to notice the insult*): Do you know what the law lays down?

JEAN: Unfortunately the law lays down no penalty for the woman who seduces a man!

JULIE: Do you see any way out other than going abroad, marrying, and then getting a divorce?

JEAN: And suppose I refuse to enter into this *mésalliance*?

JULIE: *Mésalliance* . . .

JEAN: Yes, for me! For, mark you! I'm better bred than you are; my pedigree contains no woman guilty of arson!

JULIE: Can you be sure of that?

JEAN: You can't be sure of the opposite, since we have no family records—except at the police-station! But your family records I have seen in a book on the drawing-room table. Do you know who the founder of your family was? A miller who let the king sleep with his wife one night during the Danish war. I have no ancestors of that sort! I haven't any ancestors at all, but I can become one myself!

JULIE: That's what I get for opening my heart to one who is unworthy of it, for sacrificing the honour of my family.

JEAN: Dishonour!—Now what did I tell you? People shouldn't drink—it makes them garrulous! And one must *not* be garrulous!

JULIE: Oh, how I regret what has happened!—how bitterly I regret it!—And if you had only loved me!

JEAN: For the last time—what do you mean? Do you want me to weep, to jump over your riding-whip, to kiss you? Do you want me to lure you away to Lake Como for three weeks, and then? . . . What am I to do? What do you want? This is getting rather painful! It always does when one goes and sticks one's nose into women's affairs! Miss Julie! I can see that you're unhappy: I know that you're suffering: but I cannot understand you. *We* don't have any of these whims; *we* don't hate one another! We make love for fun when our work gives us time; but we don't have time all day and all night, as you do! I think you're ill; I'm sure you're ill.

JULIE: Then you must be kind to me; and now you *are* talking like a human being.

JEAN: Yes, but be human yourself! You spit on me, and then forbid me to wipe it off—on you!

JULIE: Help me, help me! Only tell me what to do—where to go!

JEAN: O Lord! if I only knew myself!

JULIE: I've been mad—raving mad! But is there no possible escape?

JEAN: Keep still and be calm! Nobody knows anything.

JULIE: Impossible! The people know, and Kristin knows!

JEAN: They don't know: they could never believe such a thing!

JULIE (*hesitating*): But—it might happen again!

JEAN: That is true!

JULIE: And the consequences?

JEAN (*frightened*): The consequences?—Where *were* my wits, that I never thought of that? Yes, there's only one thing to do—you must go! At once! I shan't go with you or all would be lost. You must travel alone—abroad—anywhere!

JULIE: Alone? Where?—I can't do that!

JEAN: You must! And before the Count comes back! If you stay here you know what will happen! Once one has done wrong one wants to go on with it, since the harm is already done. . . . So one gets more and more reckless and—at last one is found out! So you must go! Afterwards, you can write to the Count and confess everything, except that it was me! And that I don't think he'd guess! Nor do I think he'd be very pleased to know it!

JULIE: I'll go if you come with me!

JEAN: Are you mad, woman? Miss Julie running away with her valet! I would be in the papers the next day, and the Count would never survive it! →CAUGHT BET. TWO

JULIE: I can't go! I can't stay here! Help me! I am so tired, so unutterably tired. Order me! Set me in motion! I can no longer think, nor act! . . . WORLD

JEAN: There, now! What a wretched creature you are! Why do you give yourselves airs and turn up your noses as if you were the lords of creation? Very well then—I'll give you your orders! Go upstairs and dress; provide yourself with money for the journey, and then come down again!

JULIE (*half whispering*): Come upstairs with me!

JEAN: To your room?—Now you're mad again! (*Hesitates a moment.*) No! Go, at once! (*Takes her hand and leads her out.*)

JULIE (*on her way out*): Do speak kindly to me, Jean!

JEAN: An order always sounds unkind; you can feel that yourself now!

(*Jean alone; he gives a sigh of relief; sits down at the table; takes out a note-book and pencil; adds up figures aloud now and then. Dumb show, till* KRISTIN *comes in dressed for church, carrying a dicky and a white tie.*)

KRISTIN: Good Lord, what a state the room's in! What have you been up to?

JEAN: Oh, it's the young lady been bringing the people in. Were you so sound asleep you couldn't hear anything?

KRISTIN: I've slept like a log!

JEAN: And dressed for church already!

KRISTIN: Ye-es! Why, you promised to come to communion with me to-day!

JEAN: Why, so I did!—And I see you've got the vestments there! Come along then!

(*Sits down.* KRISTIN *begins putting on his dicky and white tie. A pause.*)

(*Sleepily*): What's the gospel for the day?

KRISTIN: Something about the beheading of John the Baptist, I expect!

JEAN: Awfully long affair that's sure to be!—Look out, you're choking me!—Oh, I'm so sleepy, so sleepy!

KRISTIN: Yes: what have you been doing, sitting up all night? Why, you're quite green in the face!

JEAN: I've been sitting here talking to Miss Julie.

KRISTIN: She doesn't know what's proper, that creature! (*A pause.*)

JEAN: I say, Kristin!

KRISTIN: Well?

JEAN: It's queer anyhow, when one comes to think of it! She!

KRISTIN: What is so queer?

JEAN: Everything! (*A pause.*)

KRISTIN (*looking at the glasses standing half empty on the table*): Have you been drinking together too?

JEAN: Yes!

KRISTIN: For shame!—Look me in the face!

JEAN: Yes!

KRISTIN: Is it possible? *Is* it possible?

JEAN (*after consideration*): Yes! It is!

KRISTIN: Faugh! I could never have believed it! Shame! Shame!

JEAN: Surely you're not jealous of her?

KRISTIN: No, not of her! If it had been Clara or Sophy I'd have scratched your eyes out!—Yes, that's how it is: why, I don't know! Oh, but it really was disgusting!

JEAN: Are you angry with her then?

KRISTIN: No, with you! It was wrong, very wrong! Poor girl! No, I tell you I won't stop in this house any longer—where one can't feel any respect for the people in it.

JEAN: Why should one feel respect for them?

KRISTIN: Yes, tell me that, my artful young fellow! But you wouldn't like to be in the service of people who don't live decently, would you? Eh! It lowers one, I think.

JEAN: Yes, but isn't it some consolation to find that the others aren't one scrap better than we are?

KRISTIN: No, I don't think so; for unless they *are* better there's no standard for us to aim at, so as to better ourselves. And think of the Count! Think of all the sorrow he's had in his life! No, I won't stay here any longer! With a fellow like you too! If it had been the district attorney: if it had been somebody a little higher.

JEAN: What's that you say?

KRISTIN: Yes, yes! You may be all right in your own way, but there *is* a difference between one class and another all the same. No, this is a thing I can never get over. To think that a young lady who was so proud, so bitter against men, should go and give herself—and to such a man! She who almost had poor Diana shot for running after the lodge-keeper's pug!— Just fancy! But I won't stay here any longer; on the twenty-fourth of October I quit.

JEAN: And then?

KRISTIN: Well, talking of that, it's about time you looked round for a job, if we are going to marry after all.

JEAN: Yes, but what sort of a job? I can't get a place like this when I'm married.

KRISTIN: Of course not! But I suppose you could take a hallporter's job, or try for a place as commissionaire in some institution. Government rations are scanty, but they're safe, and there's a pension for the widow and children . . .

JEAN (*with a grimace*): That's all very fine, but it isn't in my line to start thinking so soon about dying for the sake of wife and children. I must admit that I really had slightly higher views.

KRISTIN: Your views indeed! Yes, and your duties too! Don't you forget them!

JEAN: Don't you go irritating me, talking about duties! I know well enough what I ought to do, without your telling me! (*Listens to some sound outside.*) However, we've plenty of time to think over that. Now go and get ready and we'll go to church.

KRISTIN: Who's that walking about upstairs?

JEAN: I don't know, unless it's Clara.

KRISTIN (*going out*): Surely it can't be the Count's come home without anybody hearing him?

JEAN (*frightened*): The Count? No it can't be him, or he'd have rung.

KRISTIN (*going out*): God help us! I've never seen the like.

(*The sun has now risen and is shining on the tree-tops in the park; the light moves slowly till it falls obliquely through the windows.* JEAN *goes to the doorway and makes a sign.*

JULIE *comes in in travelling dress, carrying a small birdcage covered with a towel. She places it on a chair.*)

JULIE: I'm ready now.

JEAN: Hush! Kristin's awake.

JULIE: (*extremely nervous during the following scene*): Did she suspect anything?

JEAN: She knows absolutely nothing! But, good heavens, what a sight you are!

JULIE: A sight? In what way?

JEAN: You're as pale as a corpse, and—pardon me, but your face is dirty.

JULIE: Let me wash then!—There! (*Goes to the basin and washes her hands and face.*) Give me a towel! Oh—there's the sun rising!

JEAN: And then the troll bursts!

JULIE: Yes, there've been trolls about to-night! Now, Jean! Come with me: I've got the money.

JEAN (*doubtfully*): Enough?

JULIE: Enough to begin with! Come with me! I can't travel alone to-day. Think of it—Midsummer Day, in a stuffy train, crowded with masses of people all staring at once; standing at stations when one wants to fly. No, I can't do it, I can't do it! And then memories will rise: childhood's memories of midsummer days with the church decked in green—birch leaves and lilac: dinner at the table spread for relations and friends: after dinner the park, with dancing, music, flowers, and games! Ah, one may fly and fly, but one's memories follow in the luggage van and remorse, and the pangs of conscience.

JEAN: I'll come with you—but at once, before it's too late. This moment!

JULIE: Go and get ready then! (*Takes up the cage.*)

JEAN: No luggage though! That would betray us!

JULIE: No, nothing at all! Only what we can take in the carriage with us.

JEAN (*who has got his hat*): What on earth have you got there? What is it?

JULIE: Only my greenfinch. I don't want to leave her behind!

JEAN: Well, I'm blowed! So we're to take a bird-cage with us, are we? You must be mad! Drop that cage!

JULIE: The only thing of mine I'm taking with me from my home: the only living creature that loves me since Diana proved faithless! Don't be cruel! Let me take her with me!

JEAN: Drop that cage, I tell you—and don't talk so loud! Kristin can hear us!

JULIE: No, I can't leave her in strange hands! I'd rather you killed her!

JEAN: Give me the little beast, then, and I'll wring its neck!

JULIE: Very well, but don't hurt her! Don't—no, I cannot!

JEAN: Bring it here; I can!

JULIE (*takes the bird out of the cage and kisses it*): Oh, my little Serine, must you die then and leave your mistress?

JEAN: Please don't let's have any scenes; your life, your whole future is at stake! Quick now! (*Snatches the bird from her; carries it to the chopping-block, and picks up the kitchen chopper.* MISS JULIE *turns her head away.*) You should have learnt how to kill chickens instead of revolver-shooting. (*Brings down the chopper.*) Then you wouldn't faint at the sight of a drop of blood!

JULIE (*screaming*): Kill me too! Kill me! You who can butcher an innocent creature without a quiver. Oh, how I hate you, how I loathe you! There is blood between us! I curse the hour when I first saw you; I curse the hour when I was conceived in my mother's womb!

JEAN: Oh, what's the good of your cursing? Let's go!

JULIE (*goes to the chopping-block, as though she were dragged there against her will*): No, I won't go yet; I cannot ... I must see ... Hush! There's a carriage outside. (*Listens to the sounds outside, without taking her eyes off the block and the chopper.*) So you think I can't bear the sight of blood! You think I'm so weak. . . . Oh, how I should love to see your blood, your brains on a chopping-block—to see your whole sex swimming in a sea of blood, like that poor creature. . . . I believe I could drink out of your skull; I would gladly bathe my feet in your breast; I could eat your heart roasted whole! You think I am weak; you think I love you because the fruit of my womb thirsted for your seed; you think I want to carry your offspring beneath my heart, to nourish it with my blood—to bear your child and take your name! By the way, what *is* your name! I've never heard your surname—probably you haven't got one. I should be "Mrs. Gatekeeper," or "Madam Dunghill"—you dog who wear my collar; you lackey with my crest on your buttons! I to share you with my own cook, to be the rival of my own servant! Oh! Oh! Oh! You think I'm a coward and want to run away! No, now I'm going to stay—blow wind, come wrack! My father will come home ... find his desk broken open ... his money gone! Then he'll ring—that bell there . . . twice for the valet—and then he'll send for the police . . . and I shall tell everything! Everything! Oh, how lovely to have an end to it all—if only it could be the end! And then he'll get a stroke and die! And that will be the end of all of us ... and then there will be quiet ... peace! ... eternal rest! ... And then the coat of arms will be broken on the coffin—the Count's line is extinct—but the valet's line will continue, in an orphan asylum . . . win laurels in a gutter, and end in a prison!

JEAN: There speaks the royal blood! Bravo, Miss Julie! Now cram the miller into his sack!

(KRISTIN *comes in, dressed for church, with a hymn-book in her hand.*

JULIE *hastens up to her and throws herself into her arms, as though seeking protection.*)

JULIE: Help me, Kristin! Help me against this man!

KRISTIN (*coldly and unmoved*): What a sight for a holiday morning! (*Looks at the chopping-block.*) And what a filthy mess! What does it all mean? And all this shrieking and hullabaloo!

JULIE: Kristin! You're a woman, and you're my friend! Beware of that scoundrel!

JEAN (*rather awkward and embarrassed*): While the ladies are discussing things I'll go and shave. (*Slips out to the right.*)

JULIE: *You* will understand me; *you* will listen to me!

KRISTIN: No, I really don't understand this sort of underhand business! Where are you off to, dressed up for a journey like that? And he with his hat on! What is it? What is it?

JULIE: Listen, Kristen; listen to me and I'll tell you everything ...

KRISTIN: I don't want to know anything ...

JULIE: You *shall* hear me ...

KRISTIN: What is it about? Is it about your folly with Jean? Well, I don't worry about that at all; I've nothing to do with all that. But if you're thinking of fooling him into running off with you, why, we'll soon put a stopper on that!

JULIE (*extremely nervous*): Now try to be calm, Kristin, and listen to me! I can't stay here, and Jean can't stay here—so we must go abroad. ...

KRISTIN: H'm, h'm!

JULIE (*brightening up*): I've just got an idea, though—suppose we all three went off—abroad—to Switzerland, and started a hotel together. ... I've got money, you see, and Jean and I would be responsible for everything—and you, I thought, could look after the kitchen. ... Won't that be splendid? ... Say yes, now! And come with us, then everything will be settled! ... Now do say yes! (*Embraces* KRISTIN *and pats her on the shoulder.*)

KRISTIN (*coldly and thoughtfully*): H'm, h'm!

JULIE (*presto tempo*): You've never been abroad, Kristin—you must have a look round the world. You can't imagine what fun it is travelling by train—new people continually—new countries—and then we'll go to Hamburg and have a look at the Zoological Gardens on our way—you'll like that—and go to the theatre and hear the opera—and when we get to Munich we shall have the picture galleries! There are Rubenses and Raphaels there—the great painters, you know. You've heard of Munich, where King Ludwig lived—the king who went mad, you know.—And then we'll see his castle—he still has castles furnished just like they are in fairy tales—and from there it's not far to Switzerland—and the Alps! Think of the Alps covered with snow in the middle of summer—and oranges grow there, and laurels that are green all the year round. . .

(JEAN *is seen in the right wing, stropping his razor on a strop which he holds between his teeth and his left hand; he listens amused to the conversation and nods approval now and then.)*

The disintegration of Miss Julie

(*Tempo prestissimo*). And then we'll take a hotel—and I shall sit in the office while Jean stands and receives the guests . . . goes out shopping . . . writes letters.—There's life for you! Whistling trains, omnibuses driving up, bells ringing in the bedrooms and the restaurant—and I shall make out the bills—and I know how to salt them too. . . . You can't imagine how timid travellers are when it comes to paying bills! And you—you will sit in the kitchen as housekeeper in chief. Of course you won't do any cooking yourself—and you'll have to dress neatly and stylishly when you see people—and you, with your looks—no, I'm not flattering you—why, you'll be able to catch a husband one fine day! A rich Englishman, I shouldn't wonder—they're the easy ones to—(*slackens her pace*) catch—and then we'll get rich—and build ourselves a villa on Lake Como—of course it rains there a little occasionally—but—(*slower*) I suppose the sun shines sometimes—however gloomy it seems—and—then—otherwise we can come home again—and come back—(*a pause*) here—or somewhere else——

KRISTIN: Now do you believe all that yourself?

JULIE (*crushed*): Do I believe it myself?

KRISTIN: Yes!

JULIE (*wearily*): I don't know; I don't believe anything now. (*Sinks down on the bench; puts her head between her arms on the table.*) I believe in nothing! Nothing whatever!

KRISTIN (*turning towards the right, where* JEAN *is standing*): Aha, so you were going to run away!

JEAN (*disconcerted, putting the razor on the table*): Run away? That's putting it rather strong! You've heard the young lady's plan, and though she's tired now after being up all night, the plan can quite well be carried out!

KRISTIN: Listen to me now! Did you think I was going to be cook to that—

JEAN (*sharply*): Kindly use decent language when you're speaking to your mistress! Do you understand?

KRISTIN: Mistress!

JEAN: Yes!

KRISTIN: Listen! Just listen to thé man!

JEAN: Yes, listen yourself—it would do you good—and talk a little less! Miss Julie *is* your mistress; you ought to despise yourself for the same reason that you despise her now!

KRISTIN: I've always had so much self-respect—

JEAN: That you were able to despise other people!—

KRISTIN: That I have never sunk below my station. You can't say that the Count's cook has had any dealings with the groom or the swineherd! You can't say that!

JEAN: No, you've had to do with a fine fellow—luckily for you!

KRISTIN: Yes, he must be a fine fellow to sell the oats from the Count's stable!

JEAN: You're a nice one to talk about that—getting a commission on the groceries and accepting bribes from the butcher! The CORRUPTION of THE

KRISTIN: What do you mean? LOWER CLASSES

JEAN: So you can't feel any respect for your mistress now! *You* indeed!

KRISTIN: Are you coming to church now? A good sermon on your fine deeds might do you good!

JEAN: No, I'm not going to church to-day; you can go alone and confess your own misdeeds.

KRISTIN: Yes, I shall; and I shall come back with enough forgiveness to cover yours too! Our Redeember suffered and died on the Cross for our sins, and if we draw nigh to Him in faith and with a penitent heart He will take all our guilt upon Himself.

JEAN: Including grocery peculations?

JULIE: Do you believe that, Kristin?

KRISTIN: That is my living faith, as sure as I'm standing here; it's the faith which I learnt as a child, which I have kept from my youth upwards, Miss Julie. Moreover, where sin aboundeth, grace aboundeth also!

JULIE: Oh, if I only had your faith! Oh, if—

KRISTIN: Ah, but you see one can't get that without God's especial grace, and it is not given to all men to obtain that.

JULIE: Who do obtain it then?

KRISTIN: That is the great secret of the operation of grace, Miss Julie. God is no respecter of persons, but the last there shall be first. . . .

JULIE: Well, but in that case He must have respect for the last?

KRISTIN (*continuing*): And it is easier for a camel to go through the eye of a needle than for a rich man to enter the kingdom of heaven! Yes, there you have it, Miss Julie! However, I'm going now—by myself, and on my way I shall tell the groom not to let anybody have the horses, just in case they should want to get away before the Count comes back! Good-bye! (*Goes.*)

JEAN: What a little devil! And all this because of a greenfinch!

JULIE (*wearily*): Never mind the greenfinch!—Can you see any way out of this? Any end to it?

JEAN (*after consideration*): No!

JULIE: What would you do in my place?

JEAN: In your place? Let me think!—A woman, of noble birth, fallen! I don't know—yes, now I know!

JULIE (*takes the razor and makes a gesture*): Like this?

JEAN: Yes. But I shouldn't myself—note that! There's a difference between us!

JULIE: Because you're a man and I'm a woman? What difference does that make?

JEAN: The same difference—as—between a man and a woman!

JULIE (*still holding the razor*): I should like to! But I can't! My father couldn't either, that time when he should have done it.

JEAN: No, he should *not* have done it! He had to get his revenge first.

JULIE: And now my mother gets her revenge, through me.

JEAN: Have you never loved your father, Miss Julie?

JULIE: Yes, most dearly, but I think I must have hated him too! I must have done so without being aware of it! But it was he who brought me up to despise my own sex, as half a woman and half a man! Whose fault is it—what has happened? My father's, my mother's, or my own? My own? But I *have* no own! I haven't a thought that I didn't get from my father, one passion that I didn't get from my mother, and this last idea—about all men being equal—that I got from *him*, my affianced husband—for that reason I call him a scoundrel! How can it be my own fault? To put the blame on Jesus, as Kristin did—no, I'm too proud to do that, and—

Julie wants to save the family honor

thanks to my father's teaching—too sensible. And as to a rich man not being able to go to heaven—that is a lie; anyhow Kristin, who has money in the savings-bank, will certainly never get there!—What does it matter whose fault is it? Whose fault is it? After all, it is I who have to bear the blame, to bear the consequences. . . .

JEAN: Yes, but—

(*Two sharp rings on the bell,* JULIE *starts to her feet;* JEAN *changes his coat.*)

The Count is back! Suppose Kristin——(*Goes to the speaking-tube, taps it and listens.*)

JULIE: Has he been to his desk yet?

JEAN: It's Jean, my Lord! (*Listens. The audience cannot hear what the* COUNT *says.*) Yes, my Lord! (*Listens.*) Yes, my Lord! In one moment! (*Listens.*) At once, my Lord! (*Listens.*) Very good! In half an hour!

JULIE (*extremely anxious*): What did he say? My God! What did he say?

JEAN: He wants his boots and his coffee in half an hour.

JULIE: In half an hour then! Oh, I'm so tired; I haven't the strength to do anything; I can't repent, can't run away, can't stay, can't live, can't die! Help me now! Order me, and I'll obey you like a dog! Do me this last service, save my honour, save his name! You know what I *ought* to will, but cannot. . . . Will it yourself, and command me to carry it out!

JEAN: I don't know—but now *I* can't either—I don't understand—it's just as if this coat made me—I cannot order you—and now, since the Count spoke to me—why—I can't really explain it—but—oh, it's that devil the lackey working in my backbone!—I really believe if the Count came down now and ordered me to cut my throat I'd do it on the spot.

JULIE: Then pretend you're he, and I you!—You showed me how well you could act just now, when you were on your knees—you were the aristocrat then—or—have you never been to the theatre and seen the mesmerist? (JEAN *nods.*) He says to his subject: Fetch the broom, and he fetches it. Then he says: sweep, and the man sweeps—

JEAN: The other man has to be asleep, though!

JULIE (*as if in a trance*): I am asleep already—the whole room seems like smoke to me . . . and you look like an iron stove . . . a stove like a man in black clothes and a tall hat—and your eyes are shining like coals when the fire is going out—and your face is a white patch like the ashes—(*the sunlight has now reached the floor and is shining upon* JEAN) it's

self hypnosis

so warm and lovely—(*she rubs her hands as if she were warming them before a fire*) and so light—and so peaceful!

JEAN (*takes the razor and puts it into her hand*): There is the broom! Now go, while it's light—out to the barn—and ... (*whispers in her ear.*)

JULIE (*waking up*): Thank you! Now I am going, to rest! But just say—that the first can also obtain the gift of grace. Say it, even if you don't believe it.

JEAN: The first? No, I can't say that!—But stay—Miss Julie—now I know! You're no longer among the first—you're among the—last!

JULIE: That is true.—I'm among the very last: I *am* the last! Oh!—But now I can't go—tell me once more that I'm to go!

JEAN: No, now I can't either! I can't!

JULIE: And the first shall be the last!

JEAN: Don't think! Don't think! Why, you're taking away all my strength too, and making me a coward—What! I fancied I saw the bell move!—No! Shall we stuff it up with paper?—Fancy being so afraid of a bell!—Yes, but it isn't only a bell—there's someone behind it—a hand that sets it in motion—and something else that sets the hand in motion—but just stop your ears—stop your ears! Yes, and then it rings worse! Just goes on ringing till you answer it—and then it's too late! and then the police come—and then—(*The bell rings twice violently. JEAN shrinks at the sound; then straightens himself.*) It's horrible! But there's no other possible end to it!—Go!

(JULIE *walks out firmly through the door.*)

MRS. WARREN'S PROFESSION

George Bernard Shaw

Characters

PRAED
VIVIE WARREN
MRS. WARREN
SIR GEORGE CROFTS
FRANK
THE REV. SAMUEL GARDNER

ACT 1

Summer afternoon in a cottage garden on the eastern slope of a hill a little south of Haslemere in Surrey. Looking up the hill, the cottage is seen in the left hand corner of the garden, with its thatched roof and porch, and a large latticed window to the left of the porch. Farther back a little wing is built out, making an angle with the right side wall. From the end of this wing a paling curves across and forward, completely shutting in the garden, except for a gate on the right. The common rises uphill beyond the paling to the sky line. Some folded canvas garden chairs are leaning against the side bench in the porch. A lady's bicycle is propped against the wall, under the window. A little to the right of the porch a hammock is slung from two posts. A big canvas umbrella, stuck in the ground, keeps the sun off the hammock, in which a young lady lies reading and making notes, her head towards the cottage and her feet towards the gate. In front of the hammock, and within reach of her hand, is a common kitchen chair, with a pile of serious-looking books and a supply of writing paper upon it.

A gentleman walking on the common comes into sight from behind the cottage. He is hardly past middle age, with something of the artist about him, unconventionally but carefully dressed, and clean-shaven except for a moustache, with an eager, susceptible face and very amiable and considerate manners. He has silky black hair, with waves of grey and white in it. His eyebrows are white, his moustache black. He seems not certain of his way. He looks over the paling; takes stock of the place; and sees the young lady.

THE GENTLEMAN (*taking off his hat*): I beg your pardon. Can you direct me to Hindhead View—Mrs. Alison's?

THE YOUNG LADY (*glancing up from her book*): This is Mrs. Alison's. (*She resumes her work.*)

THE GENTLEMAN. Indeed! Perhaps—may I ask are you Miss Vivie Warren?

THE YOUNG LADY (*sharply, as she turns on her elbow to get a good look at him*): Yes.

THE GENTLEMAN (*daunted and conciliatory*): I'm afraid I appear intrusive. My name is Praed. (*Vivie at once throws her books upon the chair, and gets out of the hammock.*) Oh, pray don't let me disturb you.

VIVIE (*striding to the gate and opening it for him*): Come in, Mr. Praed. (*He comes in.*) Glad to see you. (*She proffers her hand and takes his with a resolute and hearty grip. She is an attractive specimen of the sensible, able, highly-educated young middle-class Englishwoman. Age 22. Prompt, strong, confident, self-possessed. Plain, business-like dress, but not dowdy. She wears a chatelaine at her belt, with a fountain pen and a paper knife among its pendants.*)

PRAED: Very kind of you indeed, Miss Warren. (*She shuts the gate with a vigorous slam: he passes in to the middle of the garden, exercising his fingers, which are slightly numbed by her greeting.*) Has your mother arrived?

VIVIE (*quickly, evidently scenting aggression*): Is she coming?

PRAED (*surprised*): Didn't you expect us?

VIVIE: No.

PRAED: Now, goodness me, I hope I've not mistaken the day. That would be just like me, you know. Your mother arranged that she was to come down from London and that I was to come over from Horsham to be introduced to you.

VIVIE (*not at all pleased*): Did she? H'm! My mother has rather a trick of taking me by surprise—to see how I behave myself when she's away, I suppose. I fancy I shall take my mother very much by surprise one of these days, if she makes arrangements that concern me without consulting me beforehand. She hasn't come.

PRAED (*embarrassed*): I'm really very sorry.

VIVIE (*throwing off her displeasure*): It's not your fault, Mr. Praed, is it? And I'm very glad you've come, believe me. You are the only one of my mother's friends I have asked her to bring to see me.

PRAED (*relieved and delighted*): Oh, now this is really very good of you, Miss Warren!

VIVIE: Will you come indoors; or would you rather sit out here whilst we talk?

PRAED: It will be nicer out here, don't you think?

VIVIE: Then I'll go and get you a chair. (*She goes to the porch for a garden chair.*)

PRAED (*following her*): Oh, pray, pray! Allow me. (*He lays hands on the chair.*)

VIVIE (*letting him take it*): Take care of your fingers: they're rather dodgy things, those chairs. (*She goes across to the chair with the books on it; pitches them into the hammock; and brings the chair forward with one swing.*)

PRAED (*who has just unfolded his chair*): Oh, now do let me take that hard chair! I like hard chairs.

VIVIE: So do I. (*She sits down.*) Sit down, Mr. Praed. (*This invitation is given with genial peremptoriness, his anxiety to please her clearly striking her as a sign of weakness of character on his part.*)

PRAED: By the way, though, hadn't we better go to the station to meet your mother?

VIVIE (*coolly*): Why? She knows the way. (*Praed hesitates, and then sits down in the garden chair, rather disconcerted.*) Do you know, you are just like what I expected. I hope you are disposed to be friends with me?

PRAED (*again beaming*): Thank you, my dear Miss Warren; thank you. Dear me! I'm so glad your mother hasn't spoilt you!

VIVIE: How?

PRAED: Well, in making you too conventional. You know, my dear Miss Warren, I am a born anarchist. I hate authority. It spoils the relations between parent and child—even between mother and daughter. Now I was always afraid that your mother would strain her authority to make you very conventional. It's such a relief to find that she hasn't.

VIVIE: Oh! Have I been behaving unconventionally?

PRAED: Oh, no: oh, dear no. At least not conventionally unconventionally, you understand. (*She nods. He goes on, with a cordial outburst.*) But it was so charming of you to say that you were disposed to be friends with me! You modern young ladies are splendid—perfectly splendid!

VIVIE (*dubiously*): Eh? (*watching him with dawning disappointment as to the quality of his brains and character.*)

PRAED: When I was your age, young men and women were afraid of each other: There was no good fellowship—nothing real—only gallantry copied out of novels, and as vulgar and affected as it could be. Maidenly reserve!—gentlemanly chivalry!—always saying no when you meant yes!—simple purgatory for shy and sincere souls!

VIVIE: Yes, I imagine there must have been a frightful waste of time—especially women's time.

PRAED: Oh, waste of life, waste of everything. But things are improving. Do you know, I have been in a positive state of excitement about meeting you ever since your magnificent achievements at Cambridge—a thing unheard of in my day.

[handwritten marginalia: a hard business like head / The hell with the ventures re: / the honor]

It was perfectly splendid, your tieing with the third wrangler. Just the right place, you know. The first wrangler is always a dreamy, morbid fellow, in whom the thing is pushed to the length of a disease.

VIVIE: It doesn't pay. I wouldn't do it again for the same money.

PRAED (*aghast*): The same money!

VIVIE: I did it for £50. Perhaps you don't know how it was. Mrs. Latham, my tutor at Newnham, told my mother that I could distinguish myself in the mathematical tripos if I went for it in earnest. The papers were full just then of Phillipa Summers beating the senior wrangler—you remember about it; and nothing would please my mother but that I should do the same thing. I said flatly that it was not worth my while to face the grind since I was not going in for teaching; but I offered to try for fourth wrangler or thereabouts for £50. She closed with me at that, after a little grumbling; and I was better than my bargain. But I wouldn't do it again for that. £200 would have been nearer the mark.

PRAED (*much damped*): Lord bless me! That's a very practical way of looking at it.

VIVIE: Did you expect to find me an unpractical person?

PRAED: No, no. But surely it's practical to consider not only the work these honors cost, but also the culture they bring.

VIVIE: Culture! My dear Mr. Praed: do you know what the mathematical tripos means? It means grind, grind, grind, for six to eight hours a day at mathematics, and nothing but mathematics. I'm supposed to know something about science; but I know nothing except the mathematics it involves. I can make calculations for engineers, electricians, insurance companies, and so on; but I know next to nothing about engineering or electricity or insurance. I don't even know arithmetic well. Outside mathematics, lawn-tennis, eating, sleeping, cycling, and walking, I'm a more ignorant barbarian than any woman could possibly be who hadn't gone in for the tripos.

PRAED (*revolted*): What a monstrous, wicked, rascally system! I knew it! I felt at once that it meant destroying all that makes womanhood beautiful. *A CONVENTIONAL PRIG*

VIVIE: I don't object to it on that score in the least. I shall turn it to very good account, I assure you.

PRAED: Pooh! In what way?

VIVIE: I shall set up in chambers in the city and work at actuarial calculations and conveyancing. Under cover of that I shall do some law, with one eye on the Stock Exchange all the time. I've come down here by myself to read law—not for a holiday, as my mother imagines. I hate holidays.

PRAED: You make my blood run cold. Are you to have no romance, no beauty in your life?

VIVIE: I don't care for either, I assure you.

PRAED: You can't mean that.

VIVIE: Oh yes I do. I like working and getting paid for it. When I'm tired of working, I like a comfortable chair, a cigar, a little whisky, and a novel with a good detective story in it. SATIRE ON MEN —

PRAED (*in a frenzy of repudiation*): I don't believe it. I am an artist; and I can't believe it: I refuse to believe it. (*Enthusiastically.*) Ah, my dear Miss Warren, you haven't discovered yet, I see, what a wonderful world art can open up to you.

VIVIE: Yes, I have. Last May I spent six weeks in London with Honoria Fraser. Mamma thought we were doing a round of sight-seeing together; but I was really at Honoria's chambers in Chancery Lane every day, working away at actuarial calculations for her, and helping her as well as a greenhorn could. In the evenings we smoked and talked, and never dreamt of going out except for exercise. And I never enjoyed myself more in my life. I cleared all my expenses and got initiated into the business without a fee into the bargain.

PRAED: But bless my heart and soul, Miss Warren, do you call that trying art?

VIVIE: Wait a bit. That wasn't the beginning. I went up to town on an invitation from some artistic people in Fitzjohn's Avenue: one of the girls was a Newnham chum. They took me to the National Gallery, to the Opera, and to a concert where the band played all the evening—Beethoven and Wagner and so on. I wouldn't go through that experience again for anything you could offer me. I held out for civility's sake until the third day; and then I said, plump out, that I couldn't stand any more of it, and went off to Chancery Lane. Now you know the sort of perfectly splendid modern young lady I am. How do you think I shall get on with my mother?

PRAED (*startled*): Well, I hope—er—

VIVIE: It's not so much what you hope as what you believe, that I want to know.

PRAED: Well, frankly, I am afraid your mother will be a little disappointed. Not from any shortcoming on your part—I don't mean that. But you are so different from her ideal.

VIVIE: What is her ideal like?

PRAED: Well, you must have observed, Miss Warren, that people who are dissatisfied with their own bringing up generally think that the world would be all right if everybody were to be brought up quite differently. Now your mother's life has been—er—I suppose you know—

VIVIE: I know nothing. (*Praed is appalled. His consternation grows as she continues.*) That's exactly my difficulty. You forget, Mr. Praed, that I hardly know my mother. Since I was a child I have lived in England, at school or college, or with people paid to take charge of me. I have been boarded out all my life; and my mother has lived in Brussels or Vienna and never let me go to her. I only see her when she visits England for a few days. I don't complain; it's been very pleasant; for people have been very good to me; and there has always been plenty of money to make things smooth. But don't imagine I know anything about my mother. I know far less than you do.

PRAED (*very ill at ease*): In that case—(*He stops, quite at a loss. Then, with a forced attempt at gaiety.*) But what nonsense we are talking! Of course you and your mother will get on capitally. (*He rises, and looks abroad at the view.*) What a charming little place you have here!

VIVIE (*unmoved*): If you think you are doing anything but confirming my worst suspicions by changing the subject like that, you must take me for a much greater fool than I hope I am. HER DIRECTNESS

PRAED: Your worst suspicions! Oh, pray don't say that. Now don't.

VIVIE: Why won't my mother's life bear being talked about?

PRAED: Pray think, Miss Vivie. It is natural that I should have a certain delicacy in talking to my old friend's daughter about her behind her back. You will plenty of opportunity of talking to her about it when she comes. (*Anxiously.*) I wonder what is keeping her.

VIVIE: No: She won't talk about it either. (*Rising.*) However, I won't press you. Only mind this, Mr. Praed. I strongly suspect there will be a battle royal when my mother hears of my Chancery Lane project.

PRAED (*ruefully*): I'm afraid there will.

VIVIE: I shall win the battle, because I want nothing but my fare to London to start there to-morrow earning my own living by devilling for Honoria. Besides, I have no mysteries to keep up; and it seems she has. I shall use that advantage over her if necessary.

PRAED (*greatly shocked*): Oh, no. No, pray. You'd not do such a thing.

VIVIE: Then tell me why not.

PRAED: I really cannot. I appeal to your good feeling. (*She smiles at his sentimentality.*) Besides, you may be too bold, Your mother is not to be trifled with when she's angry.

VIVIE: You can't frighten me, Mr. Praed. In that month at Chancery Lane I had opportunities of taking the measure of one or two women very like my mother who came to consult Honoria. You may back me to win. But if I hit harder in my ignorance than I need, remember that it is you who refuse to enlighten me. Now let us drop the subject.

(*She takes her chair and replaces it near the hammock with the same vigorous swing as before.*)

PRAED (*taking a desperate resolution*): One word, Miss Warren. I had better tell you. It's very difficult; but—

(*Mrs. Warren and Sir George Crofts arrive at the gate. Mrs. Warren is a woman between 40 and 50, good-looking, showily dressed in a brilliant hat and a gay blouse fitting tightly over her bust and flanked by fashionable sleeves. Rather spoiled and domineering, but, on the whole, a genial and fairly presentable old blackguard of a woman.*
Crofts is a tall, powerfully-built man of about 50, fashionably dressed in the style of a young man. Nasal voice, reedier than might be expected from his strong frame. Clean-shaven, bull-dog jaws, large flat ears, and thick neck, gentlemanly combination of the most brutal types of city man, sporting man, and man about town.)

VIVIE: Here they are. (*Coming to them as they enter the garden.*) How do, mater. Mr. Praed's been here this half hour, waiting for you.

MRS. WARREN: Well, if you've been waiting, Praddy, it's your own fault: I thought you'd have had the gumption to know I was coming by the 3:10 train. Vivie, put your hat on, dear: you'll get sunburnt. Oh, forgot to introduce you. Sir George Crofts, my little Vivie.

(*Crofts advances to Vivie with his most courtly manner. She nods, but makes no motion to shake hands.*)

CROFTS: May I shake hands with a young lady whom I have known by reputation very long as the daughter of one of my oldest friends?

VIVIE (*who has been looking him up and down sharply*): If you like. (*She takes his tenderly proffered hand and gives it a squeeze that makes him open his eyes; then turns away and says to her mother*) Will you come in, or shall I get a couple more chairs? (*She goes into the porch for the chairs.*)

MRS. WARREN: Well, George, what do you think of her?

CROFTS (*ruefully*): She has a powerful fist. Did you shake hands with her, Praed? [SOMEWHAT CORNLY JOKE]

PRAED: Yes it will pass off presently. [ON SHAWS PART]

CROFTS: I hope so. (*Vivie reappears with two more chairs. He hurries to her assistance.*) Allow me.

MRS. WARREN (*patronizingly*): Let Sir George help you with the chairs, dear. [phony courtly manners]

VIVIE (*almost pitching two into his arms*): Here you are. (*She dusts her hands and turns to Mrs. Warren.*) You'd like some tea, wouldn't you?

MRS. WARREN (*sitting in Praed's chair and fanning herself*): I'm dying for a drop to drink.

VIVIE: I'll see about it. (*She goes into the cottage. Sir George has by this time managed to unfold a chair and plant it beside Mrs. Warren, on her left. He throws the other on the grass and sits down, looking dejected and rather foolish, with the handle of his stick in his mouth. Praed, still very uneasy, fidgets about the garden on their right.*)

MRS. WARREN (*to Praed, looking at Crofts*): Just look at him, Praddy: he looks cheerful, don't he? He's been worrying my life out these three years to have that little girl of mine shewn to him; and now that I've done it, he's quite out of countenance. (*Briskly.*) Come! sit up, George; and take your stick out of your mouth. (*Crofts sulkily obeys.*)

PRAED: I think, you know—if you don't mind my saying so—that we had better get out of the habit of thinking of her as a little girl. You see she has really distinguished herself; and I'm not sure, from what I have seen of her, that she is not older than any of us.

MRS. WARREN (*greatly amused*): Only listen to him, George! Older than any of us! Well, she has been stuffing you nicely with her importance.

PRAED: But young people are particularly sensitive about being treated in that way.

MRS. WARREN: Yes; and young people have to get all that nonsense taken out of them, and a good deal more besides. Don't you interfere, Praddy. I know how to treat my own child as well as you do. (*Praed, with a grave shake of his head, walks up the garden with his hands behind his back. Mrs. Warren pretends to laugh, but looks after him with perceptible concern. Then she whispers to Crofts.*) What's the matter with him? What does he take it like that for?

CROFTS (*morosely*): You're afraid of Praed.

MRS. WARREN: What! Me! Afraid of dear old Praddy! Why, a fly wouldn't be afraid of him.

CROFTS: You're afraid of him.

MRS. WARREN (*angry*): I'll trouble you to mind your own business, and not try any of your sulks on me. I'm not afraid of you, anyhow. If you can't make yourself agreeable, you'd better go home. (*She gets up, and, turning her back on him, finds herself face to face with Praed.*) Come, Praddy, I know it was only your tender-heartedness. You're afraid I'll bully her.

PRAED: My dear Kitty: you think I'm offended. Don't imagine that: pray don't. But you know I often notice things that escape you; and though you never take my advice, you sometimes admit afterwards that you ought to have taken it.

MRS. WARREN: Well, what do you notice now?

PRAED: Only that Vivie is a grown woman. Pray, Kitty, treat her with every respect.

MRS. WARREN (*with genuine amazement*): Respect! Treat my own daughter with respect! What next, pray!

VIVIE (*appearing at the cottage door and calling to Mrs. Warren*): Mother: will you come up to my room and take your bonnet off before tea?

MRS. WARREN: Yes, dearie. (*She laughs indulgently at Praed and pats him on the cheek as she passes him on her way to the porch. She follows Vivie into the cottage.*)

CROFTS (*furtively*): I say, Praed.

PRAED: Yes.

CROFTS: I want to ask you a rather particular question.

PRAED: Certainly. (*He takes Mrs. Warren's chair and sits close to Crofts.*)

CROFTS: That's right: they might hear us from the window. Look here: did Kitty ever tell you who that girl's father is?

PRAED: Never.

CROFTS: Have you any suspicion of who it might be?

PRAED: None.

CROFT: (*not believing him*): I know, of course, that you perhaps might feel bound not to tell if she had said anything to you. But it's very awkward to be uncertain about it now

that we shall be meeting the girl every day. We don't exactly
know how we ought to feel towards her.

PRAED: What difference can that make? We take her on her
own merits. What does it matter who her father was?

CROFTS (*suspiciously*): Then you know who he was?

PRAED (*with a touch of temper*): I said no just now. Did
you not hear me?

CROFTS: Look here, Praed. I ask you as a particular favor.
If you do know (*movement of protest from Praed*)—I only
say, if you know, you might at least set my mind at rest
about her. The fact is I feel attracted towards her. Oh, don't
be alarmed: it's quite an innocent feeling. That's what puz-
zles me about it. Why, for all I know, I might be her father.

PRAED: You! Impossible! Oh, no nonsense!

CROFTS (*catching him up cunningly*): You know for certain that I'm not?

PRAED: I know nothing about it, I tell you, any more than
you. But really, Crofts—oh, no, it's out of the question.
There's not the least resemblance.

CROFTS: As to that, there's no resemblance between her
and her mother that I can see. I suppose she's not your
daughter, is she?

PRAED (*He meets the question with an indignant stare;
then recovers himself with an effort and answers gently and
gravely*): Now listen to me, my dear Crofts. I have nothing
to do with that side of Mrs. Warren's life, and never had. She
has never spoken to me about it; and of course I have never
spoken to her about it. Your delicacy will tell you that a
handsome woman needs some friends who are not—well, not
on that footing with her. The effect of her own beauty would
become a torment to her if she could not escape from it occasionally. You are probably on much more confidential
terms with Kitty than I am. Surely you can ask her the question yourself.

CROFTS (*rising impatiently*): I have asked her often
enough. But she's so determined to keep the child all to herself that she would deny that it ever had a father if she
could. No: there's nothing to be got out of her—nothing that
one can believe, anyhow. I'm thoroughly uncomfortable
about it, Praed.

PRAED (*rising also*): Well, as you are, at all events, old
enough to be her father, I don't mind agreeing that we both
regard Miss Vivie in a parental way, as a young girl whom
we are bound to protect and help. All the more, as the real
father, whoever he was, was probably a blackguard. What do
you say?

CROFTS (*aggressively*): I'm no older than you, if you come to that.

PRAED: Yes, you are, my dear fellow: you were born old. I was born a boy: I've never been able to feel the assurance of a grown-up man in my life.

MRS. WARREN (*calling from within the cottage*): Prad-dee! George! Tea-ea-ea-ea!

CROFTS (*hastily*): She's calling us. (*He hurries in. Praed shakes his head bodingly, and is following slowly when he is hailed by a young gentleman who has just appeared on the common, and is making for the gate. He is a pleasant, pretty, smartly dressed, and entirely good-for-nothing young fellow, not long turned 20, with a charming voice and agreeably disrespectful manner. He carries a very light sporting magazine rifle.*)

THE YOUNG GENTLEMAN: Hallo, Praed!

PRAED: Why, Frank Gardner! (*Frank comes in and shakes hands cordially.*) What on earth are you doing here?

FRANK: Staying with my father.

PRAED: The Roman father?

FRANK: He's rector here. I'm living with my people this autumn for the sake of economy. Things came to a crisis in July: the Roman father had to pay my debts. He's stony broke in consequence; and so am I. What are you up to in these parts? Do you know the people here?

PRAED: Yes: I'm spending the day with a Miss Warren.

FRANK (*enthusiastically*): What! Do you know Vivie? Isn't she a jolly girl! I'm teaching her to shoot—you see (*shewing the rifle.*) I'm so glad she knows you: you're just the sort of fellow she ought to know. (*He smiles, and raises the charming voice almost to a singing tone as he exclaims*) It's ever so jolly to find you here, Praed. Ain't it, now?

PRAED: I'm an old friend of her mother's. Mrs. Warren brought me over to make her daughter's acquaintance.

FRANK: The mother! Is she here?

PRAED: Yes—inside at tea.

MRS. WARREN (*calling from within*): Prad-dee-ee-ee-eee! The tea-cake'll be cold.

PRAED (*calling*): Yes, Mrs. Warren. In a moment. I've just met a friend here.

MRS. WARREN: A what?

PRAED (*louder*): A friend.

MRS. WARREN: Bring him up.

PRAED: All right. (*To Frank.*) Will you accept the invitation?

FRANK (*incredulous, but immensely amused*): Is that Vivie's mother?

PRAED: Yes.

FRANK: By Jove! What a lark! Do you think she'll like me?

PRAED: I've no doubt you'll make yourself popular, as usual. Come in and try (*moving towards the house*).

FRANK: Stop a bit. (*Seriously.*) I want to take you into my confidence.

PRAED: Pray don't. It's only some fresh folly, like the barmaid at Redhill.

FRANK: It's ever so much more serious than that. You say you've only just met Vivie for the first time?

PRAED: Yes.

FRANK (*rhapsodically*): Then you can have no idea what a girl she is. Such character! Such sense! And her cleverness! Oh, my eye, Praed, but I can tell you she is clever! And the most loving little heart that—

CROFT: (*putting his head out of the window*): I say, Praed: what are you about? Do come along. (*He disappears.*)

FRANK: Hallo! Sort of chap that would take a prize at a dog show, ain't he? Who's he?

PRAED: Sir George Crofts, an old friend of Mrs. Warren's. I think we had better come in.

(*On their way to the porch they are interrupted by a call from the gate. Turning, they see an elderly clergyyman looking over it.*)

THE CLERGYMAN (*calling*): Frank!

FRANK: Hallo! (*To Praed.*) The Roman father. (*To the clergyman.*) Yes, gov'nor: all right: presently. (*To Praed.*) Look here, Praed: you'd better go in to tea. I'll join you directly.

PRAED: Very good. (*He raises his hat to the clergyman, who acknowledges the salute distantly. Praed goes into the cottage. The clergyman remains stiffly outside the gate, with his hands on the top of it. The Rev. Samuel Gardner, a beneficed clergyman of the Established Church, is over 50. He is a pretentious, booming, noisy person, hopelessly asserting himself as a father and a clergyman without being able to command respect in either capacity.*)

REV. S.: Well, sir. Who are your friends here, if I may ask?

FRANK: Oh, it's all right, gov'nor! Come in.

REV. S.: No, sir; not until I know whose garden I am entering.

FRANK: It's all right. It's Miss Warren's.

REV. S.: I have not seen her at church since she came.

FRANK: Of course not: she's a third wrangler—ever so intellectual!—took a higher degree than you did; so why should she go to hear you preach?

REV. S.: Don't be disrespectful, sir.

FRANK: Oh, it don't matter: nobody hears us. Come in. (*He opens the gate, unceremoniously pulling his father with it into the garden.*) I want to introduce you to her. She and I get on rattling well together: she's charming. Do you remember the advice you gave me last July, gov'nor?

REV. S. (*severely*): Yes. I advised you to conquer your idleness and flippancy, and to work your way into an honorable profession and live on it and not upon me.

FRANK: No: that's what you thought of afterwards. What you actually said was that since I had neither brains nor money, I'd better turn my good looks to account by marrying somebody with both. Well, look here. Miss Warren has brains: you can't deny that.

REV. S.: Brains are not everything.

FRANK: No, of course not: there's the money—

REV. S. (*interrupting him austerely*): I was not thinking of money, sir. I was speaking of higher things—social position, for instance.

FRANK: I don't care a rap about that.

REV. S.: But I do, sir.

FRANK: Well, nobody wants you to marry her. Anyhow, she has what amounts to a high Cambridge degree; and she seems to have as much money as she wants.

REV. S. (*sinking into a feeble vein of humor*): I greatly doubt whether she has as much money as you will want.

FRANK: Oh, come: I haven't been so very extravagant. I live ever so quietly; I don't drink; I don't bet much; and I never go regularly on the razzle-dazzle as you did when you were my age.

REV. S. (*booming hollowly*): Silence, sir.

FRANK: Well, you told me yourself, when I was making ever such an ass of myself about the barmaid at Redhill, that you once offered a woman £50 for the letters you wrote to her when—

REV. S. (*terrified*): Sh-sh-sh, Frank, for Heaven's sake! (*He looks round apprehensively. Seeing no one within earshot he plucks up courage to boom again, but more subduedly.*) You are taking an ungentlemanly advantage of what

I confided to you for your own good, to save you from an error you would have repented all your life long. Take warning by your father's follies, sir; and don't make them an excuse for your own.

FRANK: Did you ever hear the story of the Duke of Wellington and his letters?

REV. S.: No, sir; and I don't want to hear it.

FRANK: The old Iron Duke didn't throw away £50—not he. He just wrote: "My dear Jenny: Publish and be damned! Yours affectionately, Wellington." That's what you should have done.

REV. S. (*piteously*): Frank, my boy: when I wrote those letters I put myself into that woman's power. When I told you about her I put myself, to some extent, I am sorry to say, in your power. She refused my money with these words, which I shall never forget: "Knowledge is power," she said; "and I never sell power." That's more than twenty years ago; and she has never made use of her power or caused me a moment's uneasiness. You are behaving worse to me than she did, Frank.

FRANK: Oh, yes, I dare say! Did you ever preach at her the way you preach at me every day?

REV. S. (*wounded almost to tears*): I leave you, sir. You are incorrigible. (*He turns towards the gate.*)

FRANK (*utterly unmoved*): Tell them I shan't be home to tea, will you, gov'nor, like a good fellow? (*He goes towards the cottage door and is met by Vivie coming out, followed by Praed, Crofts, and Mrs. Warren.*)

VIVIE (*to Frank*): Is that your father, Frank? I do so want to meet him.

FRANK: Certainly. (*Calling after his father.*) Gov'nor. (*The Rev. S. turns at the gate, fumbling nervously at his hat. Praed comes down the garden on the opposite side, beaming in anticipation of civilities. Crofts prowls about near the hammock, poking it with his stick to make it swing. Mrs. Warren halts on the threshold, staring hard at the clergyman.*) Let me introduce—my father: Miss Warren.

VIVIE (*going to the clergyman and shaking his hand*): Very glad to see you here, Mr. Gardner. Let me introduce everybody. Mr. Gardner—Mr. Frank Gardner—Mr. Praed—Sir George Crofts, and—(*As the men are raising their hats to one another, Vivie is interrupted by an exclamation from her mother, who swoops down on the Reverend Samuel*).

MRS. WARREN: Why, it's Sam Gardner, gone into the

church! Don't you know us, Sam? <u>This is George Crofts, as large as life and twice as natural.</u> Don't you remember me?

REV. S. (*very red*): I really—er—

MRS. WARREN: Of course you do. Why, I have a whole <u>album of your letters still: I came across them only the other</u> day.

REV. S. (*miserably confused*): Miss Vavasour, I believe.

MRS. WARREN (*correcting him quickly in a loud whisper*): Tch! Nonsense—Mrs. Warren: don't you see my daughter there? FINE THEATRICAL SENSE! CURTAIN

ACT 2

Inside the cottage after nightfall. Looking eastward from within instead of westward from without, the latticed window, with its curtains drawn, is now seen in the middle of the front wall of the cottage, with the porch door to the left of it. In the left-hand side wall is the door leading to the wing. Farther back against the same wall is a dresser with a candle and matches on it, and Frank's rifle standing beside them, with the barrel resting in the plate-rack. In the centre a table stands with a lighted lamp on it. Vivie's books and writing materials are on a table to the right of the window, against the wall. The fireplace is on the right, with a settle: there is no fire. Two of the chairs are set right and left of the table.

The cottage door opens, shewing a fine starlit night without; and Mrs. Warren, her shoulders wrapped in a shawl borrowed from Vivie, enters, followed by Frank. She has had enough of walking, and gives a gasp of relief as she unpins her hat; takes it off; sticks the pin through the crown; and puts it on table.

MRS. WARREN: O Lord! I don't know which is the worst of the country, the walking or the sitting at home with nothing to do: I could do a whisky and soda now very well, if only they had such a thing in this place.

FRANK (*helping her to take off her shawl, and giving her shoulders the most delicate possible little caress with his fingers as he does so*): Perhaps Vivie's got some.

MRS. WARREN (*glancing back at him for an instant from the corner of her eye as she detects the pressure*): Nonsense! What would a young girl like her be doing with such things! Never mind: it don't matter. (*She throws herself wearily into*

all of this is very bad, very modern —

a chair at the table.) I wonder how she passes her time here! I'd a good deal rather be in Vienna.

FRANK: Let me take you there. (*He folds the shawl neatly; hangs it on the back of the other chair; and sits down opposite Mrs. Warren.*)

MRS. WARREN: Get out! I'm beginning to think you're a chip of the old block.

FRANK: Like the gov'nor, eh?

MRS. WARREN: Never you mind. What do you know about such things? You're only a boy.

FRANK: Do come to Vienna with me? It'd be ever such larks.

MRS. WARREN: No, thank you. Vienna is no place for you—at least not until you're a little older. (*She nods at him to emphasize this piece of advice. He makes a mockpiteous face, belied by his laughing eyes. She looks at him; then rises and goes to him.*) Now, look here, little boy (*taking his face in her hands and turning it up to her*): I know you through and through by your likeness to your father, better than you know yourself. Don't you go taking any silly ideas into your head about me. Do you hear?

FRANK (*gallantly wooing her with his voice*): Can't help it, my dear Mrs. Warren: it runs in the family. (*She pretends to box his ears; then looks at the pretty, laughing, upturned face for a moment, tempted. At last she kisses him and immediately turns away, out of patience with herself.*)

MRS. WARREN: There! I shouldn't have done that. I am wicked. Never you mind, my dear: its' only a motherly kiss. Go and make love to Vivie.

FRANK: So I have.

MRS. WARREN (*turning on him with a sharp note of alarm in her voice*): What!

FRANK: Vivie and I are ever such chums.

MRS. WARREN: What do you mean? Now, see here: I won't have any young scamp tampering with my little girl. Do you hear? I won't have it.

FRANK (*quite unabashed*): My dear Mrs. Warren: don't you be alarmed. My intentions are honorable—ever so honorable; and your little girl is jolly well able to take care of herself. She don't need looking after half so much as her mother. She ain't so handsome, you know.

MRS. WARREN (*taken aback by his assurance*): Well, you have got a nice, healthy two inches thick of cheek all over you. I don't know where you got it—not from your father, anyhow. (*Voices and footsteps in the porch*). Sh! I hear the others coming in. (*She sits down hastily.*) Remember: you've

Marvelous satire on Xian charity

got your warning. (*The Rev. Samuel comes in, followed by Crofts.*) Well, what became of you two? And where's Praddy and Vivie?

CROFTS (*putting his hat on the settle and his stick in the chimney corner*): They went up the hill. We went to the village. I wanted a drink. (*He sits down on the settle, putting his legs up along the seat.*)

MRS. WARREN: Well, she oughtn't to go off like that without telling me. (*To Frank.*) Get your father a chair, Frank: where are your manners? (*Frank springs up and gracefully offers his father his chair; then takes another from the wall and sits down at the table, in the middle, with his father on his right and Mrs. Warren on his left.*) George: where are you going to stay to-night? You can't stay here. And what's Praddy going to do?

CROFTS: Gardner'll put me up.

MRS. WARREN: Oh, no doubt you've taken care of yourself! but what about Praddy?

CROFTS: Don't know. I suppose he can sleep at the inn.

MRS. WARREN: Haven't you room for him, Sam?

REV. S.: Well, er—you see, as rector here, I am not free to do as I like exactly. Er—what is Mr. Praed's social position?

MRS. WARREN: Oh, he's all right: he's an architect. What an old-stick-in-the-mud you are, Sam!

FRANK: Yes, its' all right, gov'nor. He built that place down in Monmouthshire for the Duke of Beaufort—Tintern Abbey they call it. You must have heard of it. (*He winks with lightning smartness at Mrs. Warren, and regards his father blandly.*)

REV. S.: Oh, in that case, of course we shall only be too happy. I suppose he knows the Duke of Beaufort personally.

FRANK: Oh, ever so intimately! We can stick him in Georgina's old room.

MRS. WARREN: Well, that's settled. Now, if those two would only come in and let us have supper. They've no right to stay out after dark like this.

CROFTS (*aggressively*): What harm are they doing you?

MRS. WARREN: Well, harm or not, I don't like it.

FRANK: Better not wait for them, Mrs. Warren. Praed will stay out as long as possible. He has never known before what it is to stray over the heath on a summer night with my Vivie.

CROFTS (*sitting up in some consternation*): I say, you know. Come!

REV. S. (*startled out of his professional manner into real*

*Rev Sam says there are reasons Vivie can't marry Frank—
But Mrs. W's reaction is IMPT.*

force and sincerity): Frank, once for all, it's out of the question. Mrs. Warren will tell you that it's not to be thought of.

CROFTS: Of course not.

FRANK (*with enchanting placidity*): Is that so, Mrs. Warren?

MRS. WARREN (*reflectively*): Well, Sam, I don't know. If the girl wants to get married, no good can come of keeping her unmarried.

REV. S. (*astounded*): But married to him!—your daughter to my son! Only think: it's impossible.

CROFTS: Of course it's impossible. Don't be a fool, Kitty.

MRS. WARREN (*nettled*): Why not? Isn't my daughter good enough for your son?

REV. S.: But surely, my dear Mrs. Warren, you know the reason—

MRS. WARREN (*defiantly*): I know no reasons. If you know any, you can tell them to the lad, or to the girl, or to your congregation, if you like.

REV. S.: (*helplessly*): You know very well that I couldn't tell anyone the reasons. But my boy will believe me when I tell him there are reasons.

FRANK: Quite right, Dad: he will. But has your boy's conduct ever been influenced by your reasons?

CROFTS: You can't marry her; and that's all about it. (*He gets up and stands on the hearth, with his back to the fireplace, frowning determinedly.*) *BECAUSE HE WANTS TO*

MRS. WARREN (*turning on him sharply*): What have you got to do with it, pray?

FRANK (*with his prettiest lyrical cadence*): Precisely what I was going to ask, myself, in my own graceful fashion.

CROFTS (*to Mrs. Warren*): I suppose you don't want to marry the girl to a man younger than herself and without either a profession or twopence to keep her on. Ask Sam, if you don't believe me. (*To the Rev. S.*) How much more money are you going to give him?

REV. S.: Not another penny. He has had his patrimony; and he spent the last of it in July. (*Mrs. Warren's face falls.*)

CROFTS (*watching her*): There! I told you (*He resumes his place on the settle and puts up his legs on the seat again, as if the matter were finally disposed of.*)

FRANK (*plaintively*): This is ever so mercenary. Do you suppose Miss Warren's going to marry for money? If we love one another—

MRS. WARREN: Thank you. Your love's a pretty cheap commodity, my lad. If you have no means of keeping a wife, that settles it: you can't have Vivie.

Everyone talks in the tradional way as if Vivie had nothing to say about it herself—

FRANK (*much amused*): What do you say, gov'nor, eh?

REV. S.: I agree with Mrs. Warren.

FRANK: And good old Crofts has already expressed his opinion.

CROFTS (*turning angrily on his elbow*): Look here: I want none of your cheek.

FRANK (*pointedly*): I'm ever so sorry to surprise you, Crofts; but you allowed yourself the liberty of speaking to me like a father a moment ago. One father is enough, thank you.

CROFTS (*contemptuously*): Yah! (*He turns away again.*)

FRANK (*rising*): Mrs. Warren: I cannot give my Vivie up even for your sake.

MRS. WARREN (*muttering*): Young scamp!

FRANK (*continuing*): And as you no doubt intend to hold out other prospects to her, I shall lose no time in placing my case before her. (*They stare at him; and he begins to declaim gracefully*)

> He either fears his fate too much,
>   Or his deserts are small,
> That dares not put it to the touch
>   To gain or lose it all.

(*The cottage door opens whilst he is reciting; and Vivie and Praed come in. He breaks off. Praed puts his hat on the dresser. There is an immediate improvement in the company's behaviour. Crofts takes down his legs from the settle and pulls himself together as Praed joins him at the fireplace. Mrs. Warren loses her ease of manner, and takes refuge in querulousness.*)

MRS. WARREN: Wherever have you been, Vivie?

VIVIE (*taking off her hat and throwing it carelessly on the table*): On the hill.

MRS. WARREN: Well, you shouldn't go off like that without letting me know. How could I tell what had become of you—and night coming on, too!

VIVIE (*going to the door of the inner room and opening it, ignoring her mother*): Now, about supper? We shall be rather crowded in here, I'm afraid.

MRS WARREN: Did you hear what I said, Vivie?

VIVIE (*quietly*): Yes, mother. (*Reverting to the supper difficulty.*) How many are we? (*Counting.*) One, two, three, four, five, six. Well, two will have to wait until the rest are done: Mrs. Alison has only plates and knives for four.

PRAED: Oh, it doesn't matter about me. I—

VIVIE: You have had a long walk and are hungry, Mr. Praed: you shall have your supper at once. I can wait myself. I want one person to wait with me. Frank: are you hungry?

FRANK: Not the least in the world—completely off my peck, in fact.

MRS. WARREN (to Crofts): Neither are you, George. You can wait.

CROFTS: Oh, hang it, I've eaten nothing since tea-time. Can't Sam do it?

FRANK: Would you starve my poor father?

REV. S. (testily): Allow me to speak for myself, sir. I am perfectly willing to wait.

VIVIE (decisively): There's no need. Only two are wanted. (She opens the door of the inner room.) Will you take my mother in, Mr. Gardner. (The Rev. S. takes Mrs. Warren; and they pass into the next room. Praed and Crofts follow. All except Praed clearly disapprove of the arrangement, but do not know how to resist it. Vivie stands at the door looking in at them.) Can you squeeze past to that corner, Mr. Praed: it's rather a tight fit. Take care of your coat against the white-wash—that's right. Now, are you all comfortable?

PRAED (within): Quite, thank you.

MRS. WARREN (within): Leave the door open, dearie. (Frank looks at Vivie; then steals to the cottage door and softly sets it wide open.) Oh, Lor', what a draught! You'd better shut it, dear. (Vivie shuts it promptly. Frank noiselessly shuts the cottage door.)

FRANK (exulting): Aha! Got rid of 'em. Well, Vivvums: what do you think of my governor!

VIVIE (preoccupied and serious): I've hardly spoken to him. He doesn't strike me as being a particulary able person.

FRANK: Well, you know, the old man is not altogether such a fool as he looks. You see, he's rector here; and in trying to live up to it he makes a much bigger ass of himself than he really is. No, the gov'nor ain't so bad, poor old chap; and I don't dislike him as much as you might expect. He means well. How do you think you'll get on with him?

VIVIE (rather grimly): I don't think my future life will be much concerned with him, or with any of that old circle of my mother's, except perhaps Praed. What do you think of my mother?

FRANK: Really and truely?

VIVIE: Yes, really and truly.

FRANK: Well, she's ever so jolly. But she's rather a caution, isn't she? And Crofts! Oh, my eye, Crofts!

VIVIE: What a lot, Frank!

FRANK: What a crew! *A SHOW OF MORAL KRTR*

VIVIE (*with intense contempt for them*): If I thought that I was like that—that I was going to be a waster, shifting along from one meal to another with no purpose, and no character, and no grit in me, I'd open an artery and bleed to death without one moment's hesitation.

FRANK: Oh, no, you wouldn't. Why should they take any grind when they can afford not to? I wish I had their luck. No: what I object to is their form. It isn't the thing: it's slovenly, ever so slovenly. *REALITY RE FRANK*

VIVIE: Do you think your form will be any better when you're as old as Crofts, if you don't work?

FRANK: Of course I do—ever so much better. Vivvums mustn't lecture: her little boy's incorrigible. (*He attempts to take her face caressingly in his hands.*)

VIVIE (*striking his hands down sharply*): Off with you: Vivvums is not in a humor for petting her little boy this evening.

FRANK: How unkind!

VIVIE (*stamping at him*): Be serious. I'm serious.

FRANK: Good. Let us talk learnedly. Miss Warren: do you know that all the most advanced thinkers are agreed that half the diseases of modern civilization are due to starvation of the affections in the young. Now, I—

VIVIE (*cutting him short*): You are getting tiresome. (*She opens the inner door.*) Have you room for Frank there? He's complaining of starvation.

MRS. WARREN (*within*): Of course there is (*clatter of knives and glasses as she moves the things on the table*). Here: there's room now beside me. Come along, Mr. Frank.

FRANK (*aside to Vivie, as he goes*): Her little boy will be ever so even with his Vivvums for this. (*He goes into the other room.*)

MRS. WARREN (*within*): Here, Vivie: come on, you too, child. You must be famished. (*She enters, followed by Crofts, who holds the door open for Vivie with marked deference. She goes out without looking at him; and he shuts the door after her.*) Why, George, you can't be done; you've eaten nothing.

CROFTS: Oh, all I wanted was a drink. (*He thrusts his hands in his pockets and begins prowling about the room, restless and sulky.*)

MRS. WARREN: Well, I like enough to eat. But a little of

that cold beef and cheese and lettuce goes a long way. (*With a sigh of only half repletion she sits down lazily at the table.*)

CROFTS: What do you go encouraging that young pup for?

MRS. WARREN (*on the alert at once*): Now see here, George: what are you up to about that girl? I've been watching your way of looking at her. Remember: I know you and what your looks mean.

CROFTS: There's no harm in looking at her, is there?

MRS. WARREN: I'd put you out and pack you back to London pretty soon if I saw any of your nonsense. My girl's little finger is more to me than your whole body and soul. (*Crofts receives this with a sneering grin. Mrs. Warren, flushing a little at her failure to impose on him in the character of a theatrically devoted mother, adds in a lower key.*) Make your mind easy: the young pup has no more chance than you have.

CROFTS: Mayn't a man take an interest in a girl?

MRS. WARREN: Not a man like you.

CROFTS: How old is she?

MRS. WARREN: Never you mind how old she is.

CROFTS: Why do you make such a secret of it?

MRS. WARREN: Because I choose.

CROFTS: Well, I'm not fifty yet; and my property is as good as it ever was—

MRS. WARREN (*interrupting him*): Yes; because you're as stingy as you're vicious.

CROFT: (*continuing*): And a baronet isn't to be picked up every day. No other man in my position would put up with you for a mother-in-law. Why shouldn't she marry me?

MRS. WARREN: You!

CROFTS: We three could live together quite comfortably. I'd die before her and leave her a bouncing widow with plenty of money. Why not? It's been growing in my mind all the time I've been walking with that fool inside there.

MRS. WARREN (*revolted*): Yes; it's the sort of think that would grow in your mind. (*He halts in his prowling; and the two look at one another, she steadfastly, with a sort of awe behind her contemptuous disgust: he stealthily, with a carnal gleam in his eye and a loose grin, tempting her.*)

CROFTS (*suddenly becoming anxious and urgent as he sees no sign of sympathy in her*): Look here, Kitty: you're a sensible woman: you needn't put on any moral airs. I'll ask no more questions; and you need answer none. I'll settle the whole property on her; and if you want a cheque for yourself on the wedding day, you can name any figure you like—in reason.

(handwritten: The CONFRONTATION BETWEEN MRS. W. & CROFTS OVER VIVIE)

MRS. WARREN: Faugh! So it's come to that with you, George, like all the other worn out old creatures.

CROFTS (*savagely*): Damn you! (*She rises and turns fiercely on him; but the door of the inner room is opened just then; and the voices of the others are heard returning. Crofts, unable to recover his presence of mind, hurries out of the cottage. The clergyman comes back.*)

REV. S: (*looking around*): Where is Sir George?

MRS. WARREN: Gone out to have a pipe. (*She goes to the fireplace, turning her back on him to compose herself. The clergyman goes to the table for his hat. Meanwhile Vivie comes in, followed by Frank, who collapses into the nearest chair with an air of extreme exhaustion. Mrs. Warren looks round at Vivie and says, with her affectation of maternal patronage even more forced than usual.*) Well, dearie: have you had a good supper?

VIVIE: You know what Mrs. Alison's suppers are. (*She turns to Frank and pets him.*) Poor Frank! was all the beef gone? did it get nothing but bread and cheese and ginger beer? (*Seriously, as if she had done quite enough trifling for one evening.*) Her butter is really awful. I must get some down from the stores.

FRANK: Do, in Heaven's name!

(*Vivie goes to the writing-table and makes a memorandum to order the butter. Praed comes in from the inner room, putting up his handkerchief, which he has been using as a napkin.*)

REV. S.: Frank, my boy: it is time for us to be thinking of home. Your mother does not know yet that we have visitors.

PRAED: I'm afraid we're giving trouble.

FRANK: Not the least in the world, Praed: my mother will be delighted to see you. She's a genuinely intellectual, artistic woman; and she sees nobody here from one year's end to another except the gov'nor; so you can imagine how jolly dull it pans out for her. (*To the Rev. S.*) You're not intellectual or artistic, are you, pater? So take Praed home at once; and I'll stay here and entertain Mrs. Warren. You'll pick up Crofts in the garden. He'll be excellent company for the bull-pup.

PRAED (*taking his hat from the dresser, and coming close to Frank*): Come with us, Frank. Mrs. Warren has not seen Miss Vivie for a long time; and we have prevented them from having a moment together yet.

FRANK (*quite softened, and looking at Praed with romantic admiration*): Of course: I forgot. Ever so thanks for reminding me. Perfect gentleman, Praddy. Always were—my ideal through life. (*He rises to go, but pauses a moment between the two older men, and puts his hand on Praed's shoulder.*) Ah, if you had only been my father instead of this unworthy old man! (*He puts his other hand on his father's shoulder.*)

REV. S. (*blustering*): Silence, sir, silence: you are profane.

MRS. WARREN (*laughing heartily*): You should keep him in better order, Sam. Good-night. Here: take George his hat and stick with my compliments.

REV. S. (*taking them*): Good-night. (*They shake hands. As he passes Vivie he shakes hands with her also and bids her good-night. Then, in booming command, to Frank.*) Come along, sir, at once. (*He goes out. Meanwhile Frank has taken his cap from the dresser and his rifle from the rack. Praed shakes hands with Mrs. Warren and Vivie and goes out, Mrs. Warren accompanying him idly to the door, and looking out after him as he goes across the garden. Frank silently begs a kiss from Vivie; but she, dismissing him with a stern glance, takes a couple of books and some paper from the writing-table, and sits down with them at the middle table, so as to have the benefit of the lamp.*)

FRANK (*at the door, taking Mrs. Warren's hand*): Good night, dear Mrs. Warren. (*He squeezes her hand. She snatches it away, her lips tightening, and looks more than half disposed to box his ears. He laughs mischievously and runs off, clapping-to the door behind him.*)

MRS. WARREN (*coming back to her place at the table, opposite Vivie, resigning herself to an evening of boredom now that the men are gone*): Did you ever in your life hear anyone rattle on so? Isn't he a tease? (*She sits down.*) Now that I think of it, dearie, don't you go encouraging him. I'm sure he's a regular good-for-nothing.

VIVIE: Yes: I'm afraid poor Frank is a thorough good-for-nothing. I shall have to get rid of him; but I shall feel sorry for him, though he's not worth it, poor lad. That man Crofts does not seem to me to be good for much either, is he?

MRS. WARREN (*galled by Vivie's cool tone*): What do you know of men, child, to talk that way about them? You'll have to make up your mind to see a good deal of Sir George Crofts, as he's a friend of mine.

VIVIE (*quite unmoved*): Why? Do you expect that we shall be much together—you and I, I mean?

MRS WARREN (*staring at her*): Of course—until you're married. You're not going back to college again.

VIVIE: Do you think my way of life would suit you? I doubt it.

MRS. WARREN: Your way of life! What do you mean?

VIVIE (*cutting a page of her book with the paper knife on her chatelaine*): Has it really never occurred to you, mother, that I have a way of life like other people?

MRS. WARREN: What nonsense is this you're trying to talk? Do you want to shew your independence, now that you're a great little person at school? Don't be a fool, child.

VIVIE (*indulgently*): That's all you have to say on the subject, is it, mother?

MRS. WARREN (*puzzled, then angry*): Don't you keep on asking me questions like that. (*Violently.*) Hold your tongue. (*Vivie works on, losing no time, and saying nothing.*) You and your way of life, indeed! What next? (*She looks at Vivie again. No reply.*) Your way of life will be what I please, so it will. (*Another pause.*) I've been noticing these airs in you ever since you got that tripos or whatever you call it. If you think I'm going to put up with them you're mistaken; and the sooner you find it out, the better. (*Muttering.*) All I have to say on the subject, indeed! (*Again raising her voice angrily.*) Do you know who you're speaking to, Miss?

VIVIE (*looking across at her without raising her head from her book*): No. Who are you? What are you? DEMANDS THE RIGHT

MRS. WARREN (*rising breathless*): You young imp! TO KNOW

VIVIE: Everybody knows my reputation, my social standing, and the profession I intend to pursue. I know nothing about you. What is that way of life which you invite me to share with you and Sir George Crofts, pray?

MRS. WARREN: Take care. I shall do something I'll be sorry for after, and you, too.

VIVIE (*putting aside her books with cool decision*): Well, let us drop the subject until you are better able to face it. (*Looking critically at her mother.*) You want some good walks and a little lawn tennis to set you up. You are shockingly out of condition: you were not able to manage twenty yards uphill to-day without stopping to pant; and your wrists are mere rolls of fat. Look at mine. (*She holds out her wrists.*)

MRS. WARREN (*after looking at her helplessly, begins to whimper*): Vivie—

VIVIE (*springing up sharply*): Now pray don't begin to cry. Anything but that. I really cannot stand whimpering. I will go out of the room if you do.

MRS. WARREN (*piteously*): Oh, my darling, how can you

Act 2

be so hard on me? Have I no rights over you as your mother?

VIVIE: Are you my mother?

MRS. WARREN (_appalled_): Am I your mother! Oh, Vivie!

VIVIE: Then where are our relatives—my father—our family friends? You claim the rights of a mother: the right to call me fool and child; to speak to me as no woman in authority over me at college dare speak to me; to dictate my way of life; and to force on me the acquaintance of a brute whom anyone can see to be the most vicious sort of London man about town. Before I give myself the trouble to resist such claims, I may as well find out whether they have any real existence.

MRS. WARREN (_distracted, throwing herself on her knees_): Oh, no, no. Stop, stop. I am your mother: I swear it. Oh, you can't mean to turn on me—my own child: it's not natural. You believe me, don't you? Say you believe me.

VIVIE: Who was my father?

MRS. WARREN: You don't know what you're asking. I can't tell you.

VIVIE (_determinedly_): Oh, yes, you can, if you like. I have a right to know; and you know very well that I have that right. You can refuse to tell me, if you please; but if you do, you will see the last of me to-morrow morning.

MRS. WARREN: Oh, it's too horrible to hear you talk like that. You wouldn't—you couldn't leave me.

VIVIE (_ruthlessly_): Yes, without a moment's hesitation, if you trifle with me about this. (_Shivering with disgust._) How can I feel sure that I may not have the contaminated blood of that brutal waster in my veins?

MRS. WARREN: No, no. On my oath it's not he, nor any of the rest that you have ever met. I'm certain of that, at least. (_Vivie's eyes fasten sternly on her mother as the significance of this flashes on her._) RULES OUT REV. S.

VIVIE (_slowly_): You are certain of that, at least. Ah! You mean that that is all you are certain of. (_Thoughtfully._) I see. (_Mrs. Warren buries her face in her hands._) Don't do that, mother: you know you don't feel it a bit. (_Mrs. Warren takes down her hands and looks up deplorably at Vivie, who takes out her watch and says_) Well, that is enough for to-night. At what hour would you like breakfast? Is half-past eight too early for you?

MRS. WARREN (_wildly_): My God, what sort of woman are you?

VIVIE (_coolly_): The sort the world is mostly made of, I should hope. Otherwise I don't understand how it gets its

Doesn't know who Vivies father I

business done. Come (*taking her mother by the wrist, and pulling her up pretty resolutely*): pull yourself together. That's right.

MRS. WARREN (*querulously*): You're very rough with me, Vivie.

VIVIE: Nonsense. What about bed? It's past ten.

MRS. WARREN (*passionately*): What's the use of my going to bed? Do you think I could sleep?

VIVIE: Why not? I shall.

MRS. WARREN: You! you've no heart. (*She suddenly breaks out vehemently in her natural tongue—the dialect of a woman of the people—with all her affectations of maternal authority and conventional manners gone, and an overwhelming inspiration of true conviction and scorn in her.*) Oh, I won't bear it: I won't put up with the injustice of it. What right have you to set yourself up above me like this? You boast of what you are to me—to me, who gave you the chance of being what you are. What chance had I? Shame on you for a bad daughter and a stuck-up prude!

VIVIE (*cool and determined, but no longer confident; for her replies, which have sounded convincingly sensible and strong to her so far, now begin to ring rather woodenly and even priggishly against the new tone of her mother*): Don't think for a moment I set myself above you in any way. You attacked me with the conventional authority of a mother: I defended myself with the conventional superiority of a respectable woman. Frankly, I am not going to stand any of your nonsense; and when you drop it I shall not expect you to stand any of mine. I shall always respect your right to your own opinions and your own way of life.

MRS. WARREN: My own opinions and my own way of life! Listen to her talking! Do you think I was brought up like you—able to pick and choose my own way of life? Do you think I did what I did because I liked it, or thought it right, or wouldn't rather have gone to college and been a lady if I'd had the chance?

VIVIE: Everybody has some choice, mother. The poorest girl alive may not be able to choose between being Queen of England or Principal of Newnham; but she can choose between ragpicking and flowerselling, according to her taste. People are always blaming their circumstances for what they are. I don't believe in circumstances. The people who get on in this world are the people who get up and look for the circumstances they want, and, if they can't find them, make them. IGNORANT PIOUS SELF RIGHTEOUS

MRS. WARREN: Oh, it's easy to talk, very easy, isn't it?

Here!—would you like to know what my circumstances
were?

VIVIE: Yes: you had better tell me. Won't you sit down?

MRS. WARREN: Oh, I'll sit down: don't you be afraid. (*She
plants her chair farther forward with brazen energy, and sits
down. Vivie is impressed in spite of herself.*) D'you know
what your gran'mother was?

VIVIE: No.

MRS. WARREN: No, you don't. I do. She called herself a
widow and had a fried-fish shop down by the Mint, and kept
herself and four daughters out of it. Two of us were sisters:
that was me and Liz; and we were both good-looking and
well made. I suppose our father was a well-fed man: mother
pretended he was a gentleman; but I don't know. The other
two were only half sisters—undersized, ugly, starved looking,
hard working, honest poor creatures: Liz and I would have
half-murdered them if mother hadn't half-murdered us to
keep our hands off them. They were the respectable ones.
Well, what did they get by their respectability? I'll tell you.
One of them worked in a whitelead factory twelve hours a
day for nine shillings a week until she died of lead poisoning.
She only expected to get her hands a little paralyzed; but she
died. The other was always held up to us as a model because
she married a Government laborer in the Deptford victual-
ling yard, and kept his room and the three children neat and
tidy on eighteen shillings a week—until he took to drink.
That was worth being respectable for, wasn't it?

VIVIE (*now thoughtfully attentive*): Did you and your sister think so?

MRS. WARREN: Liz didn't, I can tell you: she had more
spirit. We both went to a church school—that was part of
the ladylike airs we gave ourselves to be superior to the children that knew nothing and went nowhere—and we stayed
there until Liz went out one night and never came back. I
know the schoolmistress thought I'd soon follow her example;
for the clergyman was always warning me that Lizzie'd end
by jumping off Waterloo Bridge. Poor fool: that was all he
knew about it! But I was more afraid of the whitelead factory than I was of the river; and so would you have been in
my place. That clergyman got me a situation as scullery maid
in a temperance restaurant where they sent out for anything
you liked. Then I was a waitress; and then I went to the bar
at Waterloo station—fourteen hours a day serving drinks
and washing glasses for four shillings a week and my board.
That was considered a great promotion for me. Well, one
cold, wretched night, when I was so tired I could hardly keep

myself awake, who should come up for a half of Scotch but Lizzie, in a long fur cloak, elegant and comfortable, with a lot of sovereigns in her purse.

VIVIE (*grinly*): My aunt Lizzie!

MRS. WARREN: Yes: and a very good aunt to have, too. She's living down at Winchester now, close to the cathedral, one of the most respectable ladies there—chaperones girls at the county ball, if you please. No river for Liz, thank you! You remind me of Liz a little: she was a first-rate business woman—saved money from the beginning—never let herself look too like what she was—never lost her head or threw away a chance. When she saw I'd grown up good-looking she said to me across the bar: "What are you doing there, you little fool? wearing out your health and your appearance for other people's profit!" Liz was saving money then to take a house for herself in Brussels: and she thought we two could save faster than one. So she lent me some money and gave me a start; and I saved steadily and first paid her back, and then went into business with her as her partner. Why shouldn't I have done it? The house in Brussels was real high class—a much better place for a woman to be in than the factory where Anne Jane got poisoned. None of our girls were ever treated as I was treated in the scullery of that temperance place, or at the Waterloo bar, or at home. Would you have had me stay in them and become a worn out old drudge before I was forty?

VIVIE (*intensely interested by this time*): No; but why did you choose that business? Saving money and good management will succed in any business.

MRS. WARREN: Yes, saving money. But where can a woman get the money to save in any other business? Could you save out of four shillings a week and keep yourself dressed as well? Not you. Of course, if you're a plain woman and can't earn anything more; or if you have a turn for music, or the stage, or newspaper-writing: that's different. But neither Liz nor I had any turn for such things: all we had was our appearance and our turn for pleasing men. Do you think we were such fools as to let other people trade in our good looks by employing us as shopgirls, or barmaids, or waitresses, when we could trade in them ourselves and get all the profits instead of starvation wages? Not likely.

VIVIE: You were certainly quite justified—from the business point of view.

MRS. WARREN: Yes; or any other point of view. What is any respectable girl brought up to do but to catch some rich man's fancy and get the benefit of his money by marrying

> prostitution is not much different from marriage

him?—as if a marriage ceremony could make any difference in the right or wrong of the thing! Oh, the hypocrisy of the world makes me sick! Liz and I had to work and save and calculate just like other people; elseways we should be as poor as any good-for-nothing, drunken waster of a woman that thinks her luck will last for ever. (*With great energy*.) I despise such people: they've no character: and if there's a thing I hate in a woman, it's want of character.

VIVIE: Come, now, mother: frankly! Isn't it part of what you call character in a woman that she should greatly dislike such a way of making money?

MRS. WARREN: Why, of course. Everybody dislikes having to work and make money; but they have to do it all the same. I'm sure I've often pitied a poor girl, tired out and in low spirits, having to try to please some man that she doesn't care two straws for—some half-drunken fool that thinks he's making himself agreeable when he's teasing and worrying and disgusting a woman so that hardly any money could pay her for putting up with it. But she has to bear with disagreeables and take the rough with the smooth, just like a nurse in a hospital or anyone else. It's not work that any woman would do for pleasure, goodness knows: though to hear the pious people talk you would suppose it was a bed of roses.

VIVIE: Still you consider it worth while. It pays.

MRS. WARREN: Of course it's worth while to a poor girl, if she can resist temptation and is good-looking and well conducted and sensible. It's far better than any other employment open to her. I always thought that oughtn't to be. It can't be right, Vivie, that there shouldn't be better opportunities for women. I stick to that: it's wrong. But it's so, right or wrong; and a girl must make the best of it. But, of course, it's not worth while for a lady. If you took to it you'd be a fool; but I should have been a fool if I'd taken to anything else.

VIVIE (*more and more deeply moved*): Mother: suppose we were both as poor as you were in those wretched old days, are you quite sure that you wouldn't advise me to try the Waterloo bar, or marry a labourer, or even go into the factory?

MRS. WARREN (*indignantly*): Of course not. What sort of mother do you take me for! How could you keep your self-respect in such starvation and slavery? And what's a woman worth? what's life worth? without self-respect! Why am I independent and able to give my daughter a first-rate education, when other women that had just as good opportunities are in the gutter? Because I always knew how to respect myself and control myself. Why is Liz looked up to in a cathedral town? The same reason. Where would we be now if we'd minded the clergyman's foolishness? Scrubbing floors for one and sixpence a day and nothing to look forward to but the workhouse infirmary. Don't you be led astray by people who don't know the world, my girl. The only way for a woman to provide for herself decently is for her to be good to some man that can afford to be good to her. If she's in his own station of life, let her make him marry her; but if she's far beneath him she can't expect it—why should she? It wouldn't be for her own happiness. Ask any lady in London society that has daughters; and she'll tell you the same, except that I tell you straight and she'll tell you crooked. That's all the difference.

VIVIE (*fascinated, gazing at her*): My dear mother: you are a wonderful woman—you are stronger than all England. And are you really and truly not one wee bit doubtful—or—or—ashamed?

MRS. WARREN: Well, of course, dearie, it's only good manners to be ashamed of it, it's expected from a woman. Women have to pretend to feel a great deal that they don't feel. Liz used to be angry with me for plumping out the truth about it. She used to say that when every woman could learn enough from what was going on in the world before her eyes, there was no need to talk about it to her. But then Liz was such a perfect lady! She had the true instinct of it: while I was always a bit of vulgarian. I used to be so pleased when you sent me your photographs to see that you were growing up like Liz: you've just her ladylike, determined way. But I can't stand saying one thing when everyone knows I mean another. What's the use in such hypocrisy? If people arrange the world that way for women, there's no good pretending that it's arranged the other way. I never was a bit ashamed really. I consider that I had a right to be proud that we managed everything so respectably, and never had a word against us, and that the girls were so well taken care of. Some of them did very well: one of them married an ambassador. But of course now I daren't talk about such things: whatever would they think of us! (*She yawns.*) Oh, dear! I do believe I'm getting sleepy after all. (*She stretches herself lazily, thoroughly relieved by her explosion, and placidly ready for her night's rest.*)

VIVIE: I believe it is I who will not be able to sleep now. (*She goes to the dresser and lights the candle. Then she extinguishes the lamp, darkening the room a good deal.*) Better let in some fresh air before locking up. (*She opens the cottage door, and finds that it is broad moonlight.*) What a beautiful night! Look! (*She draws aside the curtains of the window. The landscape is seen bathed in the radiance of the harvest moon rising over Blackdown.*)

MRS. WARREN (*with a perfunctory glance at the scene*): Yes, dear: but take care you don't catch your death of cold from the night air.

VIVIE (*contemptuously*): Nonsense.

MRS. WARREN (*querulously*): Oh, yes: everything I say is nonsense, according to you.

VIVIE (*turning to her quickly*): No: really that is not so, mother. You have got completely the better of me to-night, though I intended it to be the other way. Let us be good friends now. VIVIE IS WONDERFUL

MRS. WARREN (*shaking her head a little ruefully*): So it has been the other way. But I suppose I must give in to it. I always got the worst of it from Liz; and now I suppose it'll be the same with you.

VIVIE: Well, never mind. Come; good-night, dear old mother. (*She takes her mother in her arms.*)

MRS. WARREN (*fondly*): I brought you up well, didn't I, dearie?

VIVIE: You did.

MRS. WARREN: And you'll be good to your poor old mother for it, won't you?

VIVIE: I will, dear. (*Kissing her.*) Good-night.

MRS. WARREN (*with unction*): Blessings on my own dearie darling—a mother's blessing! (*She embraces her daughter protectingly, instinctively looking upward as if to call down a blessing.*)

The union & the understanding, love & respect between mother & daughter

ACT 3

In the Rectory garden next morning, with the sun shining and the birds in full song. The garden wall has a five-barred wooden gate, wide enough to admit a carriage, in the middle. Beside the gate hangs a bell on a coiled spring, communicating with a pull outside. The carriage drive comes down the middle of the garden and then swerves to its left, where it ends in a little gravelled circus opposite the rectory porch. Beyond the gate is seen the dusty high road, parallel with the wall, bounded on the farther side by a strip of turf and an unfenced pine wood. On the lawn, between the house and the

*drive, is a clipped yew tree, with a garden bench in its shade.
On the opposite side the garden is shut in by a box hedge;
and there is a sundial on the turf, with an iron chair near
it. A little path leads off through the box hedge, behind the
sundial.*

*Frank, seated on the chair near the sundial, on which he
has placed the morning papers, is reading the* Standard. *His
father comes from the house, red-eyed and shivery, and
meets Frank's eyes with misgiving.*

FRANK (*looking at his watch*): Half-past eleven. Nice hour
for a rector to come down to breakfast!

REV. S.: Don't mock, Frank: don't mock. I'm a little—er-
(*Shivering.*)——

FRANK: Off colour?

REV. S. (*repudiating the expression*): No, sir: unwell this
morning. Where's your mother?

FRANK: Don't be alarmed: she's not here. Gone to town
by the 11:13 with Bessie. She left several messages for you.
Do you feel equal to receiving them now, or shall I wait till
you've breakfasted?

REV. S.: I have breakfasted, sir. I am surprised at your
mother going to town when we have people staying with us.
They'll think it very strange.

FRANK: Possibly she has considered that. At all events, if
Crofts is going to stay here, and you are going to sit up
every night with him until four, recalling the incidents of
your fiery youth, it is clearly my mother's duty, as a prudent housekeeper, to go up to the stores and order a barrel of whisky and a few hundred siphons.

REV. S.: I did not observe that Sir George drank exces-
sively.

FRANK: You were not in a condition to, gov-nor.

REV. S.: Do you mean to say that *I*—

FRANK (*calmly*): I never saw a beneficed clergyman less
sober. The anecdotes you told about your past career were so
awful that I really don't think Praed would have passed the
night under your roof if it hadn't been for the way my
mother and he took to one another.

REV. S.: Nonsense, sir. I am Sir George Crofts' host. I
must talk to him about something; and he has only one subject. Where is Mr. Praed now?

FRANK: He is driving my mother and Bessie to the station.

REV. S.: Is Crofts up yet?

FRANK: Oh, long ago. He hasn't turned a hair: he's in
much better practice than you—has kept it up ever since,

probably. He's taken himself off somewhere to smoke. (*Frank resumes his paper. The Rev. S. turns disconsolately towards the gate; then comes back irresolutely.*)

REV. S.: Er—Frank.

FRANK: Yes.

REV. S.: Do you think the Warrens will expect to be asked here after yesterday afternoon?

FRANK: They've been asked already. Crofts informed us at breakfast that you told him to bring Mrs. Warren and Vivie over here to-day, and to invite them to make this house their home. It was after that communication that my mother found she must go to town by the 11:13 train.

REV. S. (*with despairing vehemence*): I never gave any such invitation. I never thought of such a thing.

FRANK (*compassionately*): How do you know, gov'nor, what you said and thought last night? Hallo! here's Praed back again.

PRAED (*coming in through the gate*): Good morning.

REV. S.: Good morning. I must apologize for not having met you at breakfast. I have a touch of—of—

FRANK: Clergyman's sore throat, Praed. Fortunately not chronic.

PRAED (*changing the subject*): Well, I must say your house is in a charming spot here. Really most charming.

REV. S.: Yes: it is indeed. Frank will take you for a walk, Mr. Praed, if you like. I'll ask you to excuse me: I must take the opportunity to write my sermon while Mrs. Gardner is away and you are all amusing yourselves. You won't mind, will you?

PRAED: Certainly not. Don't stand on the slightest ceremony with me.

REV. S.: Thank you. I'll—er—er—(*He stammers his way to the porch and vanishes into the house.*)

PRAED (*sitting down on the turf near Frank, and hugging his ankles*): Curious thing it must be writing a sermon every week.

FRANK: Ever so curious, if he did it. He buys 'em. He's gone for some soda water.

PRAED: My dear boy: I wish you would be more respectful to your father. You know you can be so nice when you like.

FRANK: My dear Praddy: you forget that I have to live with the governor. When two people live together—it don't matter whether they're father and son, husband and wife, brother and sister—they can't keep up the polite humbug which comes so easy for ten minutes on an afternoon call. Now the governor, who unites to many admirable domestic qualities the irresoluteness of a sheep and the pompousness and aggressiveness of a jackass—

PRAED: No, pray, pray, my dear Frank, remember! He is your father.

FRANK: I give him due credit for that. But just imagine his telling Crofts to bring the Warrens over here! He must have been ever so drunk. You know, my dear Praddy, my mother wouldn't stand Mrs. Warren for a moment. Vivie mustn't come here until she's gone back to town.

PRAED: But you mother doesn't know anything about Mrs. Warren, does she?

FRANK: I don't know. Her journey to town looks as if she did. Not that my mother would mind in the ordinary way: she has stuck like a brick to lots of women who had got into trouble. But they were all nice women. That's what makes the real difference. Mrs. Warren, no doubt, has her merits; but she's ever so rowdy; and my mother simply wouldn't put up with her. So—hallo! (*This exclamation is provoked by the reappearance of the clergyman, who comes out of the house in haste and dismay.*)

REV. S.: Frank: Mrs. Warren and her daughter are coming across the heath with Crofts: I saw them from the study windows. What am I to say about your mother?

FRANK (*jumping up energetically*): Stick on your hat and go out and say how delighted you are to see them; and that Frank's in the garden; and that mother and Bessie have been called to the bedside of a sick relative, and were ever so sorry they couldn't stop; and that you hope Mrs. Warren slept well; and—and—say any blessed thing except the truth, and leave the rest to Providence.

REV. S.: But how are we to get rid of them afterwards?

FRANK: There's no time to think of that now. Here! (*He bounds into the porch and returns immediately with a clerical felt hat, which he claps on his father's head.*) Now: off with you. Praed and I'll wait here, to give the thing an unpremeditated air. (*The clergyman, dazed, but obedient, hurries off through the gate. Praed gets up from the turf, and dusts himself.*)

FRANK: We must get that old lady back to town somehow, Praed. Come! honestly, dear Praddy, do you like seeing them together—Vivie and the old lady?

PRAED: Oh, why not?

FRANK (*his teeth on edge*): Don't it make your flesh creep ever so little?—that wicked old devil, up to every villainy under the sun, I'll swear, and Vivie—ugh!

PRAED: Hush, pray. They're coming. (*The clergyman and*

VIVIE & FRANK IN THE RECTORY
GARDEN.

*Crofts are seen coming along the road, followed by Mrs.
Warren and Vivie walking affectionately together.)*

FRANK: Look: she actually has her arm round the old
woman's waist. It's her right arm: she began it. She's gone
sentimental, by God! Ugh! ugh! Now do you feel the creeps?
*(The clergyman opens the gate; and Mrs. Warren and Vivie
pass him and stand in the middle of the garden looking at
the house. Frank, in an ecstasy of dissimulation, turns gaily
to Mrs. Warren, exclaiming)* Ever so delighted to see you,
Mrs. Warren. This quiet old rectory garden becomes you
perfectly.

MRS. WARREN: Well, I never! Did you hear that, George?
He says I look well in a quiet old rectory garden.

REV. S.: *(still holding the gate for Crofts, who loafs
through it, heavily bored)*: You look well everywhere, Mrs.
Warren.

FRANK: Bravo, gov'nor! Now look here: let's have an awful jolly time of it before lunch. First let's see the church. Everyone has to do that. It's a regular old thirteenth century
church, you know: the gov'nor's ever so fond of it, because
he got up a restoration fund and had it completely rebuilt six
years ago. Praed will be able to show its points.

REV. S.: *(mooning hospitably at them)*: I shall be pleased,
I'm sure, if Sir George and Mrs. Warren really care about it.

MRS. WARREN: Oh, come along and get it over. It'll do
George good: I'll lay he doesn't trouble church much.

CROFTS *(turning back towards the gate)*: I've no objection.

REV. S.: Not that way. We go through the fields, if you
don't mind. Round here. *(He leads the way by the little path
through the box hedge.)*

CROFTS: Oh, all right. *(He goes with the parson. Praed follows with Mrs. Warren. Vivie does not stir, but watches them
until they have gone, with all the lines of purpose in her face
marking it strongly.)*

FRANK: Ain't you coming?

VIVIE: No. I want to give you a warning, Frank. You were
making fun of my mother just now when you said that about
the rectory garden. That is barred in future. Please treat my
mother with as much respect as you treat your own.

FRANK: My dear Viv: she wouldn't appreciate it. She's not
like my mother: the same treatment wouldn't do for both
cases. But what on earth has happened to you? Last night we
were perfectly agreed as to your mother and her set. This
morning I find you attitudinizing sentimentally with your arm
round your parent's waist.

VIVIE *(flushing)*: Attitudinizing!

What are we to think this?

FRANK: That was how it struck me. First time I ever saw you do a second-rate thing.

VIVIE (*controlling herself*): Yes, Frank: there has been a change; but I don't think it a change for the worse. Yesterday I was a little prig.

FRANK: And to-day?

VIVIE (*wincing; then looking at him steadily*): To-day I know my mother better than you do.

FRANK: Heaven forbid!

VIVIE: What do you mean?

FRANK: Viv: there's a freemasonry among thoroughly immoral people that you know nothing of. You've too much character. That's the bond between your mother and me: that's why I know her better than you'll ever know her.

VIVIE: You are wrong: you know nothing about her. If you knew the circumstances against which my mother had to struggle—

FRANK (*adroitly finishing the sentence for her*): I should know why she is what she is, shouldn't I? What difference would that make? Circumstances or no circumstances, Viv, you won't be able to stand your mother.

VIVIE (*very angry*): Why not?

FRANK: Because she's an old wretch, Viv. If you ever put your arm round her waist in my presence again, I'll shoot myself there and then as a protest against an exhibition which revolts me.

VIVIE: Must I choose between dropping your acquaintance and dropping my mother's?

FRANK (*gracefully*): That would put the old lady at ever such a disadvantage. No, Viv: your infatuated little boy will have to stick to you in any case. But he's all the more anxious that you shouldn't make mistakes. It's no use, Viv: your mother's impossible. She may be a good sort; but she's a bad lot, a very bad lot.

VIVIE (*hotly*): Frank—! (*He stands his ground. She turns away and sits down on the bench under the yew tree, struggling to recover her self-command. Then she says*) Is she to be deserted by all the world because she's what you call a bad lot? Has she no right to live?

FRANK: No fear of that, Viv: she won't ever be deserted. (*He sits on the bench beside her.*)

VIVIE: But I am to desert her, I suppose.

FRANK (*babyishly, lulling her and making love to her with his voice*): Mustn't go live with her. Little family group of mother and daughter wouldn't be a success. Spoil our little group.

VIVIE (*falling under the spell*): What little group?

FRANK: The babes in the wood: Vivie and little Frank. (*He slips his arm round her waist and nestles against her like a weary child.*) Let's go and get covered up with leaves.

VIVIE (*rhythmically, rocking him like a nurse.*): Fast asleep, hand in hand, under the trees.

FRANK: The wise little girl with her silly little boy.

VIVIE: The dear little boy with his dowdy little girl.

FRANK: Ever so peaceful, and relieved from the imbecility of the little boy's father and the questionableness of the little girl's—

VIVIE (*smothering the word against her breast*): Sh-sh-sh-sh! little girl wants to forget all about her mother. (*They are silent for some moments, rocking one another. Then Vivie wakes up with a shock, exclaiming*) What a pair of fools we are! Come: sit up. Gracious! your hair. (*She smooths it.*) I wonder do all grown up people play in that childish way when nobody is looking. I never did it when I was a child.

FRANK: Neither did I. You are my first playmate. (*He catches her hand to kiss it, but checks himself to look round first. Very unexpectedly he sees Crofts emerging from the box hedge.*) Oh, damn!

VIVIE: Why damn, dear?

FRANK (*whispering*): Sh! Here's this brute Crofts. (*He sits farther away from her with an unconcerned air.*)

VIVIE: Don't be rude to him, Frank. I particularly wish to be polite to him. It will please my mother. (*Frank makes a wry face.*)

CROFTS: Could I have a few words with you, Miss Vivie?

VIVIE: Certainly.

CROFT: (*to Frank*): You'll excuse me, Gardner. They're waiting for you in the church, if you don't mind.

FRANK (*rising*): Anything to oblige you, Crofts—except church. If you want anything, Vivie, ring the gate bell, and a domestic will appear. (*He goes into the house with unruffled suavity.*)

CROFT: (*watching him with a crafty air as he disappears, and speaking to Vivie with an assumption of being on privileged terms with her*): Pleasant young fellow that, Miss Vivie. Pity he has no money, isn't it?

VIVIE: Do you think so?

CROFTS: Well, what's he to do? No profession, no property. What's he good for?

VIVIE: I realize his disadvantages, Sir George.

CROFTS (*a little taken aback at being so precisely interpreted*): Oh, it's not that. But while we're in this world we're

in it; and money's money. (*Vivie does not answer.*) Nice
day, isn't it?

VIVIE (*with scarcely veiled contempt for his effort at conversation*): Very.

CROFTS (*with brutal good humor, as if he liked her
pluck*): Well, that's not what I came to say. (*Affecting
frankness.*) Now listen, Miss Vivie. I'm quite aware that I'm
not a young lady's man.

VIVIE: Indeed, Sir George?

CROFTS: No; and to tell you the honest truth, I don't want
to be either. But when I say a thing I mean it; when I feel
sentiment I feel it in earnest; and what I value I pay hard
money for. That's the sort of man I am.

VIVIE: It does you great credit, I'm sure.

CROFTS: Oh, I don't mean to praise myself. I have my
faults, Heaven knows: no man is more sensible of that than I
am. I know I'm not perfect; that's one of the advantages of
being a middle-aged man; for I'm not a young man, and I
know it. But my code is a simple one, and, I think, a good
one. Honor between man and man; fidelity between man and
woman; and no cant about this religion, or that religion, but
an honest belief that things are making for good on the
whole.

VIVIE (*with biting irony*): "A power, not ourselves, that
makes for righteousness," eh?

CROFTS (*taking her seriously*): Oh, certainly, not ourselves,
of course. You understand what I mean. (*He sits down beside her, as one who has found a kindred spirit.*) Well, now
as to practical matters. You may have an idea that I've flung
my money about; but I haven't: I'm richer today than when
I first came into the property. I've used my knowledge of the
world to invest my money in ways that other men have over-
looked; and whatever else I may be, I'm a safe man from
the money point of view.

VIVIE: It's very kind of you to tell me all this.

CROFTS: Oh, well, come, Miss Vivie: you needn't pretend
you don't see what I'm driving at. I want to settle down with
a Lady Crofts. I suppose you think me very blunt, eh?

VIVIE: Not at all: I am much obliged to you for being so
definite and business-like. I quite appreciate the offer: the
money, the position, Lady Crofts, and so on. But I think I
will say no, if you don't mind. I'd rather not. (*She rises, and
strolls across to the sundial to get out of his immediate
neighborhood.*)

CROFTS (*not at all discouraged, and taking advantage of
the additional room left him on the seat to spread himself*

comfortably, as if a few preliminary refusals were part of the inevitable routine of courtship): I'm in no hurry. It was only just to let you know in case young Gardner should try to trap you. Leave the question open.

VIVIE (*sharply*): My no is final. I won't go back from it. (*She looks authoritatively at him. He grins; leans forward with his elbows on his knees to prod with his stick at some unfortunate insect in the grass; and looks cunningly at her. She turns away impatiently.*)

CROFTS: I'm a good deal older than you—twenty-five years—quarter of a century. I shan't live for ever; and I'll take care that you shall be well off when I'm gone.

VIVIE: I am proof against even that inducement, Sir George. Don't you think you'd better take your answer? There is not the slightest chance of my altering it.

CROFTS (*rising, after a final slash at a daisy, and beginning to walk to and fro*): Well, no matter. I could tell you some things that would change your mind fast enough; but I won't, because I'd rather win you by honest affection. I was a good friend to your mother: ask her whether I wasn't. She'd never have made the money that paid for your education if it hadn't been for my advice and help, not to mention the money I advanced her. There are not many men would have stood by her as I have. I put not less than £40,000 into it, from first to last.

VIVIE (*staring at him*): Do you mean to say you were my mother's business partner?

CROFTS: Yes. Now just think of all the trouble and the explanations it would save if we were to keep the whole thing in the family, so to speak. Ask your mother whether she'd like to have to explain all her affairs to a perfect stranger.

VIVIE: I see no difficulty, since I understand that the business is wound up, and the money invested.

CROFTS (*stopping short, amazed*): Wound up! Wind up a business that's paying 35 per cent in the worst years! Not likely. Who told you that? HOPES SHES WRONG

VIVIE (*her colour quite gone*): Do you mean that it is still—? (*She stops abruptly, and puts her hand on the sundial to support herself. Then she gets quickly to the iron chair and sits down.*) What business are you talking about?

CROFTS: Well, the fact is, it's not what would be considered exactly a high-class business in my set—the county set, you know—our set it will be if you think better of my offer. Not that there's any mystery about it: don't think that. Of course you know by your mother's being in it that it's perfectly straight and honest. I've known her for many years;

and I can say of her that she'd cut off her hands sooner than touch anything that was not what it ought to be. I'll tell you all about it if you like. I don't know whether you've found in travelling how hard it is to find a really comfortable private hotel.

VIVIE (*sickened, averting her face*): Yes: go on.

CROFTS: Well, that's all it is. Your mother has a genius for managing such things. We've got two in Brussels, one in Berlin, one in Vienna, and two in Buda-Pesth. Of course there are others besides ourselves in it; but we hold most of the capital; and your mother's indispensable as managing director. You've noticed, I daresay, that she travels a good deal. But you see you can't mention such things in society. Once let out the word hotel and everybody says you keep a public-house. You wouldn't like people to say that of your mother, would you? That's why we're so reserved about it. By the bye, you'll keep it to yourself, won't you? Since it's been a secret so long, it had better remain so.

VIVIE: And this is the business you invite me to join you in?

CROFT: Oh, no. My wife shan't be troubled with business. You'll not be in it more than you've always been.

VIVIE: I always been! What do you mean?

CROFTS: Only that you've always lived on it. It paid for your education and the dress you have on your back. Don't turn up your nose at business, Miss Vivie: where would your Newnhams and Girtons be without it?

VIVIE (*rising, almost beside herself*): Take care. I know what this business is.

CROFTS (*starting, with a suppressed oath*): Who told you?

VIVIE: Your partner—my mother.

CROFTS (*black with rage*): The old—(*Vivie looks quickly at him. He swallows the epithet and stands swearing and raging foully to himself. But he knows that his cue is to be sympathetic. He takes refuge in generous indignation.*) She ought to have had more consideration for you. I'd never have told you.

VIVIE: I think you would probably have told me when we were married: it would have been a convenient weapon to break me in with.

CROFTS (*quite sincerely*): I never intended that. On my word as a gentleman I didn't.

(*Vivie wonders at him. Her sense of the irony of his protest cools and braces her. She replies with contemptuous self-possession.*)

VIVIE: It does not matter. I suppose you understand that when we leave here to-day our acquaintance ceases.

CROFTS: Why? Is it for helping your mother?

VIVIE: My mother was a very poor woman who had no reasonable choice but to do as she did. You were a rich gentleman; and you did the same for the sake of 35 per cent. You are a pretty common sort of scoundrel, I think. That is my opinion of you.

CROFTS (*after a stare—not at all displeased, and much more at his ease on these frank terms than on their former ceremonious ones*): Ha, ha, ha, ha! Go it, little missie, go it: it doesn't hurt me and it amuses you. Why the devil shouldn't I invest my money that way? I take the interest on my capital like other people: I hope you don't think I dirty my own hands with the work. Come: you wouldn't refuse the acquaintance of my mother's cousin, the Duke of Belgravia, because some of the rents he gets are earned in queer ways. You wouldn't cut the Archbishop of Canterbury, I suppose, because the Ecclesiastical Commissioners have a few publicans and sinners among their tenants? Do you remember your Crofts scholarship at Newnham? Well, that was founded by my brother the M.P. He gets his 22 per cent out of a factory with 600 girls in it, and not one of them getting wages enough to live on. How d'ye suppose most of them manage? Ask your mother. And do you expect me to turn my back on 35 per cent when all the rest are pocketing what they can, like sensible men? No such fool! If you're going to pick and choose your acquaintances on moral principles, you'd better clear out of this country, unless you want to cut yourself out of all decent society.

VIVIE (*conscience stricken*): You might go on to point out that I myself never asked where the money I spent came from. I believe I am just as bad as you.

CROFTS (*greatly reassured*): Of course you are; and a very good thing, too! What harm does it do after all? (*Rallying her jocularly.*) So you don't think me such a scoundrel now you come to think it over. Eh?

VIVIE: I have shared profits with you; and I admitted you just now to the familiarity of knowing what I think of you.

CROFT: (*with serious friendliness*): To be sure you did. You won't find me a bad sort: I don't go in for being superfine intellectually; but I've plenty of honest human feeling; and the old Crofts breed comes out in a sort of instinctive hatred of anything low, in which I'm sure you'll sympathize with me. Believe me, Miss Vivie, the world isn't such a bad place as the croakers make out. So long as you don't fly openly in the face of society, society doesn't ask any inconvenient questions; and it makes precious short work of the cads who do. There are no secrets better kept than the secrets that everybody guesses. In the society I can introduce you to, no lady or gentleman would so far forget themselves as to discuss my business affairs or your mother's. No man can offer you a safer position.

VIVI (*studying him curiously*): I suppose you really think you're getting on famously with me.

CROFTS: Well I hope I may flatter myself that you think better of me than you did at first.

VIVIE (*quietly*): I hardly find you worth thinking about at all now. (*She rises and turns towards the gate, pausing on her way to contemplate him and say almost gently, but with intense conviction.*) When I think of the society that tolerates you, and the laws that protect you—when I think of how helpless nine out of ten young girls would be in the hands of you and my mother—the unmentionable woman and her capitalist bully—

CROFTS (*livid*): Damn you!

VIVIE: You need not. I feel among the damned already. (*She raises the latch of the gate to open it and go out. He follows her and puts his hand heavily on the top bar to prevent its opening.*)

CROFTS (*panting with fury*): Do you think I'll put up with this from you, you young devil, you?

VIVIE (*unmoved*): Be quiet. Some one will answer the bell. (*Without flinching a step she strikes the bell with the back of her hand. It clangs harshly; and he starts back involuntarily. Almost immediately Frank appears at the porch with his rifle.*)

FRANK (*with cheerful politeness*): Will you have the rifle, Viv; or shall I operate?

VIVIE: Frank: have you been listening?

FRANK: Only for the bell, I assure you; so that you shouldn't have to wait. I think I showed great insight into your character, Crofts.

CROFTS: For two pins I'd take that gun from you and break it across your head.

FRANK (*stalking him cautiously*): Pray don't. I'm ever so careless in handling firearms. Sure to be a fatal accident, with a reprimand from the coroner's jury for my negligence.

VIVIE: Put the rifle away, Frank: it's quite unnecessary.

FRANK: Quite right, Viv. Much more sportsmanlike to catch him in a trap. (*Crofts, understanding the insult, makes a threatening movement.*) Crofts: there are fifteen cartridges

The shocker! But we expected perhaps

in the magazine here; and I am a dead shot at the present distance at an object of your size.

CROFTS: Oh, you needn't be afraid. I'm not going to touch you.

FRANK: Ever so magnanimous of you under the circumstances! Thank you.

CROFTS: I'll just tell you this before I go. It may interest you, since you're so fond of one another. Allow me, Mister Frank, to introduce you to your half-sister, the eldest daughter of the Reverend Samuel Gardner. Miss Vivie: your half-brother. Good morning. (*He goes out through the gate and along the road.*) *CROFTS DOES THIS MALICIOUSLY*

FRANK (*after a pause of stupefaction, raising the rifle*): You'll testify before the coroner that it's an accident, Viv. (*He takes aim at the retreating figure of Crofts. Vivie seizes the muzzle and pulls it round against her breast.*)

VIVIE: Fire now. You may.

FRANK (*dropping his end of the rifle hastily*): Stop! take care. (*She lets it go. It falls on the turf.*) Oh, you've given your little boy such a turn, Suppose it had gone off—ugh! (*He sinks on the garden seat, overcome.*)

VIVIE: Suppose it had: do you think it would not have been a relief to have some sharp physical pain tearing through me?

FRANK (*coaxingly*): Take it ever so easy, dear Viv. Remember: even if the rifle scared that fellow into telling the truth for the first time in his life, that only makes us the babes in the wood in earnest. (*He holds out his arms to her.*) Come and be covered up with leaves again.

VIVIE (*with a cry of disgust*): Ah, not that, not that. You make all my flesh creep.

FRANK: Why, what's the matter? *Good ole Frank*

VIVIE: Good-bye. (*She makes for the gate.*)

FRANK (*jumping up*): Hallo! Stop! Viv! Viv! (*She turns in the gateway.*) Where are you going to? Where shall we find you?

VIVIE: At Honoria Fraser's chambers, 67 Chancery Lane, for the rest of my life. (*She goes off quickly in the opposite direction to that taken by Crofts.*)

FRANK: But I say—wait—dash it! (*He runs after her*).

immoral — flies like Crofts —

ACT 4

Honoria Fraser's chambers in Chancery Lane. An office at the top of New Stone Buildings, with a plate-glass window, distempered walls, electric light, and a patent stove. Saturday afternoon. The chimneys of Lincoln's Inn and the western sky beyond are seen through the window. There is a double writing table in the middle of the room, with a cigar box, ash pans, and a portable electric reading lamp almost snowed up in heaps of papers and books. This table has knee holes and chairs right and left and is very untidy. The clerk's desk, closed and tidy, with its high stool, is against the wall, near a door communicating with the inner rooms. In the opposite wall is the door leading to the public corridor. Its upper panel is of opaque glass, lettered in black on the outside, "Fraser and Warren." A baize screen hides the corner between this door and the window.

Frank, in a fashionable light-colored coaching suit, with his stick, gloves, and white hat in his hands, is pacing up and down the office. Somebody tries the door with a key.

FRANK (*calling*): Come in. It's not locked. (*Vivie comes in, in her hat and jacket. She stops and stares at him.*)

VIVIE (*sternly*): What are you doing here?

FRANK: Waiting to see you. I've been here for hours. Is this the way you attend to your business? (*He puts his hat and stick on the table, and perches himself with a vault on the clerk's stool, looking at her with every appearance of being in a specially restless, teasing, flippant mood.*)

VIVIE: I've been away exactly twenty minutes for a cup of tea. (*She takes off her hat and jacket and hangs them up behind the screen.*) How did you get in?

FRANK: The staff had not left when I arrived. He's gone to play football on Primrose Hill. Why don't you employ a woman, and give your sex a chance?

VIVIE: What have you come for?

FRANK (*springing off the stool and coming close to her*): Viv: let's go and enjoy the Saturday half-holiday somewhere, like the staff. What do you say to Richmond, and then a music hall, and a jolly supper?

VIVIE: Can't afford it. I shall put in another six hours' work before I go to bed.

FRANK: Can't afford it, can't we? Aha! Look here. (*He takes out a handful of sovereigns and makes them chink.*) Gold, Viv, gold!

VIVIE: Where did you get it?

FRANK: Gambling, Viv, gambling. Poker.

VIVIE: Pah! it's meaner than stealing it. No: I'm not coming. (*She sits down to work at the table, with her back to the glass door, and begins turning over the papers.*)

FRANK (*remonstrating piteously*): But, my dear Viv, I want to talk to you ever so seriously.

VIVIE: Very well: sit down in Honoria's chair and talk here. I like ten minutes' chat after tea. (*He murmurs.*) No use groaning: I'm inexorable. (*He takes the opposite seat disconsolately.*) Pass that cigar box, will you?

FRANK (*pushing the cigar box across*): Nasty womanly habit. Nice men don't do it any longer.

VIVIE: Yes: they object to the smell in the office; and we've had to take to cigarets. See! (*She opens the box and takes out a cigaret, which she lights. She offers him one; but he shakes his head with a wry face. She settles herself comfortably in her chair, smoking.*) Go ahead.

FRANK: Well, I want to know what you've done—what arrangements you've made.

VIVIE: Everything was settled twenty minutes after I arrived here. Honoria has found the business too much for her this year; and she was on the point of sending for me and proposing a partnership when I walked in and told her I hadn't a farthing in the world. So I installed myself and packed her off for a fortnight's holiday. What happened at Haslemere when I left?

FRANK: Nothing at all. I said you'd gone to town on particular business.

VIVIE: Well?

FRANK: Well, either they were too flabbergasted to say anything, or else Crofts had prepared your mother. Anyhow, she didn't say anything; and Crofts didn't say anything; and Praddy only stared. After tea they got up and went; and I've not seen them since.

VIVIE (*nodding placidly with one eye on a wreath of smoke*): That's all right.

FRANK (*looking round disparagingly*): Do you intend to stick in this confounded place?

VIVIE (*blowing the wreath decisively away and sitting straight up*): Yes. These two days have given me back all my

strength and self-possession. I will never take a holiday again
as long as I live.

FRANK (*with a very wry face*): Mps! You look quite
happy—and as hard as nails.

VIVIE (*grimly*): Well for me that I am!

FRANK (*rising*): Look here, Viv: we must have an explanation. We parted the other day under a complete misunder-
standing.

VIVIE (*putting away the cigaret*): Well: clear it up.

FRANK: You remember what Crofts said?

VIVIE: Yes.

FRANK: That revelation was supposed to bring about a
complete change in the nature of our feeling for one another.
It placed us on the footing of brother and sister.

VIVIE: Yes.

FRANK: Have you ever had a brother?

VIVIE: No.

FRANK: Then you don't know what being brother and sister feels like? Now I have lots of sisters: Jessie and Georgina
and the rest. The fraternal feeling is quite familiar to me;
and I assure you my feeling for you is not the least in the
world like it. The girls will go their way: I will go mine: and
we shan't care if we never see one another again. That's
brother and sister. But as to you, I can't be easy if I have to
pass a week without seeing you. That's not brother and sister.
It's exactly what I felt an hour before Crofts made his revelation. In short, dear Viv, it's love's young dream.

VIVIE (*bitingly*): The same feeling, Frank, that brought
your father to my mother's feet. Is that it?

FRANK (*revolted*): I very strongly object, Viv, to have my
feelings compared to any which the Reverend Samuel is capable of harboring; and I object still more to a comparison
of you to your mother. Besides, I don't believe the story. I
have taxed my father with it, and obtained from him what I
consider tantamount to a denial.

VIVIE: What did he say?

FRANK: He said he was sure there must be some mistake.

VIVIE: Do you believe him?

FRANK: I am prepared to take his word as against Crofts'.

VIVIE: Does it make any difference? I mean in your imagination or conscience; for of course it makes no real difference.

FRANK (*shaking his head*): None whatever to me.

VIVIE: Nor to me.

FRANK (*staring*): But this is ever so surprising! I thought
our whole relations were altered in your imagination and

conscience, as you put it, the moment those words were out of that brute's muzzle.

VIVIE: No: it was not that. I didn't believe him. I only wish I could. *Then why her reaction*

FRANK: Eh?

VIVIE: I think brother and sister would be a very suitable relation for us.

FRANK: You really mean that?

VIVIE: Yes. It's the only relation I care for, even if we could afford any other. I mean that.

FRANK (*raising his eyebrows like one on whom a new light has dawned, and speaking with quite an effusion of chivalrous sentiment*): My dear Viv: why didn't you say so before? I am ever so sorry for persecuting you. I understand, of course.

VIVIE (*puzzled*): Understand what?

FRANK: Oh, I'm not a fool in the ordinary sense—only in the Scriptural sense of doing all the things the wise man declared to be folly, after trying them himself on the most extensive scale. I see I am no longer Vivvums' little boy. Don't be alarmed: I shall never call you Vivvums again—at least unless you get tired of your new little boy, whoever he may be.

VIVIE: My new little boy!

FRANK (*with conviction*): Must be a new little boy. Always happens that way. No other way, in fact.

VIVIE: None that you know of, fortunately for you. (*Someone knocks at the door.*)

FRANK: My curse upon yon caller, whoe'er he be!

VIVIE: It's Praed. He's going to Italy and wants to say good-bye. I asked him to call this afternoon. Go and let him in.

FRANK: We can continue our conversation after his departure for Italy. I'll stay him out. (*He goes to the door and opens it.*) How are you, Praddy? Delighted to see you. Come in. (*Praed, dressed for travelling, comes in, in high spirits, excited by the beginning of his journey.*)

PRAED: How do you do, Miss Warren. (*She presses his hand cordially, though a certain sentimentality in his high spirits jars on her.*) I start in an hour from Holborn Viaduct. I wish I could persuade you to try Italy.

VIVIE: What for?

PRAED: Why, to saturate yourself with beauty and romance, of course. (*Vivie, with a shudder, turns her chair to the table, as if the work waiting for her there were a consolation and support to her. Praed sits opposite to her. Frank places a chair just behind Vivie, and drops lazily and carelessly into it, talking at her over his shoulder.*)

FRANK: No use, Praddy. Viv is a little Philistine. She is indifferent to my romance, and insensible to my beauty.

VIVIE: Mr. Praed: once for all, there is no beauty and no romance in life for me. Life is what it is; and I am prepared to take it as it is. TOO HARSH?

PRAED (*enthusiastically*): You will not say that if you come to Verona and on to Venice. You will cry with delight at living in such a beautiful world.

FRANK: This is most eloquent, Praddy. Keep it up.

PRAED: Oh, I assure you *I* have cried—I shall cry again. I hope—at fifty! At your age, Miss Warren, you would not need to go so far as Verona. Your spirits would absolutely fly up at the mere sight of Ostend. You would be charmed with the gaiety, the vivacity, the happy air of Brussels. (*Vivie recoils.*) What's the matter?

FRANK: Hallo, Viv!

VIVIE (*to Praed with deep reproach*): Can you find no better example of your beauty and romance than Brussels to talk to me about?

PRAED (*puzzled*): Of course it's very different from Verona. I don't suggest for a moment that—

VIVIE (*bitterly*): Probably the beauty and romance come to much the same in both places.

PRAED (*completely sobered and much concerned*): My dear Miss Warren: I—(*looking enquiringly at Frank*) Is anything the matter?

FRANK: She thinks your enthusiasm frivolous, Praddy. She's had ever such a serious call.

VIVIE (*sharply*): Hold your tongue, Frank. Don't be silly.

FRANK (*calmly*): Do you call this good manners, Praed?

PRAED (*anxious and considerate*): Shall I take him away, Miss Warren? I feel sure we have disturbed you at your work. (*He is about to rise.*)

VIVIE: Sit down: I'm not ready to go back to work yet. You both think I have an attack of nerves. Not a bit of it. But there are two subjects I want dropped, if you don't mind. One of them (*to Frank*) is love's young dream in any shape or form: the other (*to Praed*) is the romance and beauty of life, especially as exemplified by the gaiety of Brussels. You are welcome to any illusions you may have left on these subjects: I have none. If we three are to remain friends, I must be treated as a woman of business, permanently single (*to Frank*) and permanently unromantic (*to Praed*).

FRANK: I also shall remain permanently single until you

VIVIE is tormented by the knowledge of her mother

change your mind. Praddy: change the subject. Be eloquent about something else.

PRAED (*diffidently*): I'm afraid there's nothing else in the world that I can talk about. The Gospel of Art is the only one I can preach. I know Miss Warren is a great devotee of the Gospel of Getting On; but we can't discuss that without hurting your feelings, Frank, since you are determined not to get on.

FRANK: Oh, don't mind my feelings. Give me some improving advice by all means; it does me ever so much good. Have another try to make a successful man of me, Viv. Come: let's have it all: energy, thrift, foresight, self-respect, character. Don't you hate people who have no character, Viv?

VIVIE (*wincing*): Oh, stop: stop: let us have no more of that horrible cant. Mr. Praed: if there are really only those two gospels in the world, we had better all kill ourselves; for the same taint is in both, through and through.

FRANK (*looking critically at her*): There is a touch of poetry about you to-day, Viv, which has hitherto been lacking.

PRAED (*remonstrating*): My dear Frank: aren't you a little unsympathetic?

VIVIE (*merciless to herself*): No: it's good for me. It keeps me from being sentimental.

FRANK (*bantering her*): Checks your strong natural propensity that way, don't it?

VIVIE (*almost hysterically*): Oh, yes: go on: don't spare me. I was sentimental for a moment in my life—beautifully sentimental—by moonlight; and now— *Scene w/ Mother*

FRANK (*quickly*): I say, Viv: take care. Don't give yourself away.

VIVIE: Oh, do you think Mr. Praed does not know all about my mother? (*Turning on Praed.*) You had better have told me that morning, Mr. Praed. You are very old-fashioned in your delicacies, after all.

PRAED: Surely it is you who are a little old-fashioned in your prejudices, Miss Warren. I feel bound to tell you, speaking as an artist, and believing that the most intimate human relationships are far beyond and above the scope of the law, that though I know that your mother is an unmarried woman, I do not respect her the less on that account. I respect her more.

FRANK (*airily*): Hear, hear!

VIVIE (*staring at him*): Is that all you know?

PRAED: Certainly that is all.

What are the two words?

VIVIE: Then you neither of you know anything. Your guesses are innocence itself compared to the truth.

PRAED (*startled and indignant, preserving his politeness with an effort*): I hope not. (*More emphatically.*) I hope not, Miss Warren. (*Frank's face shows that he does not share Praed's incredulity. Vivie utters an exclamation of impatience. Praed's chivalry droops before their conviction. He adds, slowly*) If there is anything worse—that is, anything else—are you sure you are right to tell us, Miss Warren?

VIVIE: I am sure that if I had the courage I should spend the rest of my life in telling it to everybody—in stamping and branding it into them until they felt their share in its shame and horror as I feel mine. There is nothing I despise more than the wicked convention that protects these things by forbidding a woman to mention them. And yet I can't tell you. The two infamous words that describe what my mother is are ringing in my ears and struggling on my tongue; but I can't utter them: my instinct is too strong for me. (*She buries her face in her hands. The two men, astonished, stare at one another and then at her. She raises her head again desperately and takes a sheet of paper and a pen.*) Here: let me draft you a prospectus.

FRANK: Oh, she's mad. Do you hear, Viv, mad. Come: pull yourself together.

VIVIE: You shall see. (*She writes.*) "Paid up capital: not less than £40,000 standing in the name of Sir George Crofts, Baronet, the chief shareholder." What comes next? I forget. Oh, yes: "Premises at Brussels, Berlin, Vienna and Buda-Pesth. Managing director: Mrs. Warren;" and now don't let us forget her qualifications: the two words. There! (*She pushes the paper to them.*) Oh, no: don't read it: don't! (*She snatches it back and tears it to pieces; then seizes her head in her hands and hides her face on the table. Frank, who has watched the writing carefully over her shoulder, and opened his eyes very widely at it, takes a card from his pocket; scribbles a couple of words; and silently hands it to Praed, who looks at it with amazement. Frank then remorsefully stoops over Vivie.*)

FRANK (*whispering tenderly*): Viv, dear: that's all right. I read what you wrote: so did Praddy. We understand. And we remain, as this leaves us at present, yours ever so devotedly. (*Vivie slowly raises her head.*)

PRAED: We do, indeed, Miss Warren. I declare you are the most splendidly courageous woman I ever met. (*This sentimental compliment braces Vivie. She throws it away from her with an impatient shake, and forces herself to stand up, though not without some support from the table.*)

FRANK: Don't stir, Viv, if you don't want to. Take it easy.

VIVIE: Thank you. You can always depend on me for two things, not to cry and not to faint. (*She moves a few steps towards the door of the inner rooms, and stops close to Praed to say*) I shall need much more courage than that when I tell my mother that we have come to the parting of the ways. Now I must go into the next room for a moment to make myself neat again, if you don't mind.

PRAED: Shall we go away?

VIVIE: No: I'll be back presently. Only for a moment. (*She goes into the other room, Praed opening the door for her.*)

PRAED: What an amazing revelation! I'm extremely disappointed in Crofts: I am indeed.

FRANK: I'm not in the least. I feel he's perfectly accounted for at last. But what a facer for me, Praddy! I can't marry her now.

PRAED (*sternly*): Frank! (*The two look at one another, Frank unruffled, Praed deeply indignant.*) Let me tell you, Gardner, that if you desert her now you will behave very despicably.

FRANK: Good old Praddy! Ever chivalrous! But you mistake: it's not the moral aspect of the case: it's the money aspect. I really can't bring myself to touch the old woman's money now.

PRAED: And was that what you were going to marry on?

FRANK: What else? *I* haven't any money, nor the smallest turn for making it. If I married Viv now she would have to support me; and I should cost her more than I am worth.

PRAED: But surely a clever, bright fellow like you can make something by your own brains.

FRANK: Oh, yes, a little. (*He takes out his money again.*) I made all that yesterday—in an hour and a half. But I made it in a highly speculative business. No, dear Praddy: even if Jessie and Georgina marry millionaires and the governor dies after cutting them off with a shilling, I shall have only four hundred a year. And he won't die until he's three score and ten: he hasn't originality enough. I shall be on short allowance for the next twenty years. No short allowance for Viv, if I can help it. I withdraw gracefully and leave the field to the gilded youth of England. So that's settled. I shan't worry her about it: I'll just send her a little note after we're gone. She'll understand.

PRAED (*grasping his hand*): Good fellow, Frank! I heartily beg your pardon. But must you never see her again?

FRANK: Never see her again! Hang it all, be reasonable. I shall come along as often as possible, and be her brother. I cannot understand the absurd consequences you romantic people expect from the most ordinary transactions. (*A knock at the door.*) I wonder who this is. Would you mind opening the door? If it's a client it will look more respectable than if I appeared.

PRAED: Certainly. (*He goes to the door and opens it. Frank sits down in Vivie's chair to scribble a note.*) My dear Kitty: come in, come in.

(*Mrs. Warren comes in, looking apprehensively round for Vivie. She has done her best to make herself matronly and dignified. The brilliant hat is replaced by a sober bonnet, and the gay blouse covered by a costly black silk mantle. She is pitiably anxious and ill at ease—evidently panic-stricken.*)

MRS. WARREN (*to Frank*): What! You're here, are you?

FRANK (*turning in his chair from his writing, but not rising*): Here, and charmed to see you. You come like a breath of spring.

MRS. WARREN: Oh, get out with your nonsense. (*In a low voice.*) Where's Vivie?

(*Frank points expressively to the door of the inner room, but says nothing.*)

MRS. WARREN (*sitting down suddenly and almost beginning to cry*): Praddy: won't she see me, don't you think?

PRAED: My dear Kitty: don't distress yourself. Why should she not?

MRS. WARREN: Oh, you never can see why not: you're too amiable. Mr. Frank: did she say anything to you?

FRANK (*folding his note*): She must see you, if (*very expressively*) you wait until she comes in.

MRS. WARREN (*frightened*): Why shouldn't I wait?

(*Frank looks quizzically at her; puts his note carefully on the ink-bottle, so that Vivie cannot fail to find it when next she dips her pen; then rises and devotes his attention entirely to her.*)

FRANK: My dear Mrs. Warren: suppose you were a sparrow—ever so tiny and pretty a sparrow hopping in the roadway—and you saw a steam roller coming in your direction, would you wait for it?

MRS. WARREN: Oh, don't bother me with your sparrows. What did she run away from Haslemere like that for?

FRANK: I'm afraid she'll tell you if you wait until she comes back.

MRS. WARREN: Do you want me to go away?

FRANK: No. I always want you to stay. But I advise you to go away.

MRS. WARREN: What! And never see her again!

FRANK: Precisely.

MRS. WARREN (*crying again*): Praddy: don't let him be cruel to me. (*She hastily checks her tears and wipes her eyes.*) She'll be so angry if she sees I've been crying.

FRANK (*with a touch of real compassion in his airy tenderness*): You know that Praddy is the soul of kindness, Mrs. Warren. Praddy: what do you say? Go or stay?

PRAED (*to Mrs. Warren*): I really should be very sorry to cause you unnecessary pain; but I think perhaps you had better not wait. The fact is—(*Vivie is heard at the inner door.*)

FRANK: Sh! Too late. She's coming.

MRS. WARREN: Don't tell her I was crying. (*Vivie comes in. She stops gravely on seeing Mrs. Warren, who greets her with hysterical cheerfulness.*) Well, dearie. So here you are at last.

VIVIE: I am glad you have come: I want to speak to you. You said you were going, Frank, I think.

FRANK: Yes. Will you come with me, Mrs. Warren? What do you say to a trip to Richmond, and the theatre in the evening? There is safety in Richmond. No steam roller there.

VIVIE: Nonsense, Frank. My mother will stay here.

MRS. WARREN (*scared*): I don't know: perhaps I'd better go. We're disturbing you at your work.

VIVIE (*with quiet decision*): Mr. Praed: please take Frank away. Sit down, mother. (*Mrs. Warren obeys helplessly.*)

PRAED: Come, Frank. Good-bye, Miss Vivie.

VIVIE (*shaking hands*): Good-bye. A pleasant trip.

PRAED: Thank you: thank you. I hope so.

FRANK (*to Mrs. Warren*): Good-bye: you'd ever so much better have taken my advice. (*He shakes hands with her. Then airily to Vivie*) Bye-bye, Viv.

VIVIE: Good-bye. (*He goes out gaily without shaking hands with her. Praed follows. Vivie, composed and extremely grave, sits down in Honoria's chair, and waits for her mother to speak. Mrs. Warren, dreading a pause, loses no time in beginning.*)

MRS. WARREN: Well, Vivie, what did you go away like that for without saying a word to me? How could you do such a thing! And what have you done to poor George? I wanted him to come with me; but he shuffled out of it. I could see that he was quite afraid of you. Only fancy: he wanted me not to come. As if (*trembling*) I should be afraid of you, dearie. (*Vivie's gravity deepens.*) But of course I told him it was all settled and comfortable between us, and that we were on the best of terms. (*She breaks down.*) Vivie: what's the meaning of this? (*She produces a paper from an envelope; comes to the table; and hands it across.*) I got it from the bank this morning.

VIVIE: It is my month's allowance. They sent it to me as usual the other day. I simply sent it back to be placed to your credit, and asked them to send you the lodgment receipt. In future I shall support myself.

MRS. WARREN (*not daring to understand*): Wasn't it enough? Why didn't you tell me? (*With a cunning gleam in her eye.*) I'll double it: I was intending to double it. Only let me know how much you want.

VIVIE: You know very well that that has nothing to do with it. From this time I go my own way in my own business and among my own friends. And you will go yours. (*She rises*) Good-bye.

MRS. WARREN (*appalled*): Good-bye?

VIVIE: Yes: good-bye. Come: don't let us make a useless scene: you understand perfectly well. Sir George Crofts has told me the whole business.

MRS. WARREN (*angrily*): Silly old— (*She swallows an epithet, and turns white at the narrowness of her escape from uttering it.*) He ought to have his tongue cut out. But I explained it all to you; and you said you didn't mind.

VIVIE (*steadfastly*): Excuse me: I do mind. You explained how it came about. That does not alter it.

(*Mrs. Warren silenced for a moment, looks forlornly at Vivie, who waits like a statue, secretly hoping that the combat is over. But the cunning expression comes back into Mrs. Warren's face; and she bends across the table, sly and urgent, half whispering.*)

MRS. WARREN: Vivie: do you know how rich I am?

VIVIE: I have no doubt you are very rich.

MRS. WARREN: But you don't know all that that means: you're too young. It means a new dress every day; it means theatres and balls every night; it means having the pick of all the gentlemen in Europe at your feet; it means a lovely house and plenty of servants; it means the choicest of eating and

the automatic pitch she SAVES young girls —

drinking; it means everything you like, everything you want, everything you can think of. And what are you here? A mere drudge, toiling and moiling early and late for your bare living and two cheap dresses a year. Think it over. (*Soothingly.*) You're shocked, I know. I can enter into your feelings; and I think they do you credit; but trust me, nobody will blame you: you may take my word for that. I know what young girls are; and I know you'll think better of it when you're turned it over in your mind.

VIVIE: So that's how it's done, is it? You must have said all that to many a woman, mother, to have it so pat.

MRS. WARREN (*passionately*): What harm am I asking you to do? (*Vivie turns away contemptuously. Mrs. Warren follows her desperately.*) Vivie: listen to me: you don't understand: you've been taught wrong on purpose: you don't know what the world is really like.

VIVIE (*arrested*): Taught wrong on purpose! What do you mean?

MRS. WARREN: I mean that you're throwing away all your chances for nothing. You think that people are what they pretend to be—that the way you were taught at school and college to think right and proper is the way things really are. But it's not: it's all only a pretence, to keep the cowardly, slavish, common run of people quiet. Do you want to find that out, like other women, at forty, when you've thrown yourself away and lost your chances; or won't you take it in good time now from your own mother, that loves you and swears to you that it's truth—gospel truth? (*Urgently.*) Vivie: the big people, the clever people, the managing people, all know it. They do as I do, and think what I think. I know plenty of them. I know them to speak to, to introduce you to, to make friends of for you. I don't mean anything wrong: that's what you don't understand: your head is full of ignorant ideas about me. What do the people that taught you know about life or about people like me? When did they ever meet me, or speak to me, or let anyone tell them about me? —the fools! Would they ever have done anything for you if you hadn't paid them? Haven't I told you that I want you to be respectable? Haven't I brought you up to be respectable? And how can you keep it up without my money, and my influence and Lizzie's friends? Can't you see that you're cutting your own throat as well as breaking my heart in turning your back on me?

VIVIE: I recognise the Crofts philosophy of life, mother. I heard it all from him that day at the Gardners'.

MRS. WARREN: You think I want to force that played-out old sot on you! I don't, Vivie: on my oath I don't.

VIVIE: It would not matter if you did: you would not succeed. (*Mrs. Warren winces, deeply hurt by the implied indifference towards her affectionate intention. Vivie, neither understanding this nor concerning herself about it, goes on calmly*) Mother: you don't at all know the sort of person I am. I don't object to Crofts more than to any other coarsely built man of his class. To tell you the truth, I rather admire him for being strong-minded enough to enjoy himself in his own way and make plenty of money instead of living the usual shooting, hunting, dining-out, tailoring, loafing life of his set merely because all the rest do it. And I'm perfectly aware that if I'd been in the same circumstances as my aunt Liz, I'd have done exactly what she did. I don't think I'm more prejudiced or straitlaced than you: I think I'm less. I'm certain I'm less sentimental. I know very well that fashionable morality is all a pretence: and that if I took your money and devoted the rest of my life to spending it fashionably, I might be as worthless and vicious as the silliest woman could possibly want to be without having a word said to me about it. But I don't want to be worthless. I shouldn't enjoy trotting about the park to advertise my dressmaker and carriage builder, or being bored at the opera to show off a shop windowful of diamonds.

MRS. WARREN (*bewildered*): But—

VIVIE: Wait a moment: I've not done. Tell me why you continue your business now that you are independent of it. Your sister, you told me, has left all that behind her. Why don't you do the same?

MRS. WARREN: Oh, it's all very easy for Liz: she likes good society, and has the air of being a lady. Imagine me in a cathedral town! Why, the very rooks in the trees would find me out even if I could stand the dulness of it. I must have work and excitement, or I should go melancholy mad. And what else is there for me to do? The life suits me: I'm fit for it and not for anything else. If I didn't do it somebody else would; so I don't do any real harm by it. And then it brings in money; and I like making money. No: it's no use: I can't give it up—not for anybody. But what need you know about it? I'll never mention it. I'll keep Crofts away. I'll not trouble you much: you see I have to be constantly running about from one place to another. You'll be quit of me altogether when I die.

VIVIE: No: I am my mother's daughter. I am like you: I

must have work, and must make more money than I spend. But my work is not your work, and my way not your way. We must part. It will not make much difference to us: instead of meeting one another for perhaps a few months in twenty years, we shall never meet: that's all.

MRS. WARREN: (*her voice stifled in tears*): Vivie: I meant to have been more with you: I did indeed.

VIVIE: It's no use, mother: I am not to be changed by a few cheap tears and entreaties any more than you are, I dare say.

MRS. WARREN (*wildly*): Oh, you call a mother's tears cheap.

VIVIE: They cost you nothing: and you ask me to give you the peace and quietness of my whole life in exchange for them. What use would my company be to you if you could get it? What have we two in common that could make either of us happy together?

MRS. WARREN (*lapsing recklessly into her dialect*): We're mother and daughter. I want my daughter. I've a right to you. Who is to care for me when I'm old? Plenty of girls have taken to me like daughters and cried at leaving me; but I let them all go because I had you to look forward to. I kept myself lonely for you. You've no right to turn on me now and refuse to do your duty as a daughter.

VIVIE (*jarred and antagonized by the echo of the slums in her mother's voice.*): My duty as a daughter! I thought we should come to that presently. Now once for all, mother, you want a daughter and Frank wants a wife. I don't want a mother; and I don't want a husband. I have spared neither Frank nor myself in sending him about his business. Do you thing I will spare you?

MRS. WARREN (*violently*): Oh, I know the sort you are—no mercy for yourself or anyone else. *I* know. My experience has done that for me anyhow: I can tell the pious, canting, hard, selfish woman when I meet her. Well, keep yourself to yourself: *I* don't want you. But listen to this. Do you know what I would do with you if you were a baby again—aye, as sure as there's a Heaven above us?

VIVIE: Strangle me, perhaps.

MR. WARREN: No: I'd bring you up to be a real daughter to me, and not what you are now, with your pride and your prejudices and the college education you stole from me—yes, stole: deny it if you can: what was it but stealing? I'd bring you up in my own house, so I would.

VIVIE (*quietly*): In one of your own houses.

Is this TRUE of Vivie?

MRS. WARREN (*screaming*): Listen to her! listen to how she spits on her mother's grey hairs! Oh, may you live to have your own daughter tear and trample on you as you have trampled on me. And you will: you will. No woman ever had luck with a mother's curse on her.

VIVIE: I wish you wouldn't rant, mother. It only hardens me. Come: I suppose I am the only young woman you ever had in your power that you did good to. Don't spoil it all now.

MRS. WARREN: Yes. Heaven forgive me, it's true; and you are the only one that ever turned on me. Oh, the injustice of it, the injustice, the injustice! I always wanted to be a good woman. I tried honest work; and I was slave-driven until I cursed the day I ever heard of honest work. I was a good mother; and because I made my daughter a good woman she turns me out as if I was a leper. Oh, if I only had my life to live over again! I'd talk to that lying clergyman in the school. From this time forth, so help me Heaven in my last hour, I'll do wrong and nothing but wrong. And I'll prosper on it.

VIVIE: Yes: it's better to choose your line and go through with it. If I had been you, mother, I might have done as you did; but I should not have lived one life and believed in another. You are a conventional woman at heart. That is why I am bidding you good-bye now. I am right, am I not?

MRS. WARREN (*taken aback*): Right to throw away all my money!

VIVIE: No: right to get rid of you? I should be a fool not to? Isn't that so?

MRS. WARREN (*sulkily*): Oh, well, yes, if you come to that, I suppose you are. But Lord help the world if everybody took to doing the right thing! And now I'd better go than stay where I'm not wanted. (*She turns to the door.*)

VIVIE (*kindly*): Won't you shake hands?

MRS. WARREN (*after looking at her fiercely for a moment with a savage impulse to strike her*): No, thank you. Good-bye.

VIVIE (*matter-of-factly*): Good-bye. (*Mrs. Warren goes out, slamming the door behind her. The strain on Vivie's face relaxes; her grave expression breaks up into one of joyous content; her breath goes out in a half sob, half laugh of intense relief. She goes buoyantly to her place at the writing table; pushes the electric lamp out of the way; pulls over a great sheaf of papers; and is in the act of dipping her pen in the ink when she finds Frank's note. She opens it unconcernedly and reads it quickly, giving a little laugh at some quaint turn of expression in it.*) And good-bye, Frank.

(*She tears the note up and tosses the pieces into the waste-paper basket without a second thought. Then she goes at her work with a plunge, and soon becomes absorbed in her figures.*)

TRIFLES

Susan Glaspell

Characters

GEORGE HENDERSON, *County Attorney*
HENRY PETERS, *Sheriff*
LEWIS HALE, *a neighboring farmer*
MRS. PETERS
MRS. HALE

The scene is the kitchen in the farmhouse of JOHN
WRIGHT, *a gloomy kitchen, abandoned without having been
put in order—the walls covered with a faded wallpaper. A
door leads to the parlor at right. On the wall near this door
is a built-in kitchen cupboard with shelves in the upper portion and drawers below. In the rear wall, up two steps, is a
door opening onto stairs leading to the second floor. In the
rear wall there is another door which leads to the shed and
from there to the outside. Between these two doors is an old-
fashioned black iron stove. Running along the wall at left from
the shed door is an old iron sink and sink shelf, in which
is set a hand pump, and an uncurtained window. Near the
window is an old wooden rocker. In the center of the room is
an unpainted wooden kitchen table with straight chairs on either side. There is a small chair near the parlor door. Un-
washed pans under the sink, a loaf of bread outside the
breadbox, a dish towel on the table—other signs of incom-
pleted work. At the rear, the shed door opens and the* SHER-
IFF *comes in, followed by the* COUNTY ATTORNEY *and* HALE, *a
neighboring farmer. The* SHERIFF *and* HALE *are men in middle life, the* COUNTY ATTORNEY *is a young man; all are much
bundled up and go at once to the stove. They are followed by
two women—the* SHERIFF'S *wife,* MRS. PETERS, *first; she is a
slight, wiry woman, a thin, nervous face.* MRS. HALE *is
larger and would ordinarily be called more comfortable looking, but she is disturbed now and looks fearfully about as she
enters. The women have come in slowly, and stand close together near the door.*

COUNTY ATTORNEY (*at stove, rubbing his hands*): This
feels good. Come up to the fire, ladies.

MRS. PETERS (*after taking a step forward*): I'm not—cold.

SHERIFF (*unbuttoning his overcoat and stepping away
from the stove to table as if to mark the beginning of official
business*): Now, Mr. Hale, before we move things about, you

explain to Mr. Henderson just what you saw when you came here yesterday morning.

COUNTY ATTORNEY: By the way, has anything been moved? Are things just as you left them yesterday?

SHERIFF (*looking about*): It's just the same. When it dropped below zero last night I thought I'd better send Frank out this morning to make a fire for us. (*Sits down.*) No use getting pneumonia with a big case on, but I told him not to touch anything except the stove—and you know Frank.

COUNTY ATTORNEY: Somebody should have been left here yesterday.

SHERIFF: Oh, yesterday. When I had to send Frank to Morris Center for that man who went crazy—I want you to know I had my hands full yesterday. I knew you could get back from Omaha by today and as long as I went over everything here myself—

COUNTY ATTORNEY: Well, Mr. Hale, tell just what happened when you came here yesterday morning.

HALE (*crossing down to above table*): Harry and I had started to town with a load of potatoes. We came along the road from my place and as I got here I said, "I'm going to see if I can't get John Wright to go in with me on a party telephone." I spoke to Wright about it once before and he put me off, saying folks talked too much anyway, and all he asked was peace and quiet—I guess you know about how much he talked himself; but I thought maybe if I went to the house and talked about it before his wife, though I said to Harry that I didn't know as what his wife wanted made much difference to John—

COUNTY ATTORNEY: Let's talk about that later, Mr. Hale. I do want to talk about that, but tell now just what happened when you got to the house.

HALE: I didn't hear or see anything; I knocked at the door, and still it was all quiet inside. I knew they must be up; it was past eight o'clock. So I knocked again, and I thought I heard somebody say, "Come in." I wasn't sure, I'm not sure yet, but I opened the door—this door (*indicating the door by which the two women are still standing*), and there in that rocker (*pointing to it*) sat Mrs. Wright.

(*They all look at the rocker near the window.*)

COUNTY ATTORNEY: What—was she doing?

HALE: She was rockin' back and forth. She had her apron in her hand and was kind of—pleating it.

COUNTY ATTORNEY: And how did she—look?

HALE: Well, she looked queer.

COUNTY ATTORNEY: How do you mean—queer?

HALE: Well, as if she didn't know what she was going to do next. And kind of done up.

COUNTY ATTORNEY (*takes out notebook and pencil and sits at table*): How did she seem to feel about your coming?

HALE: Why, I don't think she minded—one way or other. She didn't pay much attention. I said, "How do, Mrs. Wright. It's cold, ain't it?" And she said, "Is it?"—and went on kind of pleating at her apron. Well, I was surprised; she didn't ask me to come up to the stove, or to set down, but just sat there, not even looking at me, so I said, "I want to see John." And then she—laughed. I guess you would call it a laugh. I thought of Harry and the team outside, so I said a little sharp: "Can't I see John?" "No," she says, kind o' dull like. "Ain't he home?" says I. "Yes," says she, "he's home." "Then why can't I see him?" I asked her, out of patience. " 'Cause he's dead," says she. "*Dead?*" says I. She just nodded her head, not getting a bit excited, but rockin' back and forth. "Why—where is he?" says I, not knowing what to say. She just pointed upstairs—like that. (*Himself pointing to the room above.*) I started for the stairs, with the idea of going up there. I walked from there to here—then I says, "Why, what did he die of?" "He died of a rope round his neck," says she, and just went on pleatin' at her apron. Well, I went out and called Harry. I thought I might—need help. We went upstairs and there he was lyin'—

COUNTY ATTORNEY: I think I'd rather have you go into that upstairs, where you can point it all out. Just go on now with the rest of the story.

HALE: Well, my first thought was to get that rope off. It looked—(*Stops, his face twitches.*) But Harry, he went up to him, and he said, "No, he's dead, all right, and we'd better not touch anything." So we went back downstairs. She was still sitting that same way. "Has anybody been notified?" I asked. "No," says she, unconcerned. "Who did this, Mrs. Wright?" said Harry. He said it businesslike—and she stopped pleatin' of her apron. "I don't know," she says. "You don't *know?*" says Harry. "No," says she. "Weren't you sleepin' in the bed with him?" says Harry. "Yes," says she, "but I was on the inside." "Somebody slipped a rope round his neck and strangled him and you didn't wake up?" says Harry. "I didn't wake up," she said after him. We must 'a' looked as if we didn't see how that could be, for after a minute she said, "I sleep sound." Harry was going to ask her more questions but I said maybe we ought to let her tell her story first to the coroner, or the sheriff, so Harry went fast as he could to Rivers' place, where there's a telephone.

COUNTY ATTORNEY: And what did Mrs. Wright do when she knew that you had gone for the coroner?

HALE: She moved from the rocker to that chair over there (*pointing to a small chair in the corner*) and just sat there with her hands held together and looking down. I got a feeling that I ought to make some conversation, so I said I had come in to see if John wanted to put in a telephone, and at that she started to laugh, and then she stopped and looked at me—scared. (*The* COUNTY ATTORNEY, *who has had his notebook out, makes a note.*) I dunno, maybe it wasn't scared. I wouldn't like to say it was. Soon Harry got back, and then Dr. Lloyd came, and you, Mr. Peters, and so I guess that's all I know that you don't.

COUNTY ATTORNEY (*rising and looking around*): I guess we'll go upstairs first—and then out to the barn and around there. (*To the* SHERIFF.) You're convinced that there was nothing important here—nothing that would point to any motive?

SHERIFF: Nothing here but kitchen things.

(*The* COUNTY ATTORNEY, *after again looking around the kitchen, opens the door of a cupboard closet. He brings a small chair over, gets up on it, and looks on a shelf. Pulls his hand away, sticky.*)

COUNTY ATTORNEY: Here's a nice mess.

(*The women draw nearer to the stove.*)

MRS. PETERS (*to the other woman*): Oh, her fruit; it did freeze. (*To the* COUNTY ATTORNEY.) She worried about that when it turned so cold. She said the fire'd go out and her jars would break.

SHERIFF (*rises*): Well, can you beat the women! Held for murder and worryin' about her preserves.

COUNTY ATTORNEY (*getting down from chair*): I guess before we're through she may have something more serious than preserves to worry about.

HALE: Well, women are used to worrying over trifles.

(*The two women move a little closer together.*)

COUNTY ATTORNEY (*with the gallantry of a young politi-*

cian): And yet, for all their worries, what would we do without the ladies? (*The women do not unbend. He goes to the sink, takes a dipperful of water from the pail, and pouring it into a basin, washes his hands. While he is doing this the* SHERIFF *and* HALE *cross to cupboard, which they inspect. The* COUNTY ATTORNEY *starts to wipe his hands on the roller towel, turns it for a cleaner place.*) Dirty towels! (*Kicks his foot against the pans under the sink.*) Not much of a housekeeper, would you say, ladies?

MRS. HALE (*stiffly*): There's a great deal of work to be done on a farm.

COUNTY ATTORNEY: To be sure. And yet (*with a little bow to her*) I know there are some Dickson County farmhouses which do not have such roller towels. (*He gives it a pull to expose its full length again.*)

MRS. HALE: Those towels get dirty awful quick. Men's hands aren't always as clean as they might be.

COUNTY ATTORNEY: Ah, loyal to your sex, I see. But you and Mrs. Wright were neighbors. I suppose you were friends, too.

MRS. HALE (*shaking her head*): I've not seen much of her of late years. I've not been in this house—it's more than a year.

COUNTY ATTORNEY (*crossing to women*): And why was that? You didn't like her?

MRS. HALE: I like her all well enough. Farmers' wives have their hands full, Mr. Henderson. And then—

COUNTY ATTORNEY: Yes—?

MRS. HALE (*looking about*): It never seemed a very cheerful place.

COUNTY ATTORNEY: No, it's not cheerful. I shouldn't say she had the homemaking instinct.

MRS. HALE: Well, I don't know as Wright had, either.

COUNTY ATTORNEY: You mean that they didn't get on very well?

MRS. HALE: No, I don't mean anything. But I don't think a place'd be any cheerfuler for John Wright's being in it.

COUNTY ATTORNEY: I'd like to talk more of that a little later. I want to get the lay of things upstairs now. (*He goes past the women to rear wall, where steps lead to a stair door.*)

SHERIFF: I suppose anything Mrs. Peters does'll be all right. She was to take in some clothes for her, you know, and a few little things. We left in such a hurry yesterday.

COUNTY ATTORNEY: Yes, but I would like to see what you

take, Mrs. Peters, and keep an eye out for anything that might be of use to us.

MRS. PETERS: Yes, Mr. Henderson.

(The men leave. The women listen to the men's steps on the stairs, then look about the kitchen.)

MRS. HALE *(crossing to sink)*: I'd hate to have men coming into my kitchen, snooping around and criticizing. *(She arranges the pans under sink which the* COUNTY ATTORNEY *had shoved out of place.)*

MRS. PETERS: Of course it's no more than their duty. *(Crosses to cupboard.)*

MRS. HALE: Duty's all right, but I guess that deputy sheriff that came out to make the fire might have got a little of this on. *(Gives the roller towel a pull.)* Wish I'd thought of that sooner. Seems mean to talk about her for not having things slicked up when she had to come away in such a hurry. *(Crosses to* MRS. PETERS *at cupboard.)*

MRS. PETERS *(who has been looking through cupboard, lifts one end of a towel that covers a pan)*: She had bread set. *(Stands still.)*

MRS. HALE *(eyes fixed on a loaf of bread beside the breadbox, which is on a low shelf of the cupboard)*: She was going to put this in there. *(Picks up loaf, then abruptly drops it. In a manner of returning to familiar things.)* It's a shame about her fruit. I wonder if it's all gone. *(Gets up on the chair and looks.)* I think there's some here that's all right, Mrs. Peters. Yes—here. *(Holding it toward the window.)* This is cherries, too. *(Looking again.)* I declare, I believe that's the only one. *(Gets down, jar in her hand. Goes to the sink and wipes it off on the outside.)* She'll feel awful bad after all her hard work in the hot weather. I remember the afternoon I put up my cherries last summer. *(She puts the jar on the big kitchen table. With a sigh, is about to sit down in the rocking chair. Before she is seated, realizes what chair it is; with a slow look at it, steps back. The chair, which she has touched, rocks back and forth.* MRS. PETERS *moves to table and they both watch the chair rock for a moment or two.)*

MRS. PETERS *(shaking off the mood which the empty rocking chair has evoked, now, in a businesslike manner, speaks)*: Well, I must get those things from the front-room closet. *(SHE goes to the parlor door, but, after looking into the other room, steps back.)* You coming with me, Mrs. Hale? You could help me carry them. *(They go in the other room; reappear,* MRS. PETERS *carrying a dress, petticoat, and skirt,*

MRS. HALE *following with a pair of shoes.*) My, it's cold in there. (*She puts the clothes on the big table, and hurries to the stove.*)

MRS. HALE (*at table examining the skirt*): Wright was close. I think maybe that's why she kept so much to herself. She didn't even belong to the Ladies' Aid. I suppose she felt she couldn't do her part, and then you don't enjoy things when you feel shabby. She used to wear pretty clothes and be lively, when she was Minnie Foster, one of the town girls singing in the choir. But that—oh, that was thirty years ago. This all you was to take in?

MRS. PETERS; She said she wanted an apron. Funny thing to want, for there isn't much to get you dirty in jail, goodness knows. But I suppose just to make her feel more natural. (*Crosses to cupboard.*) She said they was in the top drawer in this cupboard. Yes, here. And then her little shawl that always hung behind the door. (*Opens stair door and looks.*) Yes, here it is. (*Quickly shuts door leading upstairs.*)

MRS. HALE (*abruptly moving toward her*): Mrs. Peters?

MRS. PETERS: Yes, Mrs. Hale?

MRS. HALE: Do you think she did it?

MRS. PETERS (*in a frightened voice*): Oh, I don't know.

MRS. HALE: Well, I don't think she did. Asking for an apron and her little shawl. Worrying about her fruit.

MRS. PETERS (*starts to speak, glances up, where footsteps are heard in the room above; in a low voice*): Mr. Peters says it looks bad for her. Mr. Henderson is awful sarcastic in a speech and he'll make fun of her sayin' she didn't wake up.

MRS. HALE: Well, I guess John Wright didn't wake when they was slipping that rope under his neck.

MRS. PETERS (*crossing slowly to table and placing shawl and apron on table with other clothing*): No, it's strange. It must have been done awful crafty and still. They say it was such a—funny way to kill a man, rigging it all up like that.

MRS. HALE (*crossing to* MRS. PETERS *at table*): That's just what Mr. Hale said. There was a gun in the house. He says that's what he can't understand.

MRS. PETERS: Mr. Henderson said coming out that what was needed for the case was a motive; something to show anger, or—sudden feeling.

MRS. HALE (*who is standing by the table*): Well, I don't see any signs of anger around here. (*She puts her hand on the dish towel, which lies on the table, stands looking down at table, one half of which is clean, the other half messy.*) It's wiped to here. (*Makes a move as if to finish work, then turns and looks at loaf of bread outside the breadbox. Drops towel. In the voice of coming back to familiar things.*) Wonder how they are finding things upstairs. I hope she had it a little more red-up up there. You know, it seems kind of *sneaking.* Locking her up in town and then coming out here and trying to get her own house to turn against her!

MRS. PETERS: But, Mrs. Hale, the law is the law.

MRS. HALE: I s'pose 'tis. (*Unbuttoning her coat.*) Better loosen up your things, Mrs. Peters. You won't feel them when you go out.

(MRS. PETERS *takes off her fur tippet, goes to hang it on chair back left of table, stands looking at the work basket on floor near window.*)

MRS. PETERS: She was piecing a quilt. (*She brings the large sewing basket to the center table and they look at the bright pieces.*)

MRS. HALE: It's a log-cabin pattern. Pretty, isn't it? I wonder if she was goin' to quilt it or just knot it?

(*Footsteps have been heard coming down the stairs. The* SHERIFF *enters, followed by* HALE *and the* COUNTY ATTORNEY.)

SHERIFF: They wonder if she was going to quilt it or just knot it!

(*The men laugh, the women look abashed.*)

COUNTY ATTORNEY (*rubbing his hands over the stove*): Frank's fire didn't do much up there, did it? Well, let's go out to the barn and get that cleared up.

(*The men go outside.*)

MRS. HALE (*resentfully*): I don't know as there's anything so strange, our takin' up our time with little things while we're waiting for them to get the evidence. (*She sits in chair at table, smoothing out a block with decision.*) I don't see as it's anything to laugh about.

MRS. PETERS (*apologetically*): Of course they've got awful important things on their minds. (*Pulls up a chair and joins* MRS. HALE *at the table.*)

MRS. HALE (*examining another block*): Mrs. Peters, look at this one. Here, this is the one she was working on, and look at the sewing! All the rest of it has been so nice and even. And look at this! It's all over the place! Why, it looks as if she didn't know what she was about! (*After she has said this they look at each other, then start to glance back at the door. After an instant* MRS. HALE *has pulled at a knot and ripped the sewing.*)

MRS. PETERS: Oh, what are you doing, Mrs. Hale?

MRS. HALE (*mildly*): Just pulling out a stitch or two that's not sewed very good. (*Threading a needle.*) Bad sewing always made me fidgety.

MRS. PETERS (*with a glance at door, nervously*): I don't think we ought to touch things.

MRS. HALE: I'll just finish up this end. (*Suddenly stopping and leaning forward.*) Mrs. Peters?

MRS. PETERS: Yes, Mrs. Hale?

MRS. HALE: What do you suppose she was so nervous about?

MRS. PETERS: Oh, I don't know. I don't know as she was nervous. I sometimes sew awful queer when I'm just tired. (MRS. HALE *starts to say something, looks at* MRS. PETERS, *then goes on sewing.*) Well, I must get these things wrapped up. They may be through sooner than we think. (*Putting apron and other things together.*) I wonder where I can find a piece of paper and string. (*Rises.*)

MRS. HALE: In that cupboard, maybe.

MRS. PETERS (*looking in cupboard*): Why, here's a bird cage. (*Holds it up.*) Did she have a bird, Mrs. Hale?

MRS. HALE: Why, I don't know whether she did or not— I've not been here for so long. There was a man around last year selling canaries cheap, but I don't know as she took one; maybe she did. She used to sing real pretty herself.

MRS. PETERS (*glancing around*): Seems funny to think of a bird here. But she must have had one, or why would she have a cage? I wonder what happened to it?

MRS. HALE: I s'pose maybe the cat got it.

MRS. PETERS: No, she didn't have a cat. She's got that feeling some people have about cats—being afraid of them. My cat got in her room and she was real upset and asked me to take it out.

MRS. HALE: My sister Bessie was like that. Queer, ain't it?

MRS. PETERS (*examining the cage*): Why, look at this door. It's broke. One hinge is pulled apart. (*Takes a step down to* MRS. HALE.)

MRS. HALE (*looking, too.*): Looks as if someone must have been rough with it.

MRS. PETERS: Why, yes. (*She brings the cage forward and puts it on the table.*)

MRS. HALE (*glancing toward door*): I wish if they're going to find any evidence they'd be about it. I don't like this place.

MRS. PETERS: But I'm awful glad you came with me, Mrs. Hale. It would be lonesome for me sitting here alone.

MRS. HALE: It would, wouldn't it? (*Dropping her sewing.*) But I tell you what I do wish, Mrs. Peters. I wish I had come over sometimes when *she* was here. I (*looking around the room*) wish I had.

MRS. PETERS: But of course you were awful busy, Mrs. Hale—your house and your children.

MRS. HALE (*rises and crosses to window*): I could've come. I stayed away because it weren't cheerful—and that's why I ought to have come. I—(*looking out window*)—I've never liked this place. Maybe because it's down in a hollow and you don't see the road. I dunno what it is, but it's a lonesome place and always was. I wish I had come over to see Minnie Foster sometimes. I can see now— (*Shakes her head.*)

MRS. PETERS: Well, you mustn't reproach yourself, Mrs. Hale. Somehow we just don't see how it is with other folks until—something turns up.

MRS. HALE: Not having children makes less work—but it makes a quiet house, and Wright out to work all day, and no company when he did come in. (*Turning from window.*) Did you know John Wright, Mrs. Peters?

MRS. PETERS: Not to know him; I've seen him in town. They say he was a good man.

MRS. HALE: Yes—good; he didn't drink, and kept his word as well as most, I guess, and paid his debts. But he was a hard man, Mrs. Peters. Just to pass the time of day with him—(*Shivers.*) Like a raw wind that gets to the bone. (*Pauses, her eye falling on the cage.*) I should think she would 'a' wanted a bird. But what do you suppose went with it?

MRS. PETERS: I don't know, unless it got sick and died. (*She reaches over and swings the broken door, swings it again; both women watch it.*)

MRS. HALE: You weren't raised round here, were you? (MRS. PETERS *shakes her head.*) You didn't know—her?

MRS. PETERS: Not till they brought her yesterday.

MRS. HALE: She—come to think of it, she was kind of like a bird herself—real sweet and pretty, but kind of timid and —fluttery. How—she—did—change. (*Silence; then, as if struck by a happy thought and relieved to get back to every-*

*day things, crosses to cupboard, replaces small chair used to
stand on to its original place.*) Tell you what, Mrs. Peters,
why don't you take the quilt in with you? It might take up
her mind.

MRS. PETERS: Why, I think that's a real nice idea, Mrs.
Hale. There couldn't possibly be any objection to it, could
there? Now, just what would I take? I wonder if her patches
are in here—and her things.

(*They look in the sewing basket.*)

MRS. HALE (*crosses to table*): Here's some red. I expect
this has got sewing things in it. (*Brings out a fancy box.*)
What a pretty box. Looks like something somebody would
give you. Maybe her scissors are in here. (*Opens box. Suddenly puts her hand to her nose.*) Why—(MRS. PETERS *bends
nearer, then turns her face away.*) There's something
wrapped up in this piece of silk.

MRS. PETERS: Why, this isn't her scissors.

MRS. HALE (*lifting the silk*): Oh, Mrs. Peters—it's—

(MRS. PETERS *bends closer.*)

MRS. PETERS: It's the bird.

MRS. HALE: But, Mrs. Peters—look at it! Its neck! Look at
its neck! It's all—other side to.

MRS. PETERS: Somebody—wrung—its—neck.

(*Their eyes meet. A look of growing comprehension, of
horror. Steps are heard outside.* MRS. HALE *slips box under
quilt pieces, and sinks into her chair. Enter* SHERIFF *and*
COUNTY ATTORNEY. MRS. PETERS *stands looking out of window.*)

COUNTY ATTORNEY (*as one turning from serious things to
little pleasantries*): Well, ladies, have you decided whether
she was going to quilt it or knot it? (*Crosses to table.*)

MRS. PETERS: We think she was going to—knot it.

(SHERIFF *crosses to stove, lifts stove lid, and glances at
fire, then stands warming hands at stove.*)

COUNTY ATTORNEY: Well, that's interesting, I'm sure.
(*Seeing the bird cage.*) Has the bird flown?

MRS. HALE (*putting more quilt pieces over the box*): We think the—cat got it.

COUNTY ATTORNEY (*preoccupied*): Is there a cat?

(MRS. HALE *glances in a quick, covert way at* MRS. PETERS.)

MRS. PETERS (*turning from window*): Well, not *now*. They're superstitious, you know. They leave.

COUNTY ATTORNEY (*to* SHERIFF PETERS, *continuing an interrupted conversation*): No sign at all of anyone having come from the outside. Their own rope. Now let's go up again and go over it piece by piece. (*They start upstairs.*) It would have to have been someone who knew just the—

(MRS. PETERS *sits down at the table. The two women sit there not looking at one another, but as if peering into something and at the same time holding back. When they talk now it is in the manner of feeling their way over strange ground, as if afraid of what they are saying, but as if they cannot help saying it.*)

MRS. HALE (*hesitantly and in hushed voice*): She liked the bird. She was going to bury it in that pretty box.

MRS. PETERS (*in a whisper*): When I was a girl—my kitten—there was a boy took a hatchet, and before my eyes—and before I could get there—(*Covers her face an instant.*) If they hadn't held me back I would have—(*catches herself, looks upstairs where steps are heard, falters weakly*)—hurt him.

MRS. HALE (*with a slow look around her*): I wonder how it would seem never to have had any children around. (*Pause.*) No, Wright wouldn't like the bird—a thing that sang. She used to sing. He killed that, too.

MRS. PETERS (*moving uneasily*): We don't know who killed the bird.

MRS. HALE: I knew John Wright.

MRS. PETERS: It was an awful thing was done in this house that night, Mrs. Hale. Killing a man while he slept, slipping a rope around his neck that choked the life out of him.

MRS. HALE: His neck. Choked the life out of him. (*Her hand goes out and rests on the bird cage.*)

MRS. PETERS (*with rising voice*): We don't know who killed him. We dont *know*.

MRS. HALE (*her own feeling not interrupted*): If there'd

been years and years of nothing, then a bird to sing to you, it would be awful—still, after the bird was still.

MRS. PETERS (*something within her speaking*): I know what stillness is. When we homesteaded in Dakota, and my first baby died—after he was two years old, and me with no other then—

MRS. HALE (*moving*): How soon do you suppose they'll be through looking for the evidence?

MRS. PETERS: I know what stillness is. (*Pulling herself back.*) The law has got to punish crime, Mrs. Hale.

MRS. HALE (*not as if answering that*): I wish you'd seen Minnie Foster when she wore a white dress with blue ribbons and stood up there in the choir and sang. (*A look around the room.*) Oh, I *wish* I'd come over here once in a while! That was a crime! That was a crime! Who's going to punish that?

MRS. PETERS (*looking upstairs*): We mustn't—take on.

MRS. HALE: I might have known she needed help! I know how things can be—for women. I tell you, it's queer, Mrs. Peters. We live close together and we live far apart. We all go through the same things—it's all just a different kind of the same thing. (*Brushes her eyes, noticing the jar of fruit, reaches out for it.*) If I was you I wouldn't tell her her fruit was gone. Tell her it *ain't*. Tell her it's all right. Take this in to prove it to her. She—she may never know whether it was broke or not.

MRS. PETERS (*takes the jar, looks about for something to wrap it in; takes petticoat from the clothes brought from the other room, very nervously begins winding this around the jar; in a false voice*): My, it's a good thing the men couldn't hear us. Wouldn't they just laugh! Getting all stirred up over a little thing like a—dead canary. As if that could have anything to do with—with—wouldn't they *laugh!*

(*The men are heard coming downstairs.*)

MRS. HALE (*under her breath*): Maybe they would—maybe they wouldn't.

COUNTY ATTORNEY: No, Peters, it's all perfectly clear except a reason for doing it. But you know juries when it comes to women. If there was some definite thing. (*Crosses slowly to table.* MRS. HALE *and* MRS. PETERS *remain seated at either side of table.*) Something to show—something to make a story about—a thing that would connect up with this strange way of doing it—

(*The women's eyes meet for an instant. Enter* HALE *from outer door.*)

HALE (*remaining by door*): Well, I've got the team around. Pretty cold out there.

COUNTY ATTORNEY: I'm going to stay here awhile by myself. (*To the* SHERIFF.) You can send Frank out for me, can't you? I want to go over everything. I'm not satisfied that we can't do better.

SHERIFF: Do you want to see what Mrs. Peters is going to take in?

(*The* COUNTY ATTORNEY *picks up the apron, laughs.*)

COUNTY ATTORNEY: Oh, I guess they're not very dangerous things the ladies have picked out. (*Moves a few things about, disturbing the quilt pieces which cover the box. Steps back.*) No, Mrs. Peters doesn't need supervising. For that matter, a sheriff's wife is married to the law. Ever think of it that way, Mrs. Peters?

MRS. PETERS: Not—just that way.

SHERIFF (*chuckling*): Married to the law. (*Moves to parlor door.*) I just want you to come in here a minute, George. We ought to take a look at these windows.

COUNTY ATTORNEY (*scoffingly*): Oh, windows!

SHERIFF: We'll be right out, Mr. Hale.

(HALE *goes outside. The* SHERIFF *follows the* COUNTY ATTORNEY *into the other room. Then* MRS. HALE *rises, hands tight together, looking intensely at* MRS. PETERS, *whose eyes make a slow turn, finally meeting* MRS. HALE'S. *A moment* MRS. HALE *holds her, then her own eyes point the way to where the box is concealed. Suddenly* MRS. PETERS *throws back quilt pieces and tries to put the box in the bag she is carrying. It is too big. She opens box, starts to take bird out, cannot touch it, goes to pieces, stands there helpless. Sound of a knob turning in the other room.* MRS. HALE *snatches the box and puts it in the pocket of her big coat. Enter* COUNTY ATTORNEY *and* SHERIFF.)

COUNTY ATTORNEY (*crosses to outer door facetiously:*)

Well, Henry, at least we found out that she was not going to quilt it. She was going to—what is it you call it, ladies?

MRS. HALE (*standing at table facing front, her hand against her pocket*): We call it—knot it, Mr. Henderson.

APPROACHING SIMONE

Megan Terry

Characters

SIMONE
FATHER
MOTHER
BROTHER
VISITOR
SIMONE, *a college friend of Simone's*
ALBERT
JEAN-PAUL
CAROLINA
BOARD HEAD I
BOARD HEAD II
SEVERAL FRENCH MILITARY MEN
    (all played by the same actor)
THE ENSEMBLE
QUEENS
KINGS

ACT 1

The stage of the proscenium opening should be raked at a high enough angle so that any floor movement or choreography can be seen from anywhere in the house. Throughout the auditorium should be built at least five small platforms, covering the theater seats, with stairs or ropes or bridges for the actors to reach them. There should be a balcony to stage left and stage right where the opera singers will stand and sing in spotlights when necessary. Coming out from the proscenium opening on both stage right and stage left should be two platforms against the house walls, wide enough to hold ornate chairs and from four to eight actors each. On stage right platform, which should be lower than the height of the main stage but high enough that the audience can see heads and shoulders, should be male actors, dressed in the costumes of kings, emperors, presidents, prelates, etc. They are all very very old. On stage left platform jutting out from the proscenium are female actors dressed in haute couture of the thirties. They are anybody's idea of society and culture leaders. They are very very old.

Draped above the proscenium opening are the intermingled flags of France, Nazi Germany, Russia, England, and the United States. In the center of the flags is a giant ikon, painted in muted, glowing colors and illuminated with gold leaf, of God in a flowing white beard at the top, Jesus below and to the left, a golden glow below and to the right.

In the corners of the proscenium arch where the arch and the walls of the house join, stage right and stage left, are papier-mâché cherubs painted in gold. They stand from floor to ceiling. In their belly buttons are golden rings: to the rings are attached golden cords. The cords are held by the old men and old women and will be pulled at the appropriate time.

On the ceiling is a beautiful head with an open mouth. The COMPANY enters from back of the auditorium in precession. As they reach the stage, they turn and face the audience. The woman who plays Simone takes up position at extreme stage left and silently stares at the audience. The COMPANY sings.

[359]

ALL:
THE DARKNESS, THE DARKNESS
I'M NOT AFRAID OF THE NIGHT
THE DARKNESS, THE DARKNESS
WHERE I GROPED INSIDE
I LOVED THE LIGHT ON THE SNOW
I SENT MY SUGAR TO THE WAR
I WATCHED GOOD FRENCHMEN
GO
INTO THE GROUND
BUT I PAID ATTENTION TO THE SOUND
OF THE POUNDING DARK
WITHIN MY HEAD
I FOLLOWED WHERE THE HEARTBEAT LED
AND MY MIND SEEMED TO BLEED
   BARITONE:
IF THE FOOL PERSISTS IN HIS FOLLY
HE WILL BECOME WISE
IF THE FOOL PERSISTS IN HIS FOLLY
HE WILL BECOME WISE
DESIRE! DESIRE! DESIRE! DESIRE!
ECSTASY! MIND ECSTASY! DESIRE!
DESIRE!
ECLIPSE THE FIRE OF THE SEXUAL DRIVE
REACH OUT THROUGH THE MIND
LEAVE THE SPERM BEHIND
LET THE EGG FALL WHERE SHE MAY
DRIVE, DRIVE, DRIVE
TO MIND ECSTASY

(The CHORUS keeps singing "Attention, Attention.")

   WOMAN:
ANYONE CAN BECOME
ANYONE CAN BECOME

   MAN:
ANYONE CAN KNOW TRUTH
ANYONE CAN KNOW TRUTH

   ALL:
DESIRE DESIRE!

   DUET:
ONLY MAKE THE EFFORT OF ATTENTION
ONLY MAKE THE EFFORT OF ATTENTION

STAY IN THE DARK INSIDE YOUR HEAD
(*Repeat*)
TILL IT LIGHTS YOUR WAY

    ALL:
ATTENTION, PULL WITH YOUR WILL
GENIUS IS INVISIBLE.

(*One by one everyone sings the name "Simone" on a different note, then everyone taking her or his same note sings the name "Simone" five times together.*)

ACTOR (*intones from platform*): Simone taught herself the art of perpetual attention. Simone taught herself the art of perpetual attention.

    (*Exit.*)

No matter what age SIMONE *is during a scene, she always behaves and speaks as if she were somewhere near thirty.*
SIMONE *enters running and flings herself down. Her family follows. They mime carrying luggage.*

    MOTHER: Get up, Simone. We have a long way to walk to the lodge.
    SIMONE: I have nothing to carry.
    MOTHER: You're too little.
    FATHER: You don't have to carry anything.
    BROTHER: You can't carry anything, you're only five.
    SIMONE: I can carry anything.
    MOTHER: Get up at once.
    SIMONE: I can carry as much as Brother.
    FATHER: My dear little girl. Father can carry you and the luggage too: climb on my back.
    SIMONE: I want to carry my share.
    MOTHER: There's no need.
    BROTHER: You're melting the snow.
    MOTHER: You'll catch pneumonia.
    FATHER: T.B.
    BROTHER: I'm starving. Come on, Simone.
    SIMONE: No.
    MOTHER. Simone.
    SIMONE: No.
    FATHER: Simone.

SIMONE: No.

MOTHER: You'll get bronchitis, you'll get the flu, you'll have a headache, your clothes will be wet. You'll not sleep a wink. I won't sleep a wink. I'll be up all night with you coughing. You're too frail, you were not only ill all this fall, but you were in bed most of the summer. Please, my little darling, come now and take Mama's hand.

SIMONE: No. I can carry as much as he can.

BROTHER: Let's see.

(SIMONE *stands up and* BROTHER *mimes transference of luggage on his back to Simone's back. She wobbles, gets her balance, and slowly trudges ahead.*)

MOTHER: What will we do with her, she'll break her bones before she's six.

FATHER: Let her have her way. She can't keep it up.

BROTHER (*running off*): I'll eat up all the croissants.

(MOTHER *and* FATHER *freeze.*)

This series of scenes should be played very quickly in different pools of light.

BROTHER *and* SIMONE.

BROTHER: Do you know your Racine?

SIMONE: Of course.

BROTHER: Then whoever dries up first gets slapped by the other.

(He *begins to recite* Phaedra. He *stumbles.* SIMONE *slaps him and continues the passage. She falters and he slaps her.*)

BROTHER: Continue.

(SIMONE *continues to recite; she gets slapped twice.*)

Continue. Continue.

VISITOR, MOTHER, BROTHER, SIMONE.

BROTHER: I solved all the math problems before the teacher could.

MOTHER: He's been first in his class in everything since he started school.

VISITOR: He's the genius, and (*pointing to* SIMONE) she's the beauty.

(SIMONE *turns away as if slapped by an invisible hand.*)

SIMONE, BROTHER, *and* MOTHER.

MOTHER: My dearest children, where are your stockings?
BROTHER: We gave them away.
MOTHER: It's raining and freezing out.
SIMONE: The worker's children don't wear stockings, and neither do I!
MOTHER: I won't permit this. Your father won't permit this. You're not to leave the house till I send out for more stockings for you.
SIMONE: I will never wear stockings again.

SIMONE *and* MOTHER: SIMONE *is pouring sugar into an envelope.*

MOTHER: My precious baby, my own, my darling, what are you doing with that precious sugar? It was so hard for me to get. I had the maid stand in line for three hours for it.
SIMONE: I'm mailing my sugar to the soldiers at the front.
MOTHER: But why?
SIMONE: They don't have any.

At the beach: FATHER *and* SIMONE. SIMONE *is gazing at the sunset.* (*The* ENSEMBLE *become waves, gulls, shore birds, etc.*)

FATHER: Simone, you've been sitting looking out over the water for hours—go and play with the other children.
SIMONE: It's so beautiful. I'd much rather watch the sunset than play.

(*She screams a long agonized scream. The* ENSEMBLE *rush upstage and turn with their mouths open in mirror agony.*)

Father, I have an impossible headache. I've never never known such pain. It's driving me out of my mind.

FATHER: It's probably only connected to your menstrual cycle. This often happens the first few times.

SIMONE: It's not like an ordinary pain. I'm going blind. I'm afraid I'll vomit.

FATHER (*feeling her forehead*): You don't have a fever. Where's the pain centered?

SIMONE: It started in my left eye and now has traveled to the right. I can't stand the light. I can't stand the noise. The noise in the street is trampling on my brain.

FATHER: Sounds like a migraine. I hope not, my precious child. Go and lie down in your room. I'll bring an ice cloth for your head, and make it very dark until you feel better.

(*Exit.*)

Simone at Fourteen—When and Why She Wants to Kill Herself

SIMONE *is alone in her room with the wet cloth. As her pain and anguish build, aspects of her self-doubt, self-loathing, and pain and anguish appear to torture her. Each one brings a larger and larger piece of white wet cloth until she is all wrapped up except for her head, with a piece left to strangle herself.* (*or one giant white cloth can be used*).

SIMONE: Oh Father, Father, it's unbearable. Surely it's some kind of punishment.

ONE: You have no talent, Simone.

TWO: You're stupid, Simone.

THREE: You're awkward, Simone.

FOUR: Not only is your body miserable, but your mind can't move either.

FIVE: You're nothing but a girl, Simone.

SIX: You'll never amount to anything, Simone.

SEVEN: You'll never match your brother, Simone.

EIGHT: You're only a girl, Simone.

(*Taunts from the auditorium in three languages, equivalent to "You're nothing but a stupid cunt."*)

NINE: The pain in your head is evidence.

TEN: Evidence of your lack of brains, Simone.

ELEVEN: You'll never know the truth, Simone.

TWELVE: Your mind is too dim to perceive the truth, Simone.

THIRTEEN: Put an end to your stupidity, Simone.

FOURTEEN: Beauty is useless, Simone; it isn't the path to the truth.

FIFTEEN: You're unworthy, Simone.

SIXTEEN: You're wretched, Simone.

SEVENTEEN: You're unfit for this world, Simone.

EIGHTEEN: You're arrogant, Simone.

NINETEEN: You'll never create anything, Simone.

TWENTY: You have no talent, Simone.

TWENTY-ONE: You have no genius, Simone.

TWENTY-TWO: You're a girl, Simone.

TWENTY-THREE: Your pain is your proof, Simone.

TWENTY-FOUR: You're always sick and you'll always be sick, Simone.

TWENTY-FIVE: Your head will always ache, Simone.

TWENTY-SIX: You can't even draw a straight line, Simone.

TWENTY-SEVEN: You have poor circulation, Simone.

TWENTY-EIGHT: Your hands are always swollen, Simone.

TWENTY-NINE: It takes brains to discover the truth, Simone.

SIMONE: If I can't find the way to justice and truth, then I don't want to live! I'm mediocre! Only the truly great can enter that transcendant kingdom where truth lives.

THIRTY: Kill yourself, Simone.

(THIRTY *unrolls the white sheet.* SIMONE *rolls tortuously out. As the* SINGER *sings,* SIMONE *is drawn back to the will to live. She slowly rises.*)

SINGER:
ANYONE CAN KNOW TRUTH
DESIRE, DESIRE
ONLY MAKE THE EFFORT OF ATTENTION
FOCUS ON THE DARK INSIDE YOUR HEAD
UNTIL IT LIGHTS YOUR WAY
THE SIMPLEST MAN MAY KNOW TRUTH
IF HE REACHES OUT EVERY DAY.

A nightclub. SIMONE *sits smoking buried behind the menu. Her friends* SIMONE, JEAN-PAUL, ALBERT, *and some others sit around tables. There is a small band playing in the back-ground.*

SIMONE TWO: Simone, roll me a cigarette.
JEAN-PAUL: She's too clumsy.
ALBERT: She's getting better.
SIMONE TWO: They burn longer—she packs them tight.
JEAN-PAUL: Simone, your lips.
SIMONE: Eh?
ALBERT: You're reading the script off the menu.
JEAN-PAUL: She won't order anything anyway.
ALBERT: I'll order for her. Tonight we eat.
JEAN-PAUL: Tonight we drink. Whiskey!
SIMONE TWO: Whiskey! Whiskey, Simone?
SIMONE: No.
SIMONE TWO: Here, take my tobacco.
SIMONE: Thanks.
JEAN-PAUL (*watching* SIMONE *roll cigarette*): Hey, she's doing it with one hand.
ALBERT: American.
SIMONE TWO: Twist the end, like yours. Ah.

(SIMONE *rolling cigarettes in each hand, drops them and gets tobacco all over her skirt, the table. She tries to brush it together. Everyone sputters.*)

JEAN-PAUL: Get it out of the way. Carolina is almost on.
SIMONE TWO: We were lucky to get in.
ALBERT: I'm in love with her.
SIMONE: How long has she been in France?
ALBERT: I hope she never leaves; she's promised never to leave.
SIMONE: I'd like to talk with her sometime.

(*Her friends laugh. Successfully rolling another cigarette for herself, she lights it with the stub of the one in her mouth.*)

They've been so exploited. We do the same in our colonies. How can you sit here drinking and grinning like apes when we are grinding down the blacks in Africa?

JEAN-PAUL: We'll change all that tomorrow. Tonight we have fun.
SIMONE TWO: Simone is right. Have you written a position paper on the colonies?

JEAN-PAUL: I will, I will. I have to form a coalition with the workers first.

ALBERT: It won't be hard. The monetary system is cracking. I predict within six months, a year at most, we'll have no trouble recruiting.

JEAN-PAUL: The international capitalistic beast has fed on itself so long, it won't find even a kernel of corn left in its shit to keep it going.

SIMONE: It's beginning to happen in Germany. I plan to go there to examine the new workers' alliances at first hand.

JEAN-PAUL: I'll publish anything you send back.

SIMONE: Good, but I won't have much time to write. I intend to work.

ALBERT: Work, work. Always work. Whiskey!

SIMONE: Everything begins and ends with work. Work is constant. You and I pass through, but the work is always here.

SIMONE TWO: One day the machines will do all the work.

SIMONE: If we are not careful, we will work for the machines.

JEAN-PAUL: Technology will free man from manual labor.

SIMONE: I hope not.

ALBERT: What is so sacred about working with your hands. I've never worked with my hands and I never intend to— we're freed from that.

SIMONE: You are privileged; they are not.

ALBERT: I want to think; I want to plan, create.

SIMONE: You above all should understand work. Work, in contrast to reflection, to persuasion or to magic, is a sequence of actions that have no direct connection either with the initial emotion, or the end aimed at ... Colors, sounds, dimensions can change, while the law of work, which is to be endlessly indifferent to what has preceded and what will follow, never changes. Qualities, forms, and distances change, but the law of work remains the constant factor to which qualities, forms, and distances serve only as signs. The law of exterior relations defines space. To *see* space is to grasp that work's raw material is always passive, always outside one's self...

ALBERT: Whiskey.

SIMONE TWO: Here she comes.

JEAN-PAUL: Simone. Attend her closely. Tell me if Carolina is working or creating magic.

SIMONE (*smoking again, she sits back*): Now *you're* working too hard, Jean-Paul.

WAITER: Caro—lin—A!!

(CAROLINA, *a black American entertainer, takes the stage. She sings first in a blues style that changes to a Charleston and then back to a shoutin' blues. She's backed by a mixed chorus who dance in the style of 1928–29*).

CAROLINA (*singing and dancing, blues, Charleston, tap, stomp*):
THE BLUES WAS A PASS TIME
THE BLUES WAS A PASS TIME
FOR THAT TIME
I DIDN'T HAVE NO TIME
FOR NOTHIN BUT THE BLUES

I COULD SPEND THE DAY
I COULD LAY THERE ALL THE DAY
PASSIN TIME WITH MY BLUES

THE BLUES WAS MY PASS TIME
THAT WAS THE LAST TIME THAT I
LET THE BLUES GET ME THAT WAY

MY LATEST OLD MAN LEFT ME IN MY BED
HE WALKED ON DOWN TO THE STORE
HE'D WATCHED MY RED HEART
TURN TO LEAD
HE SAID "CHILE, CHILE, CHILE,
I JES CAIN'T SLEEP WITH YOU NO MORE."

IT'S PAST TIME FOR THE BLUES
THEY DON'T GONNA GRAB ME NO MORE
I AIN'T LAYIN' WITH THE BLUES
I'M SICK OF THE HEARTSICK
I DONE LICKED THE BLUES

IT'S LONG PAST TIME FOR THE BLUES
MY RED HEART DONE TURNED TO BLUE
BUT ALONG CAME A PRETTY MAN
WHO MADE ME KNOW MY EYES WAS BLACK
HE TOLE ME, BABY, YOU IS MINE NOW AND
YORE OLD MAN AIN'T NEVER COMIN BACK

AND I'M GLAD HE'S GONE
OH YES, I'M GLAD HE'S GONE
I GOT A NEW MAN, NOT A BLUE MAN

HE GIVES ME SUGAR AT NIGHT

HE GIVES ME SUGAR AT NIGHT
HE BAKES MY BREAD
HE HOLDS ME TIGHT

HE CALLS ME HIS PEACHES
I CALLS HIM MY CREAM
HE CREAMS
MY PEACHES
HE CREAMS MY PEACHES,
AND BABY LET ME TELL YOU,
BABY LET ME TELL YOU,
THIS AIN'T NO DREAM!!

(*They applaud wildly, bang the table;* ALBERT *jumps up and invites her to the table. She comes over and he introduces her around. She shakes hands.* SIMONE *crunches down in her chair. She is very shy, lights two cigarettes at once, and starts to pick up the menu again. The band begins a mild Charleston.* CAROLINA *bends over* SIMONE.)

CAROLINA: Hello baby, give me some sugar. Hey baby, give me some sugar.

(*As* SIMONE *turns red,* CAROLINA *kisses her on the neck, and then pulls her to her feet.*)

Come on and Charleston, Charleston with me.

SIMONE: I beg your pardon?
CAROLINA: Dance, baby.
SIMONE: I don't know how.
CAROLINA: Follow me.

(SIMONE *hands notebook to* ALBERT.)

SIMONE: I'm afraid I . . .
CAROLINA: Don't work so hard . . . like this, nice and easy does it. . .

(SIMONE, *awkward, makes some attempt. Her friends are delighted.*)

SIMONE: I can't get my hands right.
CAROLINA: You'll get it, you'll get it. Let it come up through the floor. Let it creep right up ya spine. Yeah, yeah, you gettin' it. Who's buyin'?
ALBERT (*yelling*): Whiskey.

JEAN-PAUL: Work or magic, Simone?
SIMONE: It's divine, Jean-Paul.

(*They all laugh.*)

ALBERT: So are you. What do you drink, Carolina?
CAROLINA: Old Forrester, neat.

(*As they exit:*)

ALBERT: Say you will never leave France. Say you will never leave me.
CAROLINA: Anything you say, baby—it's really true what they said about Paree.

(SIMONE *remains alone onstage. The* ENSEMBLE *appears in grotesque gray bags. They move slowly to smother her. She remains in one place.*)

SIMONE (*a litany*): What I am, I endure. What I am, I endure. I suffer, I desire, I doubt, I'm stupid. I'm ignorant, I'm not well put together. What I am does not satisfy me. I have become me without my consent. Tomorrow is an I that now I cannot change. What I am, I endure, I suffer.

(*The* ENSEMBLE *covers her for an instant. Then break and dissolve upstage. Alone:*)

I desire, I am stupid! What I am, I endure.

SIMONE *and her* MOTHER *arrive in a truck made of the* EN-SEMBLE *at the rooms where Simone's first teaching post is to be.* SIMONE *is chainsmoking and reading newspapers and magazines throughout the scene. The truck is loaded with all sorts of furniture, etc. The* MOTHER *directs* TWO WORKMEN *who mime unloading and placing the articles.* SIMONE *sits, smokes, reads, and makes rapid notes.*

MOTHER: A delightful cottage. Looks tight. I shall check for drafts. Bring in the furniture.

(SIMONE *takes a fast glance and goes back to her reading; the minute a chair is placed she sits and continues.*)

The bed there, the photos there, the commode there, the bureau there, the table there, the chairs, here, the sofa there, the rug here, no the bed here out of the draft, now the rug back here, the bureau there, the desk here.

(*She pays* MOVERS. *They exit.*)

Simone, see the view from your desk. You'll be able to correct your papers while you watch the sun set. Be sure not to open the window when you work; it gives you pain in your neck. We'll all miss you and write every week. Take possession of your pupils; they're lucky to have you. I've furnished your room. It's beautiful. See how well everything fits. Be well and happy and write every week. Do you like what I've done?

SIMONE (*taking cigarette out of her mouth*): It's beautiful, darling.
MOTHER: You must keep well and let me know the minute anything happens. Don't catch cold, and try to remember to eat. Promise me you'll remember to eat.
SIMONE: I promise, my darling mother, and I promise I'll write you both every week.

(MOTHER *kisses* SIMONE, *then exits.* SIMONE *starts to speak but lights another cigarette and methodically rounds up all the furniture except desk, chair, and bed and pushes them over into the orchestra pit. Then she goes to sleep on the floor.*)

Lights dim a moment—then come up bright morning. Her first class of girls is entering, chattering, and wondering about their new teacher.

ALL: *Bonjour*, etc.

(SIMONE *rises and waves her hand at them without looking; she's deep in thought.*)

PUPIL: Does that mean we're supposed to sit down?

(*They push one another into the classroom, trying to suppress laughter and excitement. The men in the* ENSEMBLE *have assumed the position of desks—the girls each choose one and sit on his back.*)
SIMONE (*pacing*): To teach or not to teach, that is the

way to earn my bread. To teach or not to teach. That is the
way to earn my soul. I hate to eat. What is feeding?

(*During all this the* GIRLS *are secretly looking at her, making fun of her, sizing her up, passing notes and making ges-
tures.*)

Bonjour mes chers enfants. Bon. It's a good day. Did you
see the sunrise?

(CLASS *giggles.*)

It's good to get up in time to see the sunrise. You all do it.
You have to get to school on time.

CLASS (*bored*): *Bonjour, Mademoiselle.*

(*They turn off and look out at the audience and stay very
stiff while shuffling their feet and picking their ears, or
secretly scratching their crotches.*)

SIMONE: I have some new ideas.

(*Many groans from* CLASS.)

They will stimulate your minds.

(*Many more groans and stamping of feet.* SIMONE *walks
around in agitation.* STUDENTS *watch her.*)

Listen to me. If you won't bend a little, I'll have to smoke.

(CLASS *laughs and claps.*)

I'm fighting off lighting up a cigarette, because I'm trying
to teach you.

CLASS (*sighs, mocking*): Ohhh!
SIMONE: I've been educated in Paris.
CLASS (*sighs*): Oooo!
SIMONE: I've been educated by the bourgeoisie to teach
you to be like me, and if that is what you want, that is what
you'll get.
STUDENT: We knew that before we came. That's why
we're here. How else will we get good jobs?
SIMONE: At the same time that I teach you to be like what

your parents expect, because I too love and respect my parents and wish to live up to what they respect, I do wish to make some innovations.

CLASS: Not another innovation.

SIMONE: What I as a teacher would like to do with my life is to try to work out with you as I'm working out with myself some of the things important to all of us. Since this class is concerned with the philosophy syllabus, what I'd like to do is to demonstrate to you how philosophy came into being as a name, as a way of thinking; I want you to know the history and the definition of it and not just the name "philisophy" that will be found one day written in your exercise books. I care to speak to you about how to live.

STUDENT (*laughs*): But we're already alive.

SIMONE: Everywhere?

STUDENT: Where's that.

SIMONE: That is what we'll discover. Class dismissed for today.

(GIRLS *rise and exit—talking bewilderedly—then return. As they enter the classroom again, they push their desks closer to* SIMONE.)

SIMONE: *Bonjour.*

CLASS: *Bonjour* (*Hi—Hello, etc.*)

SIMONE: Who wishes to hike this weekend?

(ALL *raise hands, with exclamations.*)

We're taking a difficult trail.

(*Still* ALL *raise hands, make sounds of assurance.*)

I think we'll have good weather, and I don't want to miss it before it gets too cold. I want you to begin to take yourselves more seriously as writers. It seems to me a good way to do this would be for you to see your work in print. Therefore, I've procured a printing press, and from now on all compositions in philosophy will be printed. This will mean extra hours because you'll have to learn how to run the printing press, but that will be a good lesson in physics and mathematics as it relates to work.

(GIRLS *run out while* MEN *become a printing press.* GIRLS *slide down a ramp, into the press—*MEN *stamp them as*

GIRLS *triumphantly laugh and then run out to audience to read to them their bits of poems or philosophy. The actors should write or choose these things themselves.* Each* GIRL *finds several audience members to speak to.*

After GIRLS *have reached as many audience members as possible, they gather at back of auditorium and begin their hike—over and through the audience.)*

SIMONE *on a hike with her pupils. They carry packs. They climb and struggle forward toward the stage.*

SIMONE: Let me carry that.

ONE: I can manage.

SIMONE. No, I'll carry your pack. The way is steep. (*To another*) Give me yours, too.

TWO: Thank you, *Mademoiselle.* I don't see how you do it—you don't look that strong. (*To audience member*) Would you pass my pack across to her? Thank you.

SIMONE: This is how one becomes strong.

THREE: How does one become in love?

SIMONE: Love?

FOUR: We understand what you teach us about physics. Could you tell us about love.

SIMONE: Love?

ALL (*on stage now*): Falling in love. Loving. Being in love. Is it good or bad?

THREE: I want to know love.

SIMONE: Love?

ALL: Love!

SIMONE: I have no advice to give you about love.

ALL: Yes. Yes.

SIMONE: I have no advice to give you about love.

ALL: But you must—you know all about calculus.

SIMONE: Love? No, I have no advice to give you but I must warn you: love is a very serious thing.

ALL (*expectant*): Yes, *Mademoiselle.*

SIMONE: Love often means pledging one's own life and that of another human being forever. It always means that, unless one of the two treats the other as a plaything. In that case, a love is something odious. The essential point in love is this: one human being feels a vital need of another human being. The problem then arises of reconciling this need with

* In the Boston production the actors chose lines from the works of Simone Weil.

freedom. A problem men have struggled with from time immemorial.

THREE: But if one is in love and pledged forever, why would you want to be free?

SIMONE: When I was your age, I was tempted to try to get to know love. I decided not to. I didn't want to commit my life in a direction impossible to foresee until I was sufficiently mature to know what I wish from life and what I expect from it.

FOUR: But I want to know now.

SIMONE: I'm not offering myself as an example; every life evolves by its own laws. But you might think about it. Love seems to me to involve an even more terrifying risk than blindly pledging one's own existence. I mean the risk, if one is the object of a profound love, of having absolute power over another human being. It's not that one should avoid love, but while you're very young, don't seek it, let it come and find you. Let's say hello to the mountains. There's new snow up there.

(*They climb higher as* SIMONE *walks back down mountain to her classroom. She finds several* SCHOOL BOARD MEMBERS *waiting for her.*)

HEAD OF BOARD (*holding four other* MEMBERS *in donkey reins*): *Mademoiselle!*

(SIMONE *walks in front of them reading a newspaper and puffing cigarette smoke like crazy.*)

SIMONE: M-m-m-m-m-m-m-m. . .

BOARD: *Mademoiselle* Instructor!

SIMONE: M-m-m-m-m-m-m-m. . .(*continues to read and smoke*).

BOARD: The board finds that you are not paying attention to the board.

MEN: The board.

SIMONE: M-m-m-m-m-m-m-m. . .

BOARD: The board finds that you are not paying attention to the board.

MEN: Attention!

SIMONE: There is not enough time to pay attention to the students.

BOARD: You smoke.

MEN: Smoke!

SIMONE: Yes. . .(*starts making note and takes out a ciga-*
rette).
BOARD: You had the effrontery to print the students' work.
MEN: Work?
SIMONE: M-m-m-m-m-m-m-m. . . ?
BOARD: This is nothing but the work of students.

(*They shake printed papers in front of her.*)

MEN: Students!
SIMONE: It is the printed word.
BOARD: You were not authorized to print the work of no-
bodys.
MEN: Nobodys!
SIMONE: That is how they become somebodys.
BOARD: You are fired.
SIMONE: That is a fact I accepted in advance.

(*The* SCHOOL BOARD *exits in a chaos of entangled reins.
Blackout.*)

SIMONE *at a new school. It is a tougher school than before—the* GIRLS *pretend to be blasé—no desks. They enter
and stand around in what they think are tough, sophisticated
poses.*

SIMONE: *Bonjour, Mesdemoiselles.*
CLASS: We don't want *Bonjour.* We want life.
SIMONE: First you must learn to think.
CLASS: We want to live.
SIMONE: What is living?
CLASS: Enjoyment of the now.
SIMONE: If you cannot think, you will be robbed of the
riches of the past and the future. To live in the now is plea-
surable, but to think in the past and future is necessary to
the development of your person and your family; therefore
your roots and your country.
CLASS: Teach us to think.
SIMONE: It is hard, but if you pay attention, hard things
can bring you good. Who would like to hike with me this
weekend?

(*Some hands up.*)

I have reports that there will be a break up of the ice, and possibly a flood. Who is strong enough to swim through the ice floes?

(Rest of hands up.)

Bon, meet me at the river bank at three in the morning, with a little food for the two days, and matches wrapped carefully so that we can dry ourselves out, if we have to swim or rescue anyone. How many again wish to go on the hike?

(All hands up.)

Bon. Girls are getting stronger. It's important. It's only through hard work that one understands one's intelligence.

GIRL *(delayed reaction)*: Yeah.

(After much reluctance and teasing, they pull off their clothes and one by one dive into an ice river. One GIRL almost doesn't make it, but she's saved by another. They swim to high ground and put their clothes back on again. SIMONE dresses and walks back to the classroom area.)

SIMONE *walking and smoking in front of the* SCHOOL BOARD.

BOARD: *Mademoiselle!*
SIMONE: M-m-m-m-m-m-m-m. . .
BOARD: *Mademoiselle,* You took the students on an unauthorized hike.
SIMONE: A swim. . .
BOARD: On an unauthorized swim under the most dangerous of conditions in the middle of winter.
SIMONE: The sun was out.
BOARD: There had been no permission granted by the school board or by the parents, and in fact you are to be considered under arrest for kidnapping.
SIMONE *(reading and walking and smoking)*: M-m-m-m-m-m-m. . .
BOARD: Three people caught pneumonia.
SIMONE: Five were saved from drowning.
BOARD: Your students saved by other students.

SIMONE: An excellent experience in learning.

BOARD: You have been noticed to smoke and read and not pay attention at teachers' meetings.

SIMONE: M-m-m-m-m-m-m-m. . .

BOARD: You are hereby fired for insubordination, and endangering the lives and the moral attitudes of your pupils. You are hereby separated from us, uh fired, uh terminated.

SIMONE (*walking and smoking*): M-m-m-m-m-m-m-m. . . It is the condition of my teaching.

BOARD MEMBER (*on way out*): And remove your coffee cup from the teachers' room.

(*Exit.*)

SIMONE *meets with her old teacher and master* ALAIN.

ALAIN: I've been following your articles closely.

SIMONE: They're only beginnings—I'm so awkward and confused.

ALAIN: No, I've never had a pupil like you. Your power of thought is rare.

SIMONE: All I have so far are hazy outlines and overweening ambitions.

ALAIN: Simone, on the contrary, it's like a game for you. I want to see you turn from playing games with abstract subtleties and train yourself in direct analysis.

SIMONE: I intend to. I'm going into the fields, I'm going into the factories, I'm going to study the relationship of the worker to his work. Modern science has lost its soul because it reasons only about conventional symbols—objects, they become objects by the fact that they are black marks on white paper, but which are universal by virtue of their definition. There should be a new way of conceiving mathematics—a way that its theoretical and practical value would no longer be distinct, but would reside in analogies. In man's struggle with the universe, symbols would thus be relegated back to their rank as mere instruments, and their real function would be revealed, which is not to assist the understanding but the imagination. Scientific work would thus be seen to be in fact artistic work—namely, the training of the imagination. It would be necessary to foster and develop to the maximum the faculty of conceiving analogies without making use of algebraic symbols.

ALAIN: It sounds like an excellent project, but please, Simone, when you write about it, try to make your language more penetrable to the ordinary mind.

SIMONE: I hope you'll excuse the confusion and disorder and also the audacity of my embryo ideas. If there is any value in them, it's clear that they could only be developed in silence. (*Hurriedly*) Also, I want to do a series of studies of the various existing forms of property, related to the idea that property consists, in reality, of the power to dispose of goods.

(*Fade on* ALAIN *as* SIMONE *walks into her room.*)

1934. Several ex-pupils come to visit SIMONE *in the factory town where she works.*

SIMONE: How good to see you again.

ONE: You didn't answer our letters.

TWO: We were worried.

THREE: Have you been ill?

SIMONE: Work in a factory isn't conducive to letter writing. How did you know where I was?

FOUR: The Derieu sisters.

SIMONE: Please don't tell anyone else. Promise me. This is the "contact with real life" we often talked about together.

ONE: But you're so frail.

SIMONE: Clumsy too, and slow, and not very robust.

TWO: How did they hire you?

ONE: There's no work these days.

SIMONE: One of my best friends knows the managing director of the company.

THREE: What's it like?

SIMONE: I'm glad to be working in a factory, but I'm equally glad not to be compulsorily committed to it. It's simply a year's leave for "private study."

(*As the speech continues, the* ENSEMBLE *enters and builds and becomes the factory and machines.* SIMONE *works at her machine, and the speed of her speech builds with the speed of her work.*)

If a man is very skilled, very intelligent, and very tough, there is just a chance, in the present conditions of French industry, for him to attain a factory job,

(*Her visitors become machine parts.*)

which offers interesting and humanly satisfying work; even so, these opportunities are becoming fewer every day, thanks to technical progress. But the women! The women are restricted to purely mechanical labor—Nothing is required of them but speed...

(*The machines begin to work in earnest.*)

When I say mechanical labor, don't imagine that it allows for daydreaming, much less reflection or thought. No. No. The tragedy is that, although the work is too mechanical to engage the mind, it prevents one from thinking of anything else. If you think, you work more slowly:

(*The machines slow down and are silent.*)

BARITONE (*sings*):
SPEED, SPEED, SPEED
SPEED, SPEED, SPEED
SPEED, OR THE SACK
SPEED, DON'T TALK BACK
SPEED, SPEED, SPEED
IF YOU WISH TO FEED.
(*Speaks*) Hurry up, Simone, you made only six hundred yesterday. If you make eight hundred today, maybe I won't fire you.

(*The machines abruptly speed again.*)

SIMONE: I still can't achieve the required speeds. I'm not familiar with the work, I'm innately awkward. I'm naturally slow moving, my head aches, and then I have a peculiar inveterate habit of thinking, which I can't shake off. Believe me, they would throw me out if I wasn't protected by influence. Theoretically, with the eight-hour day, one should have leisure, but really one's leisure hours are swallowed up by fatigue which often amounts to a dazed stupor. Also, life in the factory involves a perpetual humiliating subordination, forever at the orders of foremen.
THREE: How can you stand the suffering?
SIMONE: I do suffer from it, but I'm more glad than I can say to be where I am. I've wanted it for I-don't-know-how-many years.

(*The* ENSEMBLE *slowly breaks up the giant machine and exits, but* SIMONE *continues to work as she speaks.*)

But I'm not sorry I didn't do it sooner, because it's only at my age now that I can extract all the profit there is in the experience. Above all, I feel I've escaped from a world of abstractions, to find myself among real men—some good and some bad, but with *real* goodness or badness. Goodness especially, when it exists in a factory, is something real. The least act of kindness, from a mere smile to some little service, calls for victory over fatigue and the obsession with pay—all the overwhelming influences which drive a man in on himself. Thought then calls for an almost miraculous effort of rising above the conditions of one's life. Because it's not like at a university, where one is paid to think, or pretend to think. In a factory one is paid not to think. So, if you ever recognize a gleam of intelligence, you can be sure it is genuine. Besides, I really find the machines themselves highly attractive and interesting.

(*As members of* ENSEMBLE *arrive very slowly with real machines which they carry or manipulate,* SIMONE *exits, as if in a trance. The* ENSEMBLE *members stare and work their machines as if the machines were controlling them. Slow fade.*
The OLD LADIES *pull the cord attached to one cherub. The belly opens and jewels made of jello and and candy tumble out, showering the audience.*)

ACT 2

SIMONE *enters with materials for letter. As she speaks the* ENSEMBLE *work out math forms (i.e., equations or symbols) with their bodies.*

SIMONE: I need a physicist. I really need a physicist. Dearest Brother, please ask a physicist in America the following question: Planck justifies the introduction of quanta of energy by the assimilation of entropy to a probability (strictly, the logarithm of a probability): because, in order to calculate the probability of a macroscopic state of a system, it is necessary to postulate a finite number of corresponding microscopic states (discrete states). So the justification is that the calculus of probabilities is numerical. But why was it not possible to use a continuous calculus of probabilities, with generalized number instead of discrete numbers (considering that there are games of chance in which probability is continuous)? There would then have been no need of quanta. Why couldn't this have been tried? Planck says nothing about it. T. does not know of any physicist here who could enlighten me. What do you think about this?

(*The* ENSEMBLE *recites theories, goes into the audience to lecture them. Each actor should make up his own, outrageous theories or speculations.*

The ENSEMBLE *says to each other and the audience:* "*What do you think about this?*" *as they exit.*)

SIMONE: Your reply about Planck did not satisfy me. Have you read St. John of the Cross?

(*Blackout.* ENSEMBLE *stays in auditorium aisles walking back and forth resolutely with eyes closed whispering:* "*You don't interest me.*")

SOPRANO: You don't interest me.
BARITONE: You don't interest me.
SOPRANO: I can't see me.
BARITONE: You can't see me.
SOPRANO: I look right through you. I look right through you because when I look, there is nothing there to see.
BARITONE: You don't interest me.
You don't interest me.
A Pharisee interests me more than how
Definitely
You don't interest me.

(SIMONE *on stage. This is her inside now: it slowly comes out as the* SINGERS *sing, she passes people; as she passes them, she "fixes" on them. They feel it, and begin to reach out to her as if in a trance. They stop short of touching, but their eyes stay locked.*)

CHORUS:
YOU HAVE NOTHING FOR ME.
I WALK RIGHT THROUGH YOU

YOU DON'T EVEN BORE ME
I'VE NEVER HEARD YOU.

SIMONE (*into mike*): No one cay say you don't interest me, without showing grave cruelty and profound injustice to the uniqueness of the individual soul.

(*The* ENSEMBLE *actors move up onto the stage and form moving human structures two and three people high.*)

SIMONE: There is something sacred in every person.
CHORUS: There is something sacred in every person.
SIMONE: But it is not his person.
CHORUS: But it is not his person. Not his person? Not his person? But if not his person, then what is sacred in every person, if it is not his person?
SIMONE: It isn't his personality.
CHORUS: How can we sell him.
SIMONE: It isn't his personality, the personality he carries in his person.
CHORUS: But that's the package.
SIMONE: So much baggage.
CHORUS: Give me a good personality any day, and I can come with him in every way.
SIMONE: So much baggage.
SOPRANO: I agree with the chorus.
SIMONE: So much baggage.
BARITONE: I wouldn't mind for a while to carry the chorus for an extra mile.
SIMONE: Not his person, nor his thoughts
that I don't know.
Not his person, nor the way his arms grow.
Not his person, nor the way his eye is lit.
Not his person, but his total sacredness of it.
His presence. His presence that hurts us
when we must do without it.
CHORUS: His presence when we must do without it. King, Queen, father, father, mother, mother, sister, brother, friend, friend, friend, when you are gone and we have to live without your other.
SIMONE: Personality: Human personality means nothing to me. Personality isn't what's sacred to me. If it did, I could easily put out the eyes of anyone as Oedipus did his own. He still had exactly the same personality as before. I wouldn't

have touched the person in him, I would only have destroyed his eyes. What is it? What is it that prevents me from putting out that man's eyes if I'm allowed to do it and if I feel like doing it?

CHORUS: Put out his eyes. Burn his thighs. Pull out his tongue, put it in Washington where it belongs on the heaps of the other rotting dungs of tongues.

(SIMONE *addresses audience, while human pyramids made by the actors begin slowly to revolve*:)

The whole of your being is sacred to me, each one of you. But you are not sacred in all respects nor from every point of view. You are not sacred because of your long bright hair, or your thick wrists, or your strong long arms, or your kind heart, or the twinkle in your knowing eye, or even because your thoughts don't interfere with mine—none of these facts could keep me from hurting you without the knowledge that if I were to put out your eyes, your soul would be lacerated by knowing the pain, and the fact that *harm* was being done to you.

CHORUS:
AT THE BOTTOM OF YOUR HEART
FROM THE TIME YOU'RE A BABE
THOUGH YOU GROW MILES APART
FROM THE PEOPLE THROUGH WHICH
YOU WERE MADE
  DUET:
YOU EXPECT. YOU EXPECT. YOU EXPECT.
  SOPRANO:
WITH THE CERTAINTY AND THE LIGHT
WHEN THE SPERM ENTERED THE EGG.
  BARITONE:
YOU EXPECT TO GO ON BEING REMADE
  AS THE FIRST
ECSTASY OF THE TRINITY WHEN
YOU WERE MADE.

(*Pyramids disassemble and* ENSEMBLE *goes into Dance formations.*)

CHORUS:
YOU WERE MADE

YOU WERE MADE

SOPRANO:
YOU WERE MADE IN ECSTASY

BARITONE:
LYING DOWN OR STANDING UP,
SOPRANO:
CROSSED HORIZONS OR AGAINST THE G.E.

BARITONE:
YOU WERE LAID AS YOU WERE MADE.

CHORUS:
ECSTASY. ECSTASY. ECSTASY.

SIMONE (*tough and strong*): There is something in all of
us that goes on indomitably *expecting,* in the teeth of all
experience of crimes committed, suffered, and witnessed,
that good.

CHORUS (*softly*):
GOOD. GOOD.

SIMONE: That good and not evil will be done to you.
It is this faith above all that is sacred in every human being.

ALL: WOO!
(*Begin to dance.*)

CHORUS (*like a thirties musical*):
THIS ABOVE ALL,
THIS ABOVE ALL,
THIS ABOVE ALL,
LEARN TO WALK IN HIGHER HEELS
THIS ABOVE ALL, BABY
THIS ABOVE ALL
LEARN TO WALK LIKE YOU OWN
   THE WORLD

(*Simone exits.*)

LEARN HOW TO KICK AND FLY
LEARN HOW TO FLY
   WITHOUT GETTING SICK
LEARN HOW TO THROW AWAY THE STICK

WHAT YOU DO IS SHOVE IT UP THEIR ASS
IT'S ESPECIALLY GOOD
   WHEN THEY RUN OUT OF GAS
AND YOU WANT NERVE
TO CARRY THE VERVE
AND SHOW THOSE NIPPLES
LET THEM RIPPLE
THIS ABOVE ALL
GET AS TALL AS YOU CAN BEFORE
THE GEESE BEGIN
   TO STEP ALL OVER YOU AND
WHEN YOU FALL
WHEN YOU FALL BABY
PRACTICE HOW TO DO IT WITH A SMILE.
I'D WALK A MILLION MILES
FOR ONE OF YOUR LUCKIES
MY BUCKY LITTLE RAG-TIME
   SON-OF-A-BITCH
YOU WITCH
THIS WAS THE DAYS BEFORE GARY
LEARNED TO SWITCH HIS HORSE
AND COCAINE WAS RUNNING A CLOSE
SECOND TO ANYONE'S OPIUM DREAM,
   IT'S A SCREAM
BUT THIS ABOVE ALL,
THIS ABOVE ALL, LEARN HOW
TO LOOK LIKE YOU'RE TALL.
THE FALL IS FUNNIER.
THE FALL IS FUNNIER WHEN YOU FALL
   RIGHT OFF THAT WALL.
OH BE TALL.
THERE MIGHT BE A LIGHT
   OUTSIDE THE GATE,
DON'T YOU SEE IT.
THERE MIGHT BE A LIGHT
   OUTSIDE THE GATE,
DON'T YOU SEE IT.
LET'S BURN GIN TO THAT.
WE NEED A LIGHT TO SHOW
WE'RE RIGHT,
WE'RE RIGHT
BECAUSE WE KNOW IN THE
BOTTOMS OF YOUR CUPS
THAT MIGHT CAN'T CONQUER RIGHT,
THAT MIGHT CAN'T CONQUER RIGHT, ETC.
   (softer under next two lines)

BARITONE:
THERE IS NO WAR ON.
THERE IS NO WAR ON.

(*Blackout.*)

Series of rapid scenes:

Out of work MEN *of the town are pounding huge stones with sledge hammers.*

SIMONE: Why are you cracking the rocks?
ONE: We have to.
SIMONE: Are you going to build a wall or a garden.
TWO: We're out of work.
SIMONE: What do you mean you're out of work, you're working harder than I do.
THREE: We have to do this or they won't give us our unemployment checks.

SIMONE: Give me one of those and I'll help you.

(*She stands beside the* MEN *and though she's slower, she still works. Then* ALL *run to the next scene.*)

In the factory. The WORKERS *are having a sit-in. They sit on the floor, arms linked and swaying, singing the end of "The International."* SIMONE *is there too, arms linked with the* WORKERS, *between two men.* TWO MEN *in charge of running the factory are conferring with one another as the song ends. They turn and shout at the* WORKERS.

MANAGER ONE: Seven percent increase.
WORKERS: Fifteen.
MANAGER TWO: Seven percent.
WORKERS: *Fifteen.*

(*They yell this back and forth in mounting crescendo. Moment of silence.*)

WORKERS: Fifteen and a joint committee of workers and management.

MANAGER ONE: I'll hire and fire whom I choose.

WORKERS: Joint committee or no work done. Joint committee or no work done.

MANAGER TWO: We'll close down the factory.

MANAGER ONE: We'll close down the factory—that will put some sense into you.

WORKERS: Good, good, good. Close down the factory and we'll take it over and run it ourselves. We run this factory ourselves anyway.

MANAGER ONE: This is a gross infringement of liberty.

WORKERS: We want fifteen percent more.

MANAGER TWO: You make me sick.

WORKERS: Fifteen! Fifteen! Fifteen! Fifteen! Fifteen! We'll make you sick, all right.

(*Go for the managers' throats—then immediately transform into* COMRADES *at a meeting.*)

A political meeting of leftist coalition parties.

SIMONE (*addressing the crowd*): Friends and fellow workers. Some of us have been greatly troubled and alarmed by news of the continuing purge in Russia. I'm afraid that in this struggle that begins to look like the classic struggle between the conservatives and the innovators the value of life is being forgotten. The conservatives do not know what to conserve, and the innovators do not know what to innovate—

VOICE: Revisionists! Traitorous revisionists!

SIMONE: Please, I ask you to pay one more minute of attention. It's true so far as we know it that Stalin's lieutenant S. M. Kirov was murdered. But Stalin is using this crime as a tool against many comrades who fought and sacrificed many long years to bring Marxist-Leninist concepts into being. If he is allowed to continue unchecked in this "purge," there will be no chance for the dictatorship of the proletariat, because all his brothers will have been eliminated resulting in the dictatorship of one man, Joseph Stalin. We must show him that there is a world of opinion, considered and humane opinion by his brothers in other countries that condemn his actions, that he must cease and desist in this cruel persecution—

ONE: Traitor! She's a Trotskyite.

(*Some people walk out.*)

TWO: The purge is just and moral. Those men were working with the Germans to overthrow Stalin and so are you. I denounce Simone as a Trotskyite!

THREE: Get her.

FOUR: Beat her up.

(They move slowly toward her.)

FIVE: Smash her mouth.

SIX: Don't let her open it again.

SEVEN: Kill her.

SIMONE: I'm not a Trotskyite, I belong to no party. I am against totalitarianism in all its forms. If this "purge" continues in Russia, Stalin will succeed in creating a monolithic totaliarian unity and it will be an end to Lenin's ideals and an end to people's democracy.

EIGHT: Get her. Trotskyite!

(They grab her. NINE and a small group of friends holding two guns surround SIMONE to protect her.)

TEN: I support Stalin.

ELEVEN: Shut that Trotskyite's trap.

SIMONE: I'm not a Trotskyite, I'm a Frenchman.

NINE: Simone, comrade, stay in the middle of us. We'll get you out safely.

TWELVE: You're a Trotskyite and you're a Jew!

(With some brief scuffling, they get her out of the meeting.)

Outside the meeting, SIMONE *is talking with* MAN *who rescued her.*

SIMONE: Thank you, Pierre. I'll never forget your kindness and your bravery.

PIERRE: Those Communist fanatics want to drive us into war. You know that during the general strike they were working on the side of management to *prevent our* strike!

SIMONE: I know, because they want all the armaments built as soon as possible to speed up the prospect of war. Well, I'm going off to fight in a war, a just war. I've decided to go to Spain. At least *there*, my one more pair of hands might be useful.

PIERRE: Be careful your rifle doesn't backfire on you, you're not so clever with your hands.

SIMONE: Don't worry. I'm a pacifist. I'll never carry a rifle, there's other work to do.

(*Blackout.*)

SIMONE *in Spain: on the banks of the Ebro River. The Anarchist forces she has joined are on one side and Fascist forces are on the other. Sound of airplane overhead.*

CAPTAIN: Get that plane!

(*The* SQUADRON, *including* SIMONE, *who does have a rifle in hand, begin to shoot.* SIMONE *lies on her back and shoots straight up into the air.*)

The pisser's flying too high.

(*Sound of small bomb exploding.*)

At least their bombs are getting smaller. That means we're winning.

(*A small squad of* MEN *come in dragging* TWO PRIESTS.)

ONE: Captain! Captain! Look what we found hiding in the rushes on the river bank.

CAPTAIN: This will make forty priests we've shot. (*He points at one of them*) Kneel with your head in prayer.

(*The other* MEN *laugh;* SIMONE *lowers her rifle. The* CAPTAIN *shoots the* PRIEST. *He falls forward and dies, crying out* "Jesus" *in Spanish.*)

CAPTAIN (*to the* SECOND PRIEST): We're going to let you go, so you can tell the rest of your brothers to get the hell out of our country. Get going, on the double.

(*As the* PRIEST *turns, he shoots him too. The* MEN *laugh again.* SIMONE *throws down her rifle.*)

Squadron. Attention! We're going out on patrol. The Fascists are just across the river, and at dawn we're going to start picking them off. Simone?

SIMONE: I'll stay in camp and cook.

TWO (*sotto voce, to a comrade*): Thank God, she's so awkward with a gun, she'll kill one of us one day.

CAPTAIN: Good, you stay and deep-fry me some of those chickens we commandeered. I haven't had fresh meat in two months.

(*They march off stealthily.* SIMONE *puts a pot of oil on the fire. Another* WOMAN *helps her peel vegetables to throw into the oil. They pluck chickens.*)

SIMONE: Atrocities. On both sides.

WOMAN (*laughing*): Did you see how the other thought God had saved his life?

SIMONE: How can you laugh at a thing like that?

WOMAN: It was funny. Did you see the look on his face after the bullet hit his head?

SIMONE: This isn't our war. This is nothing but a war fought by Germany against Russia. We're fools and pawns.

(*She's so angry she hits the pot of oil so hard that it spills over onto her leg. She screams and falls.*)

WOMAN: Oh, my God, your leg is burning.

(*She runs out screaming for help.*)

SIMONE *alone in a field hospital reciting math formulas to avoid the pain. Her* FATHER *and* MOTHER *rush on.*

FATHER: Simone, my precious.

MOTHER: Simone, my own.

FATHER: It's taken us a month to find you.

MOTHER (*not daring to look*): How bad?

FATHER: What butcher has been tending you? This dressing hasn't been changed in a week, half the flesh is exposed. (*He brings things out of his bag, gives her a sedative.*) Here, this will still the pain.

SIMONE: I'm getting used to it.

MOTHER: We'll take her home to recover.

SIMONE: No, no, father, I have to rejoin my unit.

FATHER: I'm your father and your doctor and you'll do as I say. Let's get a stretcher.

(MOTHER *and* FATHER *exit.*)

SIMONE *is alone in her room.*

Visitation.

SIMONE: My spirit is sick. Do I have a spirit. Pains in the throat, double pains. I can't swallow but I feel constantly that I'll vomit. My spine. My spine is sick. I can't work and that makes me sicker. Not to be able to work. No work. Work beating in my head, but my hands refuse to close around a pencil, my mind won't work for me, but something in me is working, and I'm so sick and weak. The struggle against this stupid body is getting too much to bear. I've got to think my way out of it but I can't think. My God, my God, I can't think. I can't move, out of this bed, my God I can't stand. I can't walk. I can't think, I can't think, this stupid pain. My God. My God, I need something. I need something. I need my work. I need to work. Any work. I'd cry for joy to be able to bend in the dirt and pick up potatoes till my back ached from work. Honest work, not the work of fighting this endless headache. I'll try to vomit. I'll get it out, I'll vomit out the illness. Oh my God, can't I get any light into my head? My God! My God! My God!

(*The* ENTIRE CAST *comes on stage and lifts* SIMONE *up, giving her a total caress. They hum. They take her pain into their bodies, until all but five who lift her up to God are feeling the pain that she had.*
As they lift SIMONE, *they take her clothes off, and as the clothes fall, other actors put them on, continuing a pain cennered at a point in the body the garment covers. They lift her straight up if they can, her arms outstretched, smiling with her eyes closed.*
They put her down and exit.)

LOVE III.
The Poem of George Herbert
SIMONE (*transfixed, warmed, and filled with divine love, sings*):
LOVE BADE ME WELCOME
  YET MY SOUL DREW BACK,
  GUILTY OF DUST AND SINNE.

BUT QUICK-EY'D LOVE,
   OBSERVING ME GROW SLACK
   FROM MY FIRST ENTRANCE IN,
DREW NEARER TO ME,
   SWEETLY QUESTIONING,
   IF I LACK'D ANY THING.

A GUEST, I ANSWER'D,
   WORTHY TO BE HERE:
   LOVE SAID, YOU SHALL BE HE.
I THE UNKINDE, UNGRATEFULL?
   AH MY DEARE,
   I CANNOT LOOK ON THEE.
LOVE TOOK MY HAND,
   AND SMILING DID REPLY,
   WHO MADE THE EYES BUT I?

TRUTH LORD, BUT I HAVE MARR'D THEM:
   LET MY SHAME GO WHERE
   IT DOTH DESERVE.
AND KNOW YOU NOT, SAYES LOVE,
   WHO BORE THE BLAME?
   MY DEARE, THEN I WILL SERVE.
YOU MUST SIT DOWN, SAYES LOVE,
   AND TASTE MY MEAT:
   SO I DID SIT AND EAT.

(ENSEMBLE *dancers enter and dance with* SIMONE, *while the* CHORUS *sings:*)

   Song for SIMONE, OPERA SINGERS, CHORUS *and* DANCERS.

I BELIEVE GOD CREATED
SO HE COULD BE LOVED
GOD CREATED TO BE LOVED
GOD CREATED AROUND AND ABOVE
SO THAT HE, GOD COULD BE LOVED.

BUT GOD CAN'T CREATE GOD
GOD CAN'T CREATE ANYTHING TO BE GOD

BUT GOD CANNOT BE LOVED BY ANYTHING
WHICH ISN'T GOD, GOD NEEDS
GOD TO SING
GOD NEEDS GOD TO SING TO HIM OF HIS LOVE
OF GOD FOR GOD
GOD NEEDS GOD TO LOVE HIM INTO GOD.

THIS IS A CONTRADICTION!
NOT A FICTION BUT A PERFECT
A PERFECT, AN EXACT CONTRADICTION.
I HAVE THE CONVICTION
THAT THIS CONTRADICTION
CONTAINS IN ITSELF NECESSITY ITSELF.
THIS IS NOT PERVERSITY
THIS IS NOT MIND PLAY
OR PLAY OF MIND
BUT THIS IS A PERFECT CONTRADICTION
CONTRADICTION CREATES ACTION
THIS IS A CONTRADICTION THAT DEFINES
NECESSITY. NECESSITY. *NECESSITY!*

BUT EVERY CONTRADICTION
HAS THE CONDITION OF RESOLVING
ITSELF THROUGH THE PROCESS
THROUGH THE PROCESS
THROUGH THE PROCESS OF
BECOMING, BECOMING, BECOMING,
BECOMING, *BECOMING!*

GOD CREATED ME TO SEE THE SEA
AND TO LOVE HIM
AND TO LOVE HIM
"I"—"I"—"I" THIS FINITE BEING
I THIS THIS "I"
"I" AND "I," THIS LITTLE "I"
I CAN'T LOVE GOD
UNTIL
UNTIL, THROUGH THE ACTION OF GRACE
THAT TAKES OVER THE EMPTY SPACE
OF MY TOTAL SOUL—
THE GRACE THAT FILLS MY SOUL
THE GRACE TO MAKE ME WHOLE WITH GOD.

AND AS THE LITTLE "I" DISAPPEARS
GOD LOVES HIMSELF
GOD LOVES HIMSELF

BY MY GIVING UP MY "I"
AS I BECOME NOT "I"
AS I CANNOT SEE THE SKY, NOR BE THE SKY
GOD LOVES ME AS I DISAPPEAR

I GIVE GOD TO GOD AND
AND GOD LOVES HIMSELF
AS THIS PROCESS GOES ON FOREVER
THEREFORE GOD
HAS CREATED TIME
TIME IS INDIFFERENT TO ME,
THERE IS ALL THE TIME
IN MY SHORT WORLD
FOR ME TO BECOME NOT ME

SO THAT GOD
SO THAT GOD CAN LOVE HIMSELF
THIS
THIS
THIS
THIS
THIS
THIS IS THE NECISSITY, THE NECESSITY,
THE NECESSITY.
   N E C E S S I T Y !

A police station, three POLICEMEN *and a* SECRETARY.

ONE: it's been reported that you are a Gaulliste.

TWO: You were seen distributing *Témoignage chrétien*.

THREE: An illegal paper.

SIMONE: It has a higher literary style than the government censors.

TWO: So you admit to this underground activity.

SIMONE: I admit that I read everything I can get my hands on.

ONE: If you don't tell us who the rest of your comrades are. . .

TWO: You'll go to prison.

THREE: And I'll personally see that you, a teacher of philosophy, will be put into the same cells as the prostitutes.

ONE: As the prostitutes.

SIMONE: Why I've always wanted to know about such circles of women. It will be a very good opportunity to get to know them. Yes, please do send me to jail.

TWO: She's crazy.

THREE: She's crazy, no professor of philosophy would want to associate with filthy prostitutes.

SIMONE: But I would. It's a subject I haven't had time to study yet.

ONE: Release the prisoner. She's crazy.

(*Blackout.*)

SIMONE *arrives in Marseilles and goes to the Dominican monastery where she can ask a* PRIEST *who is helping people to get out of the country for work while she waits to get out too. There are several* PEOPLE *before her, one is in his office and is just leaving.*

MAN: Thank you for getting me the passport, Father, it's saved my life.

FATHER (*a warm man with natural charm*): Safe journey and God bless, my son.

SIMONE (*enters shyly*): Excuse me, Father. I hate to take away from your valuable time, but I need some sort of work, preferably manual labor, where I can fade into a group. Is there any farm work about, perhaps the grape harvest?

FATHER: My child, you look so frail, I hardly...

SIMONE: I'm not as frail as I look—I've worked in factories.

FATHER: You don't speak like a factory worker.

SIMONE: You know about the laws: we're not allowed to work. My family and I are bound for Morocco on our way to the States. I want to work to occupy my time.

FATHER: Are you sure you can manage. The sun's hot.

SIMONE: Good.

FATHER: I have a friend, just outside of town who might take you on...

SIMONE: Thank you Father ... Father ... may I come to speak with you sometime again...

FATHER: I'm taken up with many duties besides my clerical ones—so many people are being hounded down by the police, so many people need help and advice.

SIMONE: I'd like to speak to you about Christ.

(*They freeze, walk in a circle. She hesitantly approaches him again.*)

SIMONE: After working in the factories, I finally understood affliction. I began to see myself as a slave and I was often able to rise above the physical affliction of my headaches. Then in a Chapel in Solesmes where I'd gone to hear the

Gregorian music at Easter I was able to listen to the music in spite of pain. By an extreme effort of attention I was able to get outside this miserable flesh, leaving it to suffer by itself, and I found a pure and perfect joy in the unspeakable beauty of the chanting and the words. During the time I was there I also met a young man, a messenger I think of him now, who introduced me to George Herbert's poem "Love." From then on whenever my headache would reach a painful crisis, I would recite this poem fixing all my attention on it, clinging with all my soul to the tenderness it enshrines. One day, while saying this poem with all my attention, Christ Himself came down and He took possession of me.

FATHER: Did you see Him?

SIMONE: No, it was the presence of love, of infinite love, a certainty of love, a love which I have never sought and which I'd never thought existed.

FATHER: My child, are you seeking Catholic instruction?

SIMONE: I don't wish Baptism.

FATHER: But that is complete union.

SIMONE: I prefer to stand at the door of the church.

FATHER: Then you're still a long way from Christianity.

(*Again they freeze, walk in a small circle, relax, and she approaches him again.*)

SIMONE: Every day before I go out to harvest I say the "Our Father" in Greek. I try to do this with the utmost attention and if I do, Christ comes nearer to me now than He did that first time.

FATHER: It gives me joy to see the light growing within you.

(*They freeze, she kneels and says the Pater Noster in Greek, or any language the actress would like. Then she stands. They approach each other again.*)

FATHER: My child, you suffer too much from your former intellectual life. You're confusing reality with distortions of it. I feel you're hardest and most severe in your judgments on that which could touch you the most.

SIMONE: I have to beware of you. Friendship and the power of suggestion is what I'm most susceptible to.

FATHER: But Baptism is—

SIMONE: I don't want to belong to any groups. I want to be invisible, so that I can move among all groups. I'm suspicious of structures, and especially the structure of the Catholic Church, it has been totalitarian since the time of the Roman Empire.

FATHER: You're still locked into the narrow philosophy of Spinoza.

SIMONE: I'd never read any of the mystics till my love of Christ, but now I see that Dionysus and Osiris are an early form of Christ. The *Bhagavad-Gita* when read aloud is a marvelous Christian sound. Yes, even Plato was a mystic. I see the *Iliad* now as bathed in Christian light.

FATHER: Your early intellectual training and culture are keeping you from contemplating the true mysteries of the Church dogma. Baptism is a complete union.

SIMONE: I want to thank you for bearing with me for so long. I'd never really considered the problem of Baptism as a practical one before. I'm sorry to withhold from you what would give you the greatest joy, but God has other uses for me. If I felt His command to be baptized, I would come running at once. For now I think God doesn't want me in the Church, perhaps at the moment of death. . .

FATHER: It's my only concern that you stay in readiness. . .

SIMONE: I could only say all this to you because I'm leaving tomorrow. Goodbye, you've been a father and a brother to me . . . It's impossible to think of you without thinking of God.

(*Exit.*)

Outside a Harlem church. Sounds of Gospel music.

CLAIRE: We're the only white people here. Are you sure we won't offend?

SIMONE: I've been to a different church in Harlem every Sunday since I arrived in New York.

CLAIRE: I'm a bit uneasy.

SIMONE: Are you my friend?

CLAIRE: Yes, you know it; we've talked for days and nights together.

SIMONE: Will you be my friend?

CLAIRE: We're going to get back to France together; we're going to sabotage the Nazis together.

SIMONE: Come, let's enter this church of God.

(CLAIRE *presses Simone's hand and they enter the church*

together. A song is ending and they sit in first row of auditorium.)

PREACHER: Brothers and Sisters, let us pray for our President. Let us pray for our great President Franklin Delano Roosevelt. He faces trying times in this terrible war. The people on the East is attacking us, and the people in the West is attacking us. Brothers and Sisters, let us pray to Jesus to help our President in these terrible times so that with the help of You, oh Lord, and Your chosen Son, Jesus, our President Roosevelt can make peace all over God's great, green and beautiful garden.
Give yourself up to the power of Our Lord,
Give yourself up to the power of Our Lord,
If you ever gonna find yourself
You got to give yourself up,
Give yourself up to the power of Our Lord.

PREACHER *(sings)*:
BROTHERS AND SISTERS
BROTHERS AND SISTERS
WHAT SEX IS JESUS?
WHAT SEX IS GOD?

CHORUS *(repeats and claps)*:
WHAT SEX IS JESUS:
WHAT SEX IS GOD?

PREACHER:
WHAT SEX WAS MARY?
WHAT SEX WAS SAUL
AFTER HE CHANGED HIS NAME TO PAUL?
JESUS LETS US INTO HIM
BOTH MEN AND WOMEN.
JESUS LETS US INTO HIM
BOTH SAINTS AND SINNIN'

MALE SINGER: Simone, Simone, Simone. Your body is women and your head talks to God. *(Brings* SIMONE *on stage.)*

CHORUS:
JESUS HAD A PRICK
HE DIDN'T USE TO FUCK WITH
BUT PENETRATING THE WATERS
HE MADE ENOUGH FISHES TO
FEED THE MULTITUDE
WITHOUT LICKING ESSENTIAL OILS, JESUS
MADE BREAD WITHOUT AN OVEN
HE FED A THOUSAND DOZENS

CLAIRE: Simone, I feel I have to leave. I'm overcome with emotion, I feel I might dissolve. Let's go before I can't control myself any longer.

SIMONE: Get up with the congregation. Let's go with them to Jesus.

CLAIRE: I'm afraid.

SIMONE: You're ready to face the Nazis, but you're still not ready to approach God?

(*They rise and join the congregation, who are singing and jitterbugging and throwing themselves into a trance with their closeness to the Lord.*)

(*A woman leaps up from the congregation. She is possessed and sings. The* CHORUS *echoes her.*)

WOMAN:
OH LORD, OH LORD, OH LORD
I'M OPENING UP FOR YOU
OH LORD, OH LORD,
I'M READY TO RECEIVE
MY JESUS,
OH JESUS, SON OF GOD,
I'LL DO YOU RIGHT
OH JESUS, SON OF GOD,
I'LL DO RIGHT TO YOU

MY ARMS ARE OPEN
MY ARMS ARE OPEN
OH LORD, OH JESUS,
I'LL GIVE IT ALL BACK TO YOU.
TAKE MY HANDS
TAKE MY FEET

(*Repeat all the parts of the body till end of scene.*)

CHORUS:
SHE'S A JESUS LADY
SHE'S A JESUS LADY
WHAT SEX IS JESUS?
JESUS DONE ENTERED HER
JESUS DONE ENTERED HER
JESUS DONE ENTERED HER
  PREACHER:
SHE'S A JESUS LADY

SHE'S A JESUS LADY
SHE'S A JESUS LADY
RIGHT NOW AND FOREVERMORE.

(*Exit.*)

French headquarters in England.
As this scene progresses it should be as if SIMONE *is visiting a series of offices. Each official, and, if possible, his secretary too, gets taller and fatter, until the final one is a giant figure somewhat like De Gaulle.*
On screens and slides, on scrolls, that come down, from projections, etc., we should see films and stills of people in their death agonies.

SIMONE: *Bonjour, mon cher ami*, It's good to see you again. I had no idea how long it would take me to get to London.
MAN: Did you go to America?
SIMONE: Only because I thought it would be a faster way to get here, so that I can be of service to France. It took much longer than I'd hoped.
MAN: Your parents?
SIMONE: They wanted to escape from the anti-Semitism without being separated from me. I've come to offer you my services to work for France. I distributed one of the most important clandestine publications in the free zone, *Les Cahiers du témoignage chrétien*. But when I was there, I was consoled by sharing the suffering of my country. I've come back to offer myself, because France's misfortunes hurt me much more at a distance than when I was there. Leaving was like tearing up my roots. But I only left in the hope that I could take a bigger and more effective part in the efforts, dangers and sufferings of this great struggle. I have an idea.
MAN: Perhaps you'd like to explain it to the Captain?
CAPTAIN (*enters and bows*): *Mademoiselle*.
SIMONE: I have an idea.
CAPTAIN: *Bon*, they are needed.
SIMONE: This idea will save the lives of many soldiers.
CAPTAIN: *Bon*.
SIMONE: Many needless deaths happen on the battlefield due to the lack of immediate care, cases of shock, exposure, loss of blood.
CAPTAIN: Correct.

SIMONE: Please consider it seriously. I want to work in secret operations, preferably dangerous.

CAPTAIN: Perhaps you should speak to the major. (*Exits.*)

MAJOR (*enters*): *Mademoiselle.*

SIMONE: I really believe I can be useful. I appeal to you as a comrade to get me out of this painful moral situation. A lot of people don't understand why it's a painful moral situation, but you certainly do. We had a great deal in common when we were students together. It gave me a real joy to learn that you have such an important position in London. I'm relying on you.

MAJOR: We can certainly use your brilliant mind. You were first in your class.

SIMONE: I want action. Here's the idea: create a special body of front-line nurses.

MAJOR: Of women?

SIMONE (*nods and hurries on*): It would be a very mobile organization and should always be at the points of greatest danger.

MAJOR: But the horrors of war at the front—

SIMONE:—are so disinct today in everyone's imagination that one can regard any woman who is capable of volunteering for such work as being very probably capable of performing it.

MAJOR: But they risk certain death.

SIMONE: They would need to have a good deal of courage. They would need to offer their lives as a sacrifice.

MAJOR: But we have never put our women in such danger. That's why we men leave for the front to defend our homes and families.

SIMONE: There is no reason to regard the life of a woman, especially if she has passed her first youth without marrying or having children, as more valuable than a man's life. All the less so if she has accepted the risk of death.

MAJOR: But how to regulate . . .

SIMONE: Simply make mothers, wives and girls below a certain age ineligible.

MAJOR: I'm considering the idea.

SIMONE: The moral support would be inestimable. They would comfort the men's last moments, they would mitigate by their presence and their words the agony of waiting for the arrival of the stretcher-bearers. You must understand the essential role played in the present war by moral factors. They count for very much more than in past wars. It's one of

the main reasons for Hitler's successes that he was the first to
see this.

MAJOR: I believe you should explain this to the General.
(*Exits.*)

(*General enters, only nods.*)

SIMONE (*exhorting*): Hitler has never lost sight of the essential need to strike everybody's imagination; his own people's, his enemies', and the innumerable spectators'. One of
his most effective instruments has been the SS. These men are
unmoved by suffering and death, either for themselves or for
all the rest of humanity. Their heroism originates from an extreme brutality that corresponds perfectly to the spirit of the
regime and the designs of their leader. We cannot copy these
methods of Hitler's. First, because we fight in a different
spirit and with different motives. But when it is a question of
striking the imagination, copies never succeed. Only the new
is striking. We give a lot of thought to propaganda for the
rear, yet it is just as important at the front. At the rear, propaganda is carried on by words. At the front, verbal propaganda must be replaced by the propaganda of action.

GENERAL: What do you propose?

SIMONE: A simple corps of women performing a few humane services in the very center of the battle—the climax of
inhumanity—would be a signal defiance of the inhumanity
which the enemy has chosen for himself and which he also
compels us to practice. A small group of women exerting day
after day a courage of this kind with a maternal solicitude
would be a spectacle so new, so much more striking than
Hitler's young SS fanatics. The contrast between these
women and the SS would make a more telling argument than
any propaganda slogan. I would illustrate with supreme clar-
ity the two roads between which humanity today is forced to
choose.

GENERAL: *Merci.* A very good idea. We will think about it.
In the meantime we have some essential work for you to do.

(*Typewriter and mounds of papers are wheeled out.*)

Four copies of each as soon as possible. There's a war on.

(*Blackout. The* OLD MEN *pull the cord attached to their
cherub and ashes, bones and plastic baby dolls shower the
audience.*)

SIMONE, *with a mike on a high platform, addresses a crowd. As she speaks, lights begin to go off and on. Strange noises—gunshot. Bit by bit the* PEOPLE *leave and take up sides to fight the war.*

SIMONE: We're in a conflict with no definable objective. When there is no objective, there is no common measure of proportion. Compromise is inconceivable. The only way the importance of such a battle can be measured is by the sacrifices it demands. From this it follows that the sacrifices already made are a perpetual argument for new sacrifices. There would never be any reason to stop killing and dying, except that there is fortunately a limit to human endurance.

(Silence.)

This paradox is so extreme as to defy analysis. And yet the most perfect example of it is known to every so-called educated man, but, by a sort of taboo, we read it without understanding. The Greeks and Trojans massacred one another for ten years on account of Helen. Not one of them except the dilettante warrior Paris cared two straws about her. All of them wished she'd never been born. Its importance was simply imagined as corresponding to the deaths incurred and the further massacres expected.

(Lights flicker and go out. PEOPLE *crawl in aisles and over audience. Lights—flashing; crying, running.)*

This implied an importance beyond all reckoning. Hector foresaw that his city would be destroyed, his father and brothers massacred, his wife degraded to a slavery worse than death. Achilles knew that he was condemning his father to the miseries and humiliations of a defenseless old age. All of them were aware that their long absence at the war would bring ruin on their homes; yet no one felt the cost too great, because they were all in pursuit of a literal non-entity whose only value was in the *price paid for it!*

(Silence—then the war begins again.)

For the clear-sighted, there is no more distressing symptom of this truth than the unreal character of most of the conflicts that are taking place today. They have even less reality than the war between Greeks and Trojans. At the heart of the Trojan War there was at least a woman, and what is

more, a woman of perfect beauty. For our contemporaries
the role of Helen is played by words with capital letters. If
we grasp one of these words, all swollen with blood and
tears, and squeeze it, we find it is empty.

(*Silence—then just breathing. Then war begins again.*)

Words with content and meaning are not murderous. When
empty words are given capital letters, then men on the
slightest pretext will begin shedding blood. In these conditions
the only definition of success is to crush a rival group of men
who have a hostile word on their banners. When a word is
properly defined, it loses its capital letter and can no longer
serve either as a banner or as a hostile slogan.

(*Screams. Someone is shot while pleading not to be.
Silence.*)

It becomes simply a sign, helping us to grasp some concrete
reality, concrete objective or method of activity. To clarify
thought, to discredit the intrinsically meaningless words and
to define the use of others by precise analysis—to do this,
strange though it may appear, might be a way of saving human lives.

BARITONE: How like a woman to reduce war to semantics.
SOPRANO: How like a man to reduce war to mathematics.

(*All the* MEN *are lying on stage or in aisles. The* WOMEN
drag their bodies to a pile on stage as SIMONE *speaks.*)

SIMONE: My dearest brothers, lying twenty years in your
hospital beds, you are privileged men. The present state of
the world is reality for you. You are experiencing more reality in your constant affliction than those who are dying in the
war, at this moment killing and dying, wounded and being
wounded. Because they are taken unaware. They don't know
where they are. They don't know what is happening to them.
People not in the middle of the war don't know what's real.
But you men have been repeating in thought, for twenty years,
that act which took and then released so many men. But you
were seized permanently. And now the war is here again to
kill millions of men. You are ready to think. Or if you are
still not quite ready—as I feel you are not—you only have
the thinnest shell to break before emerging from the darkness
inside the egg into the light of truth. It is a very ancient
image. The egg is this world we see. The bird in it is Love,

the Love which is God Himself and which lives in the depths
of every man, though at first as an invisible seed.

MAN: Will you help me kill myself.

SIMONE: Break your shell and you will no longer be inside.
Space is opened and torn apart.

(*Silence for a moment. In pain and twitching like the men,
Simone's voice at first mirrors migraine pain, but then rises
above the pain through the speech.*)

The spirit throws the miserable body in some corner and is
transported to a point outside space. Space has become an in-
finity. The moment stands still.

WOMEN (*singing, facing audience from stage or in position
in aisles*):
THE MOMENT STANDS STILL!
THE MOMENT STANDS STILL!
THE MOMENT STANDS STILL!
THE MOMENT STANDS STILL!
THE SILENCE IS DENSE
SOUNDS
SOUNDS
SILENCE IS
THE WHOLE OF SPACE IS FILLED
NOT AN ABSENCE OF SOUND
BUT THE MOMENT IS FILLED
WITH THE SECRET WORD
ONCE YOU BREAK OUT OF YOUR SHELL
YOU WILL KNOW WHAT IS REAL
ABOUT WAR
YOU WILL KNOW THE SECRET WORD
YOU NEVER KNEW BEFORE
NOT THE ABSENCE OF SOUND
BUT LOVE, LOVE, LOVE,LOVE, LOVE.

SIMONE (*speaking*): It is not an absence of sound, but a
positive object of sensation.

Singing:
YOU, WHEN YOU'VE EMERGED
FROM THE SHELL,
WILL KNOW THE REALITY OF WAR.
THE MOST PRECIOUS REALITY TO KNOW
IS THAT, WAR IS UNREALITY ITSELF.

Speaking: You are infinitely privileged. War has permanently lodged in your body.

WOMEN (*singing*):

WAR IS AFFLICTION,
FORTUNATE ARE YOU TO KNOW.

SIMONE: War is affliction. It isn't easy to direct one's thought toward affliction voluntarily. To think affliction, it's necessary to bear it in one's flesh, driven very far in like a nail, and for a long time, so that thought may have time to grow strong enough to regard it.

WOMEN (*singing*):
WAR IS AFFLICTION,
FORTUNATE ARE WE TO KNOW.
FORTUNATE ARE WE.
WAR IS AFFLICTION.
FORTUNATELY WE CANNOT SEE IT.
WAR IS AFFLICTION.

SIMONE: You have the opportunity and the function of knowing the truth of the world's affliction. Contemplate its reality!

(MEN *rise and take their places facing the audience.* SIMONE *begins to move through them, climbing ever higher on the platforms.*)

MAN ONE: Eat, Simone.

(*She shakes her head and moves up ramp.*)

MAN TWO: Eat, Simone.

(*She shakes head and climbs to highest platform. She's weak and must hold onto the bars to stand up.*
An ACTRESS *mounts an auditorium platform and mechanically intones.*)

WOMAN DOCTOR (*at an inquest, British accent*): I tried to persuade Simone to take some food, and she said she would try. She did not eat, however, and gave as a reason the thought of her people in France starving.

(ENSEMBLE *whispers:* "Strange suicide" *over and over.*)

She died on the twenty-fourth of August, and death was due to cardiac failure due to degeneration through starvation.

BARITONE (*singing, as a judge*): Simone, aged thirty-four, committed suicide by starvation while the balance of her mind was disturbed.

CHORUS *speaks.*

WOMEN: Strange suicide. Strange suicide.

MEN: Refused to eat.

WOMEN: Strange suicide. Strange suicide.

MEN: Refused to eat.

MEN AND WOMEN (*as lights begin to dim on* ENSEMBLE):
She refused. She refused. She refused.

WOMAN ONE: She wouldn't eat. She wouldn't eat the bombs
of the Germans, she wouldn't eat the furnaces of the Nazis.
She swallowed the pride of France, but it didn't stick to her
ribs.

CHORUS: Strange, strange, strange, strange, strange—
Simone wouldn't eat.
Simone wouldn't eat.

WOMAN TWO: Her soul was full, she didn't have to eat.
There's no such thing as a personality. There's no such thing
as a mind when the body dies. The mind can die before the
body dies.

WOMAN THREE: She wouldn't eat. She wouldn't eat. She
couldn't eat when others starved. She wouldn't eat while Hitler carved the meat of her countryside.

WOMAN FOUR: While everyone else lived on spoiled cab-
bage leaves and boiled rainwater, Simone ate nothing.

(*Blackout on* ENSEMBLE.)

WOMAN FIVE: How thin she must have been. What a tiny
coffin they must have buried her in.

(*Pin spot on* SIMONE, *dimming slowly, slowly, slowly,
slowly to black.*)

C

The SIGNET Classic Shakespeare

Ⓒ

- ☐ **THE MERRY WIVES OF WINDSOR**, William Green, ed., Queens College. (#CD318—50¢)
- ☐ **A MIDSUMMER NIGHT'S DREAM**, Wolfgang Clemen, ed., University of Munich. (#CY973—$1.25)
- ☐ **MUCH ADO ABOUT NOTHING**, David Stevenson, ed., Hunter College. (#CQ830—95¢)
- ☐ **OTHELLO**, Alvan Kernan, ed., Yale University. (#CY958—$1.25)
- ☐ **RICHARD II**, Kenneth Muir, ed., University of Liverpool. (#CY1072—$1.25)
- ☐ **ROMEO AND JULIET**, Joseph Bryant, ed., University of North Carolina. (#CY968—$1.25)
- ☐ **THE TAMING OF THE SHREW**, Robert Heilman, ed., University of Washington. (#CY1101—$1.25)
- ☐ **THE TEMPEST**, Robert Langbaum, ed., University of Virginia. (#CY994—$1.25)
- ☐ **TIMON OF ATHENS**, Maurice Charney, ed., Rutgers. (#CD289—50¢)
- ☐ **THE TWO NOBLE KINSMEN, TITUS ANDRONICUS, PERICLES**, Sylvan Barnet, general ed., Tufts. (#CE1027—$2.95)
- ☐ **TROILUS AND CRESSIDA**, Daniel Seltzer, ed., Harvard. (#CQ935—95¢)
- ☐ **TWELFTH NIGHT**, Herschel Clay Baker, ed., Harvard. (#CQ748—95¢)
- ☐ **THE TWO GENTLEMEN OF VERONA**, Bertrand Evans, ed., University of California. (#CQ805—95¢)
- ☐ **THE WINTER'S TALE**, Frank Kermode, ed., University of Bristol. (#CY966—$1.25)
- ☐ **THE SONNETS**, William Burto, ed., Introduction by W. H. Auden. (#CY1039—$1.25)
